THE MEDICINE BOOK

BIG IDEAS

SIMPLY EXPLAINED

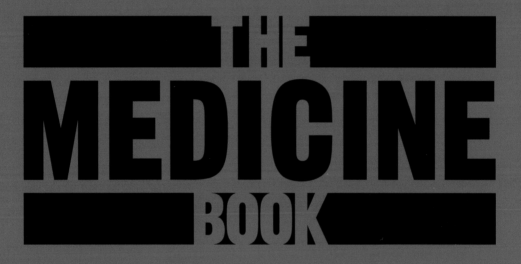

THE MEDICINE BOOK

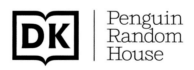

DK LONDON

SENIOR ART EDITOR
Helen Spencer

SENIOR EDITORS
Camilla Hallinan, Kathryn Hennessy,
Laura Sandford

EDITORS
Anna Cheifetz, Lydia Halliday,
Joanna Micklem, Victoria Pyke,
Dorothy Stannard, Rachel Warren Chadd

US EDITOR
Kayla Dugger

ILLUSTRATIONS
James Graham

JACKET DESIGN
DEVELOPMENT MANAGER
Sophia MTT

PRODUCTION EDITOR
George Nimmo

PRODUCER
Nancy-Jane Maun

SENIOR MANAGING ART EDITOR
Lee Griffiths

MANAGING EDITOR
Gareth Jones

ASSOCIATE PUBLISHING DIRECTOR
Liz Wheeler

ART DIRECTOR
Karen Self

DESIGN DIRECTOR
Philip Ormerod

PUBLISHING DIRECTOR
Jonathan Metcalf

DK DELHI

SENIOR ART EDITORS
Ira Sharma, Vikas Sachdeva,
Vinita Venugopal

PROJECT ART EDITOR
Sourabh Challariya

ART EDITORS
Shipra Jain, Noopur Dalal, Anukriti Arora

ASSISTANT ART EDITORS
Ankita Das, Bandana Paul, Adhithi Priya

SENIOR EDITOR
Janashree Singha

EDITORS
Nandini D. Tripathy, Rishi Bryan,
Avanika

MANAGING EDITOR
Soma B. Chowdhury

SENIOR MANAGING ART EDITOR
Arunesh Talapatra

SENIOR JACKET DESIGNER
Suhita Dharamjit

DTP DESIGNERS
Ashok Kumar, Mrinmoy Mazumdar

PICTURE RESEARCH COORDINATOR
Sumita Khatwani

ASSISTANT PICTURE RESEARCHER
Sneha Murchavade

PICTURE RESEARCH MANAGER
Taiyaba Khatoon

PRE-PRODUCTION MANAGER
Balwant Singh

PRODUCTION MANAGER
Pankaj Sharma

original styling by
STUDIO 8

First American Edition, 2021
Published in the United States by
DK Publishing
1450 Broadway, Suite 801,
New York, NY 10018

A catalog record for this book
is available from the Library of Congress.
ISBN 978-0-7440-2836-2

Printed in China

For the curious
www.dk.com

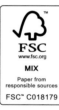

This book was made with
Forest Stewardship Council ™
certified paper—one small step in
DK's commitment to a sustainable
future. For more information go to
www.dk.com/our-green-pledge

CONTRIBUTORS

STEVE PARKER, CONSULTANT EDITOR

Steve Parker is a writer and editor of more than 300 information books specializing in science, particularly biology and medicine, and allied life sciences. He holds a BSc in Zoology, is a senior scientific fellow of the Zoological Society of London, and has authored titles for a range of ages and publishers. Among Steve's recent accolades is the British Medical Association's Award for the Public Understanding of Science for *Kill or Cure: An Illustrated History of Medicine*.

JOHN FARNDON

John Farndon is a science writer whose books have been shortlisted for the Royal Society's Young People's Science Book Prize five times, including for *The Complete Book of the Brain* and *Project Body*. A widely published author, he has written or contributed to around 1,000 books on a range of subjects, including the history of medicine, and has contributed to major books such as *Science* and *Science Year By Year* and the Nobel Prize in Physiology or Medicine website.

TIM HARRIS

Tim Harris is a widely published author on science and nature for both children and adults. He has written more than 100 mostly educational reference books and contributed to many others, including *Knowledge Encyclopedia Human Body!*, *An Illustrated History of Engineering*, *Physics Matters*, *Great Scientists*, *Exploring the Solar System*, and *Routes of Science*.

BEN HUBBARD

Ben Hubbard is an accomplished nonfiction author of books for children and adults. He has more than 120 titles to his name and has written on everything from space, the samurai, and sharks to poison, pets, and the Plantagenets. His books have been translated into more than a dozen languages and can be found in libraries around the world.

PHILIP PARKER

Philip Parker is a critically acclaimed author, award-winning editor, and historian specializing in the classical and medieval world. He is author of the *DK Companion Guide to World History*, *The Empire Stops Here: A Journey around the Frontiers of the Roman Empire*, and *A History of Britain in Maps*, and he was a contributor to DK's *Medicine*. He was previously a diplomat working on the UK's relations with Greece and Cyprus and holds a diploma in international relations from Johns Hopkins University's School of Advanced International Studies.

ROBERT SNEDDEN

Robert Snedden has been involved in publishing for over 40 years, researching and writing science and technology books for young people on topics ranging from medical ethics, autism, cell biology, nutrition, and the human body to space exploration, engineering, computers, and the internet. He has also contributed to histories of mathematics, engineering, biology, and evolution and has written books for an adult audience on breakthroughs in mathematics and medicine and the works of Albert Einstein.

CONTENTS

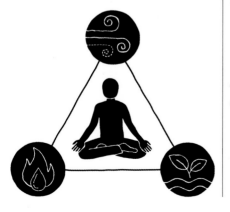

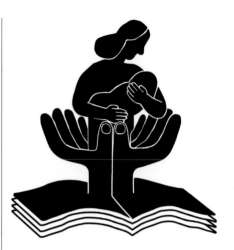

CELLS AND MICROBES
1820–1890

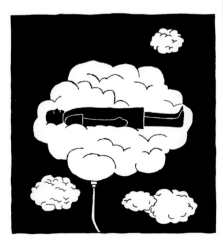

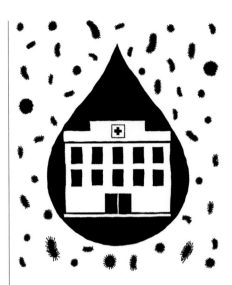

VACCINES, SERUMS, AND ANTIBIOTICS
1890–1945

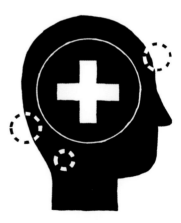
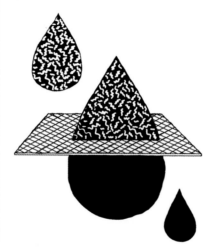

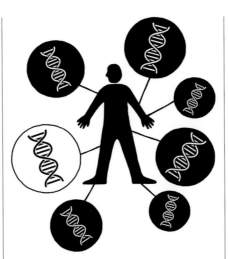
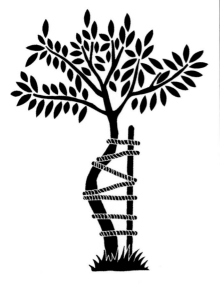

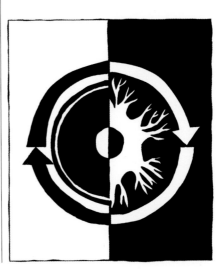

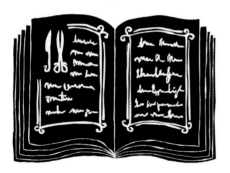

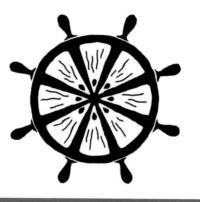

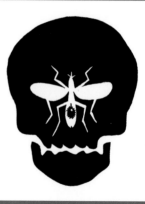

Illness and disease have always been with us, and the need to find ways to prevent and treat them can often be literally a matter of life and death. Over time, many new techniques have been tried, and a number of key discoveries, such as vaccines and antibiotics, have made a lasting impact, saved countless lives, or restored many people to health.

Early practice

In prehistoric times, people relied on traditional knowledge, healers, and even magic when they fell ill. More systematic approaches gradually evolved, with Ayurvedic healing emerging in ancient India around 3,000 BCE. It still has many adherents, as does the ancient Chinese system of medicine, which includes acupuncture. While these medical practices have endured, the ideas that led to today's science-based medicine developed in ancient Greece.

In the late 5th century BCE, the Greek physician Hippocrates insisted that illness has natural causes, so it might also have natural cures. This has been the guiding principle of medicine ever since. Hippocrates also founded a school of medicine where students undertook to act with a duty of care to patients. This ideal, enshrined in the Hippocratic Oath, continues to inform medical ethics and practice.

The Greeks had few cures and, because dissecting bodies was taboo, knew little anatomy, but the Romans' military campaigns helped physicians develop new surgical skills. The celebrated Roman physician Claudius Galen greatly advanced anatomical knowledge by learning from animal dissections and from gladiators' wounds.

Galen's medical approach was detailed and thorough, and he wrote the first great manuals of medicine. However, his theories were based on the mistaken idea, originating in ancient Greece, that illnesses are caused by an imbalance between four body fluids called humors—

> ❝
> Cure sometimes,
> treat often,
> comfort always.
> **Hippocrates**
> (c. 460–c. 375 BCE)
> ❞

blood, yellow bile, phlegm, and black bile. This idea persisted in Europe even into the 19th century.

Scientific investigation

When the Roman Empire fell, the teachings of Galen were kept alive in the Islamic world by a succession of scholar–physicians who developed new surgical skills and introduced many innovative medicines. Al-Razi pioneered chemical drug treatments and Ibn Sina wrote the definitive work *The Canon of Medicine*.

In the later medieval period, medical ideas from Islam and Galen filtered back into Europe. Dedicated medical schools, based on Galenic and Islamic practices, were set up alongside universities in cities such as Salerno and Padua. Medicine was recognized for the first time as a legitimate subject of academic study, and the Renaissance that followed ushered in a new age of discovery based on inquiry and first-hand observations.

In the mid-16th century, the detailed dissections conducted by Flemish physician Andreas Vesalius began to build an accurate picture of human anatomy. Physicians also started to learn about physiology—the science of how the body works. A major breakthrough was the demonstration by English physician

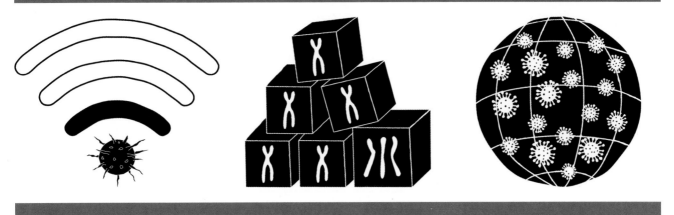

William Harvey in 1628 that the heart is a pump that circulates blood around the body.

Progress in treating disease was slow. In the 16th century, the Swiss physician and alchemist Paracelsus pioneered the idea of the body as a chemical system that could be treated with chemical cures. While his use of mercury for syphilis was a standard treatment for nearly 400 years, it took until the 20th century for his chemical approach to be applied in modern drug therapies.

Tackling disease

The fight against disease received a major boost in 1796, when British physician Edward Jenner developed a vaccination for smallpox. In 1881, French chemist Louis Pasteur showed that vaccination could work for other diseases, too, and the search for vaccines is now a major area of medical research.

Pasteur, with German physician Robert Koch, also led the way to an understanding of what disease is. They ended belief in the humors by proving germ theory—the idea that infectious diseases are caused by microscopic organisms such as bacteria. Their discovery generated a new field of research, as scientists hunted for the germ responsible for each disease. Koch's isolation of the bacteria that causes tuberculosis inspired Russian scientist Élie Metchnikoff to identify cells in the body that fight against germs. The gradual revelation of the body's intricate immune system over the last century has been one of medicine's most remarkable stories.

In the early 20th century, new approaches in microbiology and chemistry transformed ideas about how to treat disease. Identifying tiny immune particles in the body called antibodies, German scientist Paul Ehrlich developed the idea of targeted drugs, which hit germs but leave the body unharmed. His success in developing Salvarsan, the first effective drug for syphilis, in 1910 marked the beginning of a global pharmaceutical industry.

Modern medicine

Scottish bacteriologist Alexander Fleming's discovery of penicillin in 1928 marked a new era of medicine. For the first time, physicians had an effective treatment for a range of previously life-threatening diseases. Antibiotics also facilitated one of the miracles of modern surgery, organ transplants, which had often failed as a result of infection.

Since the 1950s, advances such as the deciphering of genetic code have shed new light on how diseases develop and fueled new methods to fight them. The field of biomedical engineering has also produced solutions in all areas of health care, from noninvasive imaging to robotic surgery and implantable medical devices such as pacemakers and replacement joints.

Whether a flash of individual insight or the result of several years of research and testing by large teams of people, new ideas in medicine have saved millions from suffering and death. Yet the innovations of medical science are also tempered by more caution and regulation than many other disciplines—after all, human lives are at stake. ∎

> ❝
> Advances in medicine and agriculture have saved vastly more lives than have been lost in all the wars in history.
> **Carl Sagan**
> **American scientist (1934–1996)**
> ❞

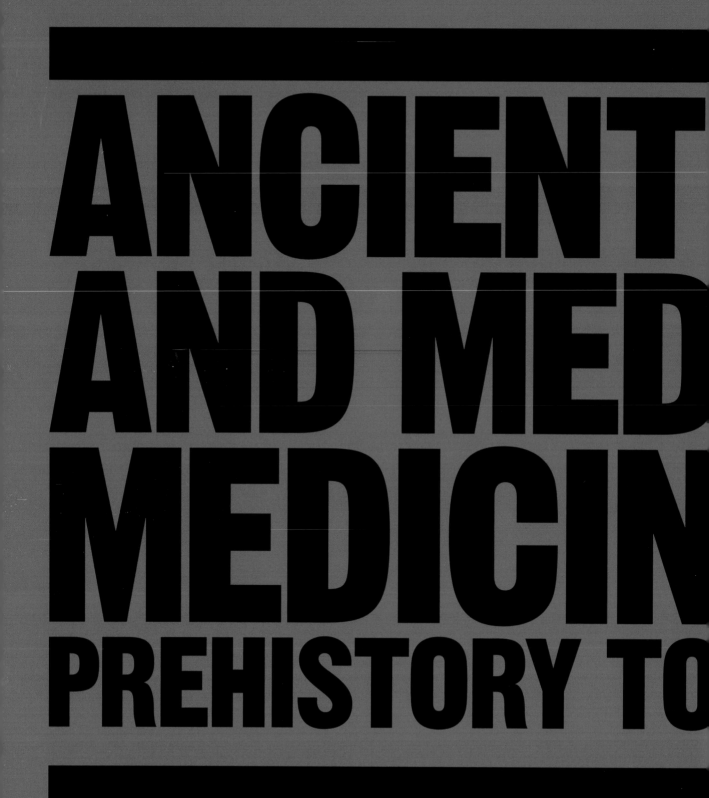

ANCIENT AND MEDICIN MEDICIN PREHISTORY TO

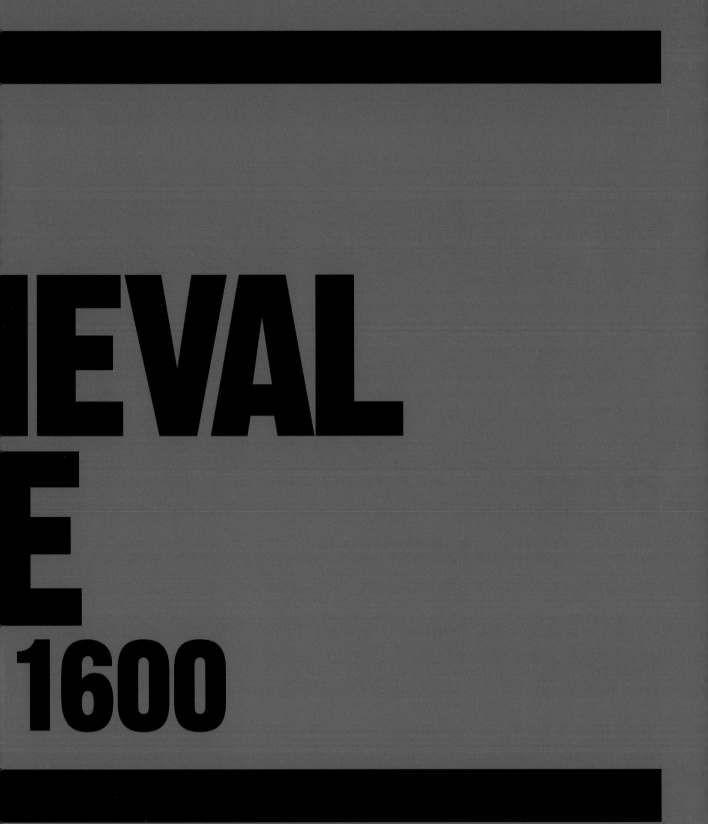

Human skulls found in Europe have holes chipped or drilled into them, a practice called **trepanning**, possibly to treat pain or let out "evil spirits."

6TH MILLENNIUM BCE

Egypt's **Edwin Smith papyrus**, one of the earliest surviving medical documents, describes 48 cases of trauma to the body.

c. 17TH CENTURY BCE

Hippocrates, a physician in **ancient Greece**, embarks on his medical career. He and his followers develop an ethical code for doctors later known as the Hippocratic Oath.

c. 440 BCE

Roman soldier–physician **Pedanius Dioscorides** compiles his **De Materia Medica (On Medicinal Substances)**, listing hundreds of herbal and other medications.

c. 70 CE

27TH CENTURY BCE

In **ancient Egypt**, the architect, high priest, vizier, and physician **Imhotep** rises to fame. Centuries later, he is deified as the god-on-Earth of medical practices.

c. 500 BCE

In **India**, the physician Sushruta begins compiling the **Sushruta Samhita**, a compendium of **Ayurvedic** surgical methods that include reconstructive procedures.

c. 300 BCE

In China, the **Huangdi Neijing (The Yellow Emperor's Classic of Internal Medicine)** sets out the principles and methods of **traditional Chinese medicine**.

Prehistoric evidence such as skeletons, tools, and rock art indicate that humans were practicing medicine more than 40,000 years ago. Early humans were aware that certain minerals, herbs, and parts of animals had health-giving properties. People who possessed such knowledge were sought-after specialists whose ability to heal was often associated with myths, magic, and the worship of supernatural powers.

Many regions—North and South America, Africa, and large parts of Asia and Australasia—cultivated spiritual practices in which individuals believed to have access to supernatural beings entered a trancelike state in order to contact and even join with those spirits. Practitioners channeled the healing powers of the spirits or bargained with them for the relief of illness and disease. Such practices still exist in some Indigenous societies.

Medical systems

Each of the ancient civilizations developed medical practices, many of them linked to religious rituals. In Egypt, in the 4th millennium BCE, serious disease was regarded as the work of the gods—probably as a punishment for a misdemeanor in the current or past life. Temple priests administered herbal medications, carried out healing rituals, and placated the gods with offerings. By the 2nd millennium BCE, there were Egyptian doctors who specialized in disorders of the eyes, digestion, joints, and teeth, and in surgery that was informed by many centuries of experience in mummification and embalming.

In India, Ayurvedic medicine developed from around 800 BCE. Still practiced by some physicians today, its central premise is that illness is caused by an imbalance between the body's three elemental *doshas*: *vata* (wind), *pitta* (bile), and *kapha* (phlegm). The task of the *vaidya*, the Ayurvedic physician, is to detect imbalances and correct them using herbal and mineral remedies, bloodletting, laxatives, enemas, emetics, and massage.

Ancient China developed a theory of health based on balance within the body between the oppositions of *yin* and *yang*; the five elements of fire, water, earth, wood, and metal; and the life-sustaining energy of *qi* flowing along the body's many meridians (channels). Chinese medicine included some remedies that were common to other ancient

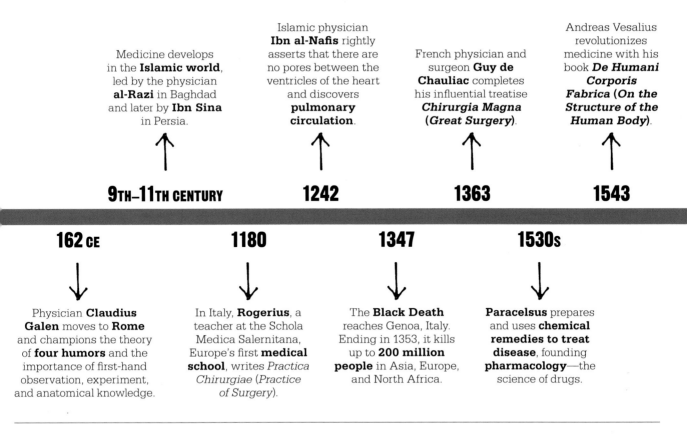

Medicine develops in the **Islamic world**, led by the physician **al-Razi** in Baghdad and later by **Ibn Sina** in Persia.

Islamic physician **Ibn al-Nafis** rightly asserts that there are no pores between the ventricles of the heart and discovers **pulmonary circulation**.

French physician and surgeon **Guy de Chauliac** completes his influential treatise *Chirurgia Magna (Great Surgery)*.

Andreas Vesalius revolutionizes medicine with his book *De Humani Corporis Fabrica (On the Structure of the Human Body)*.

9TH–11TH CENTURY   **1242**   **1363**   **1543**

162 CE   **1180**   **1347**   **1530s**

Physician **Claudius Galen** moves to **Rome** and champions the theory of **four humors** and the importance of first-hand observation, experiment, and anatomical knowledge.

In Italy, **Rogerius**, a teacher at the Schola Medica Salernitana, Europe's first **medical school**, writes *Practica Chirurgiae (Practice of Surgery)*.

The **Black Death** reaches Genoa, Italy. Ending in 1353, it kills up to **200 million people** in Asia, Europe, and North Africa.

Paracelsus prepares and uses **chemical remedies to treat disease**, founding **pharmacology**—the science of drugs.

---

civilizations, such as herbs, diets, and massage, but it also developed its own practices. It placed great emphasis on the pulse for diagnosis and on acupuncture—the insertion of needles along the meridians—to correct imbalances in the body.

New insights
Medicine flourished in ancient Greece in the 1st millennium BCE. Its many celebrated physicians included Hippocrates of Cos, whose caring attitude toward patients and rational approach to diagnosis and treatment still influence medicine today. The Romans made strides in many areas of medicine, especially surgery. They, too, believed that good health depended on balance—in this case, four bodily fluids, or humors: blood, phlegm, yellow bile, and black bile. In the 2nd century CE, physician

Claudius Galen became hugely respected, especially for anatomy, and physicians consulted his works until well into the 16th century.

As the Roman Empire declined and eventually fell in 476 CE, Europe entered a period of fragmentation. Much medical knowledge was lost, and for most of the medieval era (c. 500–1400), medical care was the preserve of monasteries. However, with the spread of Islam, the Arabic world made significant advances in many areas of science, including medicine. During Islam's Golden Age (c. 750–1258), scholars at the Abbasid court in Baghdad translated and studied the medical texts of the ancient world, and physicians such as al-Razi and Ibn Sina added influential works of their own, which were later translated into Latin by scholars in Europe.

In the 14th century, the European Renaissance ("rebirth") arose in Italy, inspired by the rediscovery of Greco–Roman culture and learning. It spread across Europe, with an explosion of new ideas in the arts, education, politics, religion, science, and medicine.

Scientists and physicians now turned to first-hand observation, experimentation, and rational analysis rather than relying solely on the pronouncements of ancient texts such as Galen's. Two towering figures of the period were the Swiss physician Paracelsus, who founded pharmacology, and Flemish anatomist Andreas Vesalius, whose masterwork *De Humani Corporis Fabrica (On the Structure of the Human Body)* transformed the medical profession's understanding of the human body. ■

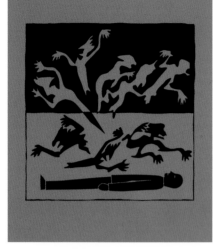

A SHAMAN TO COMBAT DISEASE AND DEATH

PREHISTORIC MEDICINE

IN CONTEXT

BEFORE

47000 BCE Evidence from the teeth of Neanderthal skeletons found at El Sidrón, a cave in northern Spain, suggests the early use of medicinal plants.

AFTER

7000–5000 BCE Cave art in Tassili n'Ajjer, Algeria, depicts shamanlike figures carrying or covered in *Psilocybe mairei* mushrooms, known for their psychedelic effects.

c. 3300 BCE Studies of the body of Ötzi the Iceman, found in the Ötztal Alps on the Austrian-Italian border in 1991, indicate that he took medicinal herbs.

c. 1000 CE Spiritual healers in southwest Bolivia use psychoactive drugs, including cocaine; chemical traces of the drugs were found in López Altiplano in 2010.

2000 Chuonnasuan, one of the last practicing shamans in Siberia, dies.

Early humans faced with injuries and disease began to self-medicate with herbs and clays, a behavior similar to that of chimpanzees or apes. They also turned to the supernatural to explain misfortune, blaming injuries and ill health on the operation of malevolent spirits.

Magical healing

Around 15,000 to 20,000 years ago, a new figure emerged in the prehistoric world. Part healer and part magician, this shape-shifter was believed to be able to access and even enter the spirit world to influence the forces there and bring peace and healing to the suffering and sick.

Prehistoric rock art in Africa and cave paintings in Europe are thought to represent ancient ritual practices, including the healer's transformation into a creature form. The burial of what may be a female spiritual healer at Hilazon Tachtit in Israel, from around 11,000 BCE, contains the wings of a golden eagle, a leopard pelvis, and a severed human foot—artifacts believed to suggest the healer's ability to

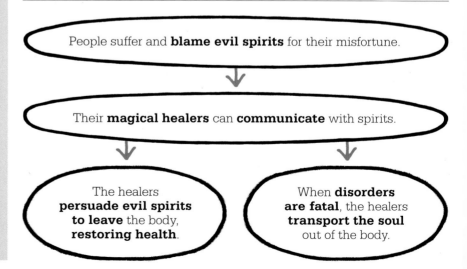

People suffer and **blame evil spirits** for their misfortune.

⬇

Their **magical healers** can **communicate** with spirits.

⬇ ⬇

The healers **persuade evil spirits to leave** the body, **restoring health**.

When **disorders are fatal**, the healers **transport the soul** out of the body.

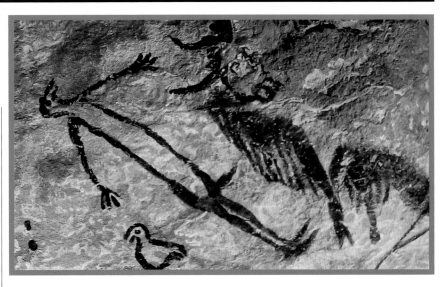

The Bird Man from the Lascaux caves in France, created c. 15000 BCE, may depict a shaman. His head, four-fingered hands, and the bird beside him suggest he can take an avian form.

transform and transcend the normal human state. Such spiritual healers may have developed practical healing skills, too, as archaeologists have found ample evidence not only of the use of medicinal plants, but also of surgical procedures such as trepanning and attempts to reset broken bones.

Meeting a need

Belief in supernatural healing gave way to other spiritual and medical practices but never died out. In the 17th century, European travelers rediscovered the Siberian spiritual healers called "shamans"—from the word *šaman* ("one who knows") in their Tungusic language—and the term shamanism was often applied to spiritual practices elsewhere.

In Siberia, a dwindling number of shamans still use hallucinogens, drumming, and chants to promote a trance state in which they receive a vision of the spirit world. The most powerful healers are thought to project themselves (often guided by a spirit animal) into the other world to persuade the evil spirit causing the disease to release the sick person and restore their health. Where healing is not possible, a shaman conducts a similar ritual to lead the soul of the dying person safely into the afterlife.

Today, varying forms of spiritual healing continue in East Asia; Africa; and among Indigenous peoples in Australia, the Arctic, and the Americas. For millennia, these beliefs have answered a primal need to explain why disease occurs and why—where the spirits prove too strong or intractable—it cannot be cured. If less widespread as populations of Indigenous people decline, the beliefs still live on. ▪

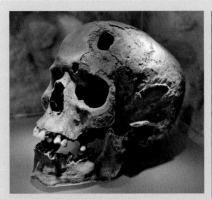

An 11th-century skull discovered below the Market Square in Krakow, Poland, indicates the therapeutic use of trepanning in the medieval era.

Prehistoric trepanning

Archaeologists have unearthed thousands of skulls with a small hole drilled or sawn into them—a practice called trepanning, dating from around 8000 BCE. Probably performed by community healers, trepanning was possibly a ritual to drive out evil spirits; the bone removed was sometimes worn as an amulet. As these skulls often show signs of earlier injuries or disease, it also seems likely that healers used the procedure to repair injuries, relieve head pain, and treat neurological diseases.

One of the earliest examples, a 7,000-year-old skull of a man unearthed at Ensisheim in France in the 1990s, had been trepanned twice. Here and elsewhere, new bone growth shows that trepanned patients often survived for some years.

Healers and physicians practiced trepanning in the ancient civilizations of Egypt, Greece, Rome, China, and South America. Later, in Europe and the US, surgeons used it to treat concussion and brain inflammation and to clean head wounds (as in the Civil War).

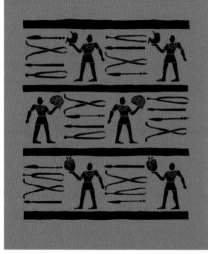

A HEALER OF ONE DISEASE AND NO MORE

ANCIENT EGYPTIAN MEDICINE

IN CONTEXT

BEFORE

c. 3500 BCE Trepanning (drilling or sawing holes in the skull) is used to relieve cranial pressure in Egypt.

c. 2700 BCE Egyptians begin the mummification of royal corpses, giving the embalmers knowledge of internal organs.

AFTER

c. 2600 BCE Death of the first known dentist, Hesy-Re, revered as "chief of the ivory cutters."

c. 17th century BCE The Edwin Smith papyrus (named after the dealer who bought it in 1862) shows a knowledge of surgery to treat wounds, fractures, and other trauma.

c. 440 BCE Herodotus notes the high level of specialization among Egyptian doctors.

1805 CE The Moorfields Eye Hospital, one of the first modern specialty hospitals, opens in London, UK.

The prevailing view in the earliest societies was that disease was caused by supernatural influence. As a result, in many cultures, healing was the domain of shamans or priests. In ancient Mesopotamia, a person afflicted by venereal disease was said to be struck "by the hand of Lilith," a storm demon, while the first Egyptian doctors were based in areas of temples known as *Per-Ankh,* or houses of healing.

In ancient Egypt, the first physician whose name survives was Imhotep, vizier to the pharaoh Djoser in the 27th century BCE. Little is known of his medical views, yet he is believed to have been a skillful practitioner, and was later deified as a god of medicine.

Egyptian specialization

Imhotep started a tradition of medicine that implemented practical measures to preserve patients' lives and marked the divergence between priests and doctors. In the 5th century BCE, the Greek historian

Surgical instruments on a wall carving in the Kom Ombo Temple near Aswan show the significance of surgery in ancient Egyptian culture.

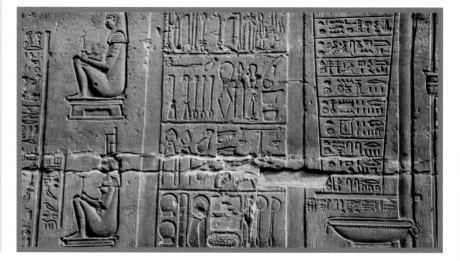

See also: Prehistoric medicine 18–19 ▪ Greek medicine 28–29 ▪ Hospitals 82–83
▪ Orthopedic surgery 260–265

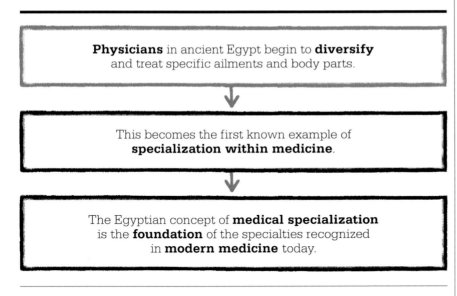

Physicians in ancient Egypt begin to **diversify** and treat specific ailments and body parts.

↓

This becomes the first known example of **specialization within medicine**.

↓

The Egyptian concept of **medical specialization** is the **foundation** of the specialties recognized in **modern medicine** today.

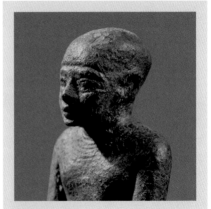

Imhotep

Most biographical information about Imhotep dates from more than 1,000 years after his death, and few details are known for certain. His name appears on a statue of the Old Kingdom pharaoh Djoser, held in the Cairo Museum. Born in the 27th century BCE, he was a commoner who rose in the service of Djoser and became his vizier (chancellor). He was believed to have been the architect of the step-pyramid at Saqqara, a style of tomb that predated the pyramids built at Giza a century later. He was also the high priest of Ra at Heliopolis.

Imhotep's reputation as a physician has led to attempts to identify him as either the author of the Edwin Smith papyrus or as the source of the surgical techniques it contains. However, there is no direct evidence to support this, and he was not associated with medicine until the 4th century BCE. After his death, Imhotep was revered as a god of medicine and as the son of Sekhmet, a healing goddess. He was sometimes associated with Asclepios, the Greek god of medicine, and also became identified with Thoth, the god of architecture and wisdom.

Herodotus wrote that Egyptian medicine was notable for the existence of specialty practitioners in various disciplines, such as dentistry, the stomach, and "hidden diseases." Egyptian documents of the time support Herodotus's view, and the tomb of Hesy-Re (an Egyptian official and contemporary of Imhotep) reveals his title "chief of dentists." Further records mention *swnw* (who practiced general medicine); others who specialized in eye or intestinal disorders; and female physicians, such as Merit-Ptah, who lived around 2700 BCE; as well as midwives and surgeons.

Egyptian surgery

Surgery was among the most developed specialties in Egypt, at least for external operations. (Operating on internal organs invariably risked fatal infections.) The oldest surviving Egyptian surgical text, the Edwin Smith papyrus written c. 17th century BCE, describes trauma surgery, detailing 48 case studies with instructions given for fractures, wounds, and dislocations. The practical approach suggests that it was composed for use by a military doctor, unlike documents such as the Ebers papyrus (c. 1550 BCE), which proposes folk remedies and healing magic for the treatment of infectious diseases.

Although they were considered specialists, Egyptian physicians' understanding of internal anatomy was rudimentary. They appreciated that the heart played a central role in the healthy workings of the body but believed that veins, arteries, and nerves operated as part of 46 "channels" allowing energy to pass through the body. However, it was their innovative specializing in medical fields that had the most lasting impact, passing from Egyptian to Roman physicians and later into Arabic and medieval European medicine. This differentiation accelerated during the 19th century with the founding of many specialty hospitals, such as London's Moorfields Eye Hospital in 1805— by the 1860s, London had more than 60 specialty centers. ▪

THE BALANCE OF THE DOSHAS IS FREEDOM FROM DISEASE

AYURVEDIC MEDICINE

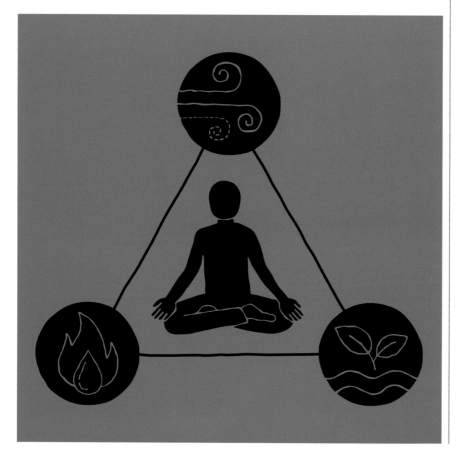

IN CONTEXT

BEFORE
c. 3000 BCE In legend, the *rishis* (seers) of India are gifted Ayurveda by Dhanvantari, the physician of the gods.

c. 1000 BCE The *Atharvaveda* is the first major Indian text to contain medical guidance.

AFTER
13th century CE The *Dhanvantari Nighantu*, a comprehensive lexicon of herbal and mineral Ayurvedic remedies, is compiled.

1971 The Central Council of Indian Medicine is established to oversee training at recognized institutions and to develop good practice.

1980s Ayurvedic practitioners Dr. Vasant Lad and Dr. Robert Svoboda and American Vedic scholar David Frawley spread the teachings of Ayurveda throughout the US.

A preventive and curative medical system infused with a strong philosophy emerged in India between 800 and 600 BCE. Called Ayurveda from the Sanskrit words for life (*ayur*) and knowledge (*veda*), it was based on the theory that disease is caused by an imbalance in the elements that make up the human body. Interventions and therapies aimed to restore and maintain the body's equilibrium and were adapted to patients' personal physical, mental, and spiritual requirements.

The roots of Ayurveda lie in the *Atharvaveda*, one of four sacred texts—the Vedas—which enshrine

See also: Greek medicine 28–29 ▪ Traditional Chinese medicine 30–35 ▪ Herbal medicine 36–37
▪ Roman medicine 38–43 ▪ Islamic medicine 44–49 ▪ Medieval medical schools and surgery 50–51

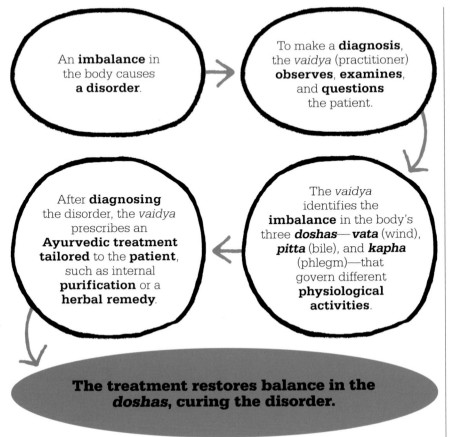

An **imbalance** in the body causes **a disorder**.

To make a **diagnosis**, the *vaidya* (practitioner) **observes**, **examines**, and **questions** the patient.

After **diagnosing** the disorder, the *vaidya* prescribes an **Ayurvedic treatment tailored** to the **patient**, such as internal **purification** or a **herbal remedy**.

The *vaidya* identifies the **imbalance** in the body's three **doshas**— **vata** (wind), **pitta** (bile), and **kapha** (phlegm)—that govern different **physiological activities**.

The treatment restores balance in the *doshas*, curing the disorder.

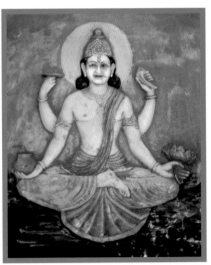

According to Hindu tradition, Ayurveda was communicated to Dhanvantari by the creator god Brahma. In India, Dhanvantari's birthday is celebrated as National Ayurveda Day.

the core beliefs of the civilization that emerged in India in the 2nd millennium BCE. Providing formulae and rituals for everyday living, the *Atharvaveda* contains a number of magico-religious prescriptions for treating disease, such as the exorcism of evil spirits, but also features less mystical cures, such as the use of herbal remedies.

Two later treatises, the *Sushruta Samhita* and the *Charaka Samhita,* further developed the key tenets of Ayurvedic medical theory and practice. The *Sushruta Samhita*— attributed to the physician Sushruta, who practiced around 500 BCE in Varanasi, northern India—is a

compendium of *shalya chikitsa* or Ayurvedic surgical methods. It includes guidance on such complex procedures as cataract removal, hernia repair, and setting broken bones, alongside hundreds of herbal remedies. The *Charaka Samhita,* compiled around 300 BCE and attributed to Charaka, a court physician, takes a more theoretical approach. Dealing with *kaya chikitsa* or "internal medicine," it focuses on the origins of disease.

In the 5th century CE, the body of Ayurvedic knowledge was increased by the creation of three more scholarly works: the *Ashtanga Sangraha* and the *Ashtanga*

Hridayam, both written by Vagbhata, a disciple of Charaka, and the Bower manuscript, named after Hamilton Bower, the British officer who acquired it in 1890. Together, all six texts constitute the Ayurvedic medical tradition that has flourished for centuries in Asia and more recently in the West.

The elements and *doshas*
At the heart of Ayurvedic medicine is the notion of harmony and balance between all components of the human body. It is the primary role of the *vaidya*, or Ayurvedic physician, to diagnose and correct any imbalances. The body (like the material world) is said to be made up of five elements: *akash* (space), *vayu* (air), *jala* (water), *prithvi* (earth), and *teja* (fire). In the body, certain combinations of these elements manifest themselves as three *doshas* (roughly analogous »

to the humors of the ancient Greek and Roman medical traditions). These *tridosha* are *vata* (wind), *pitta* (bile), and *kapha* (phlegm). A state of good health and well-being occurs when all three *doshas* are well balanced, but the ideal proportions may vary from person to person. Disease and damaging metabolic conditions occur when the *doshas* are not in balance. An excess of *vata*, for example, can cause problems such as indigestion and flatulence, while a surfeit of *kapha* may bring on lung disorders or breathing problems.

In Ayurvedic medicine, the body is viewed as a dynamic system rather than a static one, and the way energies flow through the body is as important as its anatomy. Each *dosha* is associated with a particular form of energy: *vata* with movement, governing the action of muscles, the flow of breath, and the heartbeat; *pitta* with the metabolic system, digestion, and nutrition; and *kapha* with the structure of the body, including the bones.

The *doshas* flow from one part of the body to another along porous channels known as *srotas*. There are 16 main *srotas*, three of which bring nourishment into the body in the form of breath, food, and water; three allow for the elimination of metabolic waste products; two carry breast milk and menses; one is the conduit for thought; and seven link directly to the body's tissues—the *dhatus*. The *dhatus* are *rasa* (fluids including plasma and lymph), *rakta* (blood), *mamsa* (muscle), *meda* (fat), *asthi* (bones), *majja* (marrow and nerve tissue), and *shukra* (reproductive tissue). The internal balance of the body is also controlled by *agni* ("biological fire"), the energy that fuels the body's metabolic processes. The most important aspect of *agni* is *jatharagni*, or "digestive fire," which ensures the elimination of waste products. If this is too low, urine, feces, and sweat will build up, causing issues such as urinary tract infections.

Diagnosis and treatment

Practitioners of Ayurvedic medicine evaluate the signs of disease by directly observing and questioning the patient in order to devise an appropriate treatment. The main methods of physical diagnosis are measuring the pulse; analyzing the urine and stools; inspecting the tongue; checking the voice and speech; examining the skin and eyes; and assessing the patient's overall appearance.

The physician may also examine the *marma* points on a patient's body. These 108 points are where

The seven *dhatus*, or body tissues, function sequentially. This means if one *dhatu* is affected by a disorder (caused by an imbalance in one of the three *doshas*—*vata*, *pitta*, or *kapha*), it will directly affect the nutritional support and function of the next *dhatu*.

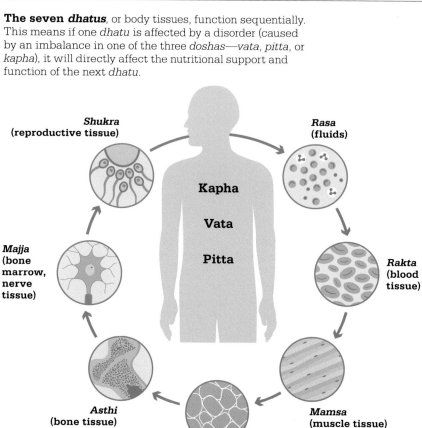

Shukra (reproductive tissue)

Rasa (fluids)

Majja (bone marrow, nerve tissue)

Kapha

Vata

Pitta

Rakta (blood tissue)

Asthi (bone tissue)

Mamsa (muscle tissue)

Meda (fat)

> " When diet is wrong, medicine is of no use. When diet is correct, medicine is of no need.
> **Ancient Ayurvedic proverb**

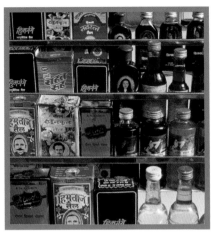

Ayurvedic medicines are widely available across India in stores and pharmacies. Over 3,000 years, around 1,500 medicinal plants have become part of Ayurveda's pharmacopeia.

body tissues (veins, muscles, joints, ligaments, tendons, and bones) intersect. They are also junctions between the physical body itself, consciousness, and the energy that flows in the body.

Following a diagnosis, Ayurvedic practitioners select from a number of therapies aimed at correcting imbalances between the *doshas* or other elements in the Ayurvedic physiological systems. Among these are *panchakarma*, a multistep purification process that employs steam treatment, massage therapy, *virechana* (the use of laxatives), *vamana* (induced vomiting), *raktamokshana* (bloodletting), *basti* (enemas), and *nasya* (a nasal treatment) to eliminate excess waste products. Also prescribed are herbal remedies, which act in a more direct way on the *doshas*. Of the numerous plant, animal, and mineral ingredients used in these, garlic is considered especially potent. It is used to treat a wide range of conditions, including colds, coughs, and digestive disorders, and as an emollient for sores, bites, and stings.

Foodstuffs, including spices, play a major role in Ayurvedic practice by supporting the body's healing processes. *Vaidya* may prescribe dietary changes as part of their holistic (whole-person) approach to restoring a balance between the body, mind, spirit, and environment. Dietary regulation considers the patient's physical and emotional makeup and their dominant *dosha*, and practitioners draw on six principal "tastes" as the basis for their recommended regimens: astringent, sour, sweet, salty, pungent, and bitter.

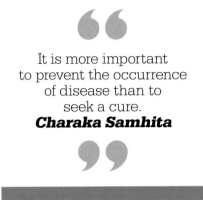

> It is more important to prevent the occurrence of disease than to seek a cure.
> **Charaka Samhita**

The 11th-century arrival of Islamic medicine (incorporating earlier Greco-Roman concepts) introduced a new approach, as did the founding of scientific medical schools and modern hospitals in the 19th and 20th centuries. Yet Ayurvedic practitioners remained the primary healthcare providers in India. Today, they cater to around 500 million patients in India alone, who use Ayurveda exclusively or along with conventional Western medicine.

Safety concerns

In the West, Ayurveda is used as a complementary therapy alongside conventional medical care. A few studies and trials have suggested that its approaches are effective, but there are concerns about the safety of Ayurvedic medicines. Sold largely as food supplements, the presence of metals in some makes them potentially harmful. A 2004 study found that 20 percent of 70 Ayurvedic medicines produced by 27 South Asian manufacturers contained toxic levels of lead, mercury, and arsenic. They have also been shown to work against the effects of Western medicines, so their use should always be supervised by a trained Ayurvedic practitioner. ∎

Other Indian medical traditions

Ayurveda is not the only traditional Indian medical system. The practice of Siddha medicine (its name derives from the Tamil *siddhi*, which means "attaining perfection") is particularly strong in South India. While also seeking to restore balance in the body, it espouses a duality of matter and energy in the Universe that needs to be kept in harmony. Siddha's treatment system has three branches: *Bala vahatam* (pediatrics), *Nanjunool* (toxicology), and *Nayan vidhi* (ophthalmology).

Unani medicine (from a Hindi word meaning "Greek") is a descendant of ancient Greek and Islamic medical practices. It aims to keep the humors (blood, phlegm, black bile, and yellow bile) in balance. Unani also places great value on the examination of the patient but regards measurement of the pulse as particularly important.

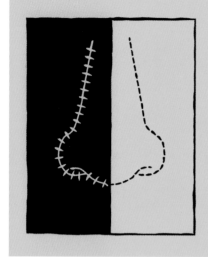

WE REBUILD WHAT FORTUNE HAS TAKEN AWAY

PLASTIC SURGERY

IN CONTEXT

BEFORE

c. 17th century BCE The Egyptian Edwin Smith papyrus shows how to treat wounds to reduce scarring.

c. 950 BCE An artificial wooden toe in an Egyptian tomb is the first known prosthesis.

AFTER

c. 40 CE In his *De Medicina*, Celsus refers to operations to repair damaged earlobes.

1460 Heinrich von Pfolspeundt describes an operation to rebuild a nose (rhinoplasty).

1814 The first rhinoplasty operation using Sushruta's techniques is carried out in Western Europe.

1914–1918 During World War I, New Zealand–born surgeon Harold Gillies specializes in performing facial repairs.

2008 French surgeon Laurent Lantieri claims to have carried out the first full face transplant.

In **accidents**, **torture**, and times of **war**, countless individuals receive **disfiguring injuries**.

↓

A disfiguring injury can have **damaging psychological** effects.

↓

Innovative, compassionate **surgeons** devise new **reconstructive** procedures.

↓

Successful plastic surgery **conceals** or **rebuilds** damaged **facial** and **other features**.

↓

These procedures help **heal** physical and psychological wounds, boost **confidence**, and **transform lives**.

For most of human history, doctors could do little for patients who suffered disfiguring accidents, disease, or congenital conditions. Minor blemishes could be concealed with cosmetics, and prostheses were used to replace missing limbs, but those more severely affected suffered social ostracism. The medical culture that arose in India in the 1st millennium BCE gave rise to techniques that offered hope to such patients.

Ayurvedic surgery

Early references to operations—alleged to have restored severed heads—feature in the Vedas, the ancient religious texts that form the basis of Hindu religion and philosophy. However, the first clear evidence of reconstructive surgery comes from the *Sushruta Samhita* (*Sushruta's Compendium*), written around 500 BCE.

Belonging to a tradition of *Shalya*, or Ayurvedic surgery, this Sanskrit text is believed to be the work of Sushruta, a physician from Varanasi, northern India. Sushruta's medical approach was advanced for his time; he urged students to gain a knowledge of internal anatomy

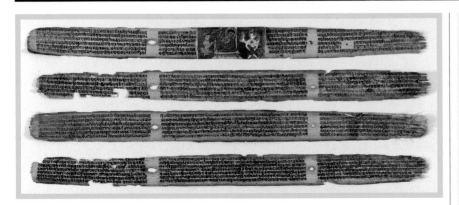

through dissecting dead bodies. His key innovation lies in his descriptions of reconstructive procedures, and he is often referred to as the "father of plastic surgery."

Among 300 surgical operations described in the *Sushruta Samhita* are instructions for *nasa sandhan* (rhinoplasty—rebuilding the nose) and *ostha sandhan* (otoplasty—reconstruction of the ear). Sushruta explains how a flap of skin should be excised from the cheek and then turned backward to cover the nose while still attached to the cheek—a technique later modified using skin from the forehead. At the time, the mutilation of the nose was a common punishment, so these

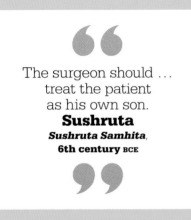

> The surgeon should ...
> treat the patient
> as his own son.
> **Sushruta**
> *Sushruta Samhita*,
> **6th century** BCE

The *Sushruta Samhita* has strikingly modern ideas about surgical training, instruments, and procedures. This 12th- or 13th-century version was found in Nepal.

operations were in great demand. Sushruta also recommended the use of wine as an anesthetic for such painful operations.

Spread of plastic surgery

Indian plastic surgery remained more advanced than anything in Europe for more than two millennia. In the 1st century CE, the Roman physician Aulus Celsus outlined how otoplasty corrected earlobes damaged by heavy earrings. In the 15th century, German surgeon Heinrich von Pfolspeundt described how to reconstruct a nose "which is off entirely." It was only when Europeans colonized India in the 17th and 18th centuries that they encountered sophisticated Indian rhinoplasty techniques. British surgeon Joseph Carpue was the first to adopt them, in 1814.

Plastic surgery progressed swiftly in the West; by 1827, the first operation to correct a cleft palate had been carried out in the US. The demands of treating severe wounds during two World Wars led

Plastic surgery and World War II

New Zealand–born plastic surgeon Archibald McIndoe became chief plastic surgery consultant to Britain's Royal Air Force in 1938. When World War II broke out in 1939, he was called to treat aircrew with severe burns.

Most burn treatments at the time used tannic jelly, resulting in severe contraction of the wound tissue, as well as permanent scarring. McIndoe devised new techniques, including saline burn baths and flap reconstruction to repair the faces and hands of injured airmen. McIndoe also understood the importance of postoperative rehabilitation, and he set up the Guinea Pig Club, a support network made up of more than 600 service personnel who had undergone operations at McIndoe's burn unit at the Queen Victoria Hospital in East Grinstead.

to the development of skin grafts. Plastic surgery techniques to fix accidental and congenital defects became increasingly sophisticated during the 1900s. Cosmetic surgery also became widespread. The first facelift was performed in 1901, and by the end of the 1900s, a range of facial and body enhancements were available. Plastic surgeons performed more than 10 million aesthetic surgical procedures in 2018. The same year, a 64-year-old Canadian Maurice Desjardins, who had suffered a shot wound to the face, became the oldest person ever to have a full facial transplant. ▪

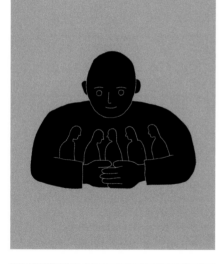

FIRST, DO NO HARM

GREEK MEDICINE

IN CONTEXT

BEFORE

c. 1750 BCE Hammurabi's Code stipulates payments for physicians and penalties for their failures.

c. 500 BCE Alcmaeon of Croton identifies the brain as the seat of intelligence.

AFTER

4th century BCE The great philosopher Aristotle expands on the humors theory, but sees the heart as the seat of vitality, intellect, and feeling.

c. 260 BCE Herophilus of Alexandria establishes the science of anatomy, describing nerves, arteries, and veins.

c. 70 BCE Asclepiades of Bithynia states the body is composed of molecules, and disease occurs if their pattern is disrupted.

c. 70 CE Dioscorides writes *De Materia Medica*, which remains the core text for plant-based medicine for 16 centuries.

Ancient medical practice was largely rooted in the belief that disease was caused by malevolent spirits or inflicted as a punishment by the gods. Most attempts to heal an illness usually involved ritual and prayer rather than any real attempt at medicinal cure. Although drug recipes using various plants had been concocted by Egyptian and Sumerian healers, their efficacy was questionable. An early attempt to regulate medical practice was set out by the Babylonian king Hammurabi around 1750 BCE. His wide-ranging law code included a scale of fees that doctors could charge—such as 10 shekels for excising a tumor from a nobleman. It also laid down harsh punishments for botched operations—a surgeon could lose his hands for causing the death of a patient. Yet Babylonian medicine

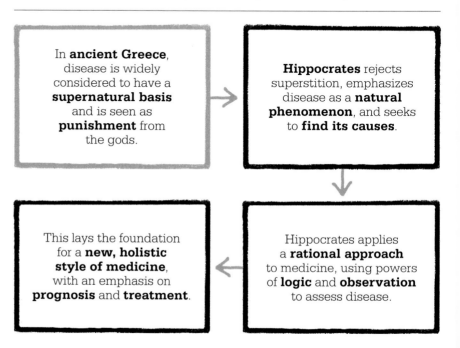

In **ancient Greece**, disease is widely considered to have a **supernatural basis** and is seen as **punishment** from the gods.

Hippocrates rejects superstition, emphasizes disease as a **natural phenomenon**, and seeks to **find its causes**.

Hippocrates applies a **rational approach** to medicine, using powers of **logic** and **observation** to assess disease.

This lays the foundation for a **new, holistic style of medicine**, with an emphasis on **prognosis** and **treatment**.

See also: Ancient Egyptian medicine 20–21 ▪ Herbal medicine 36–37
▪ Roman medicine 38–43 ▪ Pharmacy 54–59 ▪ Anatomy 60–63

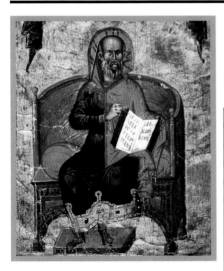

Hippocrates, the founding father of Western medicine, is depicted with a copy of his works in this 14th-century portrait. Widely translated, his theories greatly influenced medieval learning.

still employed exorcists to chase away disease-causing spirits, and it was not until the ancient Greeks began to try to explain the nature of the Universe in philosophical rather than divine terms that medical practice began to change.

Philosophy and medicine

Among the first to adopt a more rational approach to medicine was the philosopher–scientist Alcmaeon of Croton. In the 5th century BCE, he identified the brain as the seat of intelligence and also conducted scientific experiments, such as dissecting an eye to establish the structure of the optic nerve. He believed the body was governed by opposing influences (dry/hot or sweet/bitter) that must be balanced. Empedocles, another 5th-century Greek philosopher, believed that the human body was ruled by the four elements—earth, air, fire, and water.

These two theories were then synthesized by Hippocrates (c. 460 BCE–c. 375 BCE), the greatest physician in the ancient Greek world, in order to produce an all-encompassing theory of human physiology. He had founded a medical school on his native Cos, where he developed and taught the theory of the four humors (blood, phlegm, yellow bile, and black bile), whose equilibrium in the body was necessary for good health. Unlike rival medical schools such as the Cnidian school, he saw the body as a single system, not a collection of isolated parts, and insisted on observation of symptoms of disease to inform diagnosis and treatment.

A rational approach

The Hippocratic Corpus is a body of more than 60 works (including *Epidemics* and *On Fractures and Joints*) attributed to Hippocrates and his followers. Along with detailed case studies, it includes neatly defined disease categories that are still used today, such as *epidemic*, *chronic*, and *acute*. Hippocrates promoted holistic treatment of his patients, with as much emphasis placed on diet, exercise, massage, and hygiene as on drugs. This professional approach was reflected in his school's later insistence that its students take an oath promising to do patients no harm and to respect their confidentiality.

Hippocrates' rationalism laid the foundations for later physicians such as Galen and Dioscorides to establish medicine as a respected and vitally important profession. Its key advances would stem from science rather than the shady practices and old superstitions of itinerant healers and exorcists. ▪

The Hippocratic Oath

Traditionally attributed to Hippocrates and named after him, the oath required new physicians to swear to uphold a code of ethics. As a revered teacher and physician who had traveled widely, Hippocrates had great influence. The oath set a high standard of expertise and etiquette and established medicine as a profession that ordinary people could trust. It separated physicians from other "healers" and included a promise not to poison patients and to protect confidentiality. Hippocrates himself insisted that physicians be of a good appearance, as patients could not trust a doctor who did not look capable of taking care of himself. According to the oath, the physician must be calm, honest, and understanding.

The oath became a basis for medical ethics in the Western world, and many of its clauses are still relevant today, such as patient confidentiality and respect for patients.

A medieval Greek copy of the Hippocratic Oath. The original was probably written by a follower of Hippocrates, *c.* 400 BCE or later.

A BODY IN BALANCE

TRADITIONAL CHINESE MEDICINE

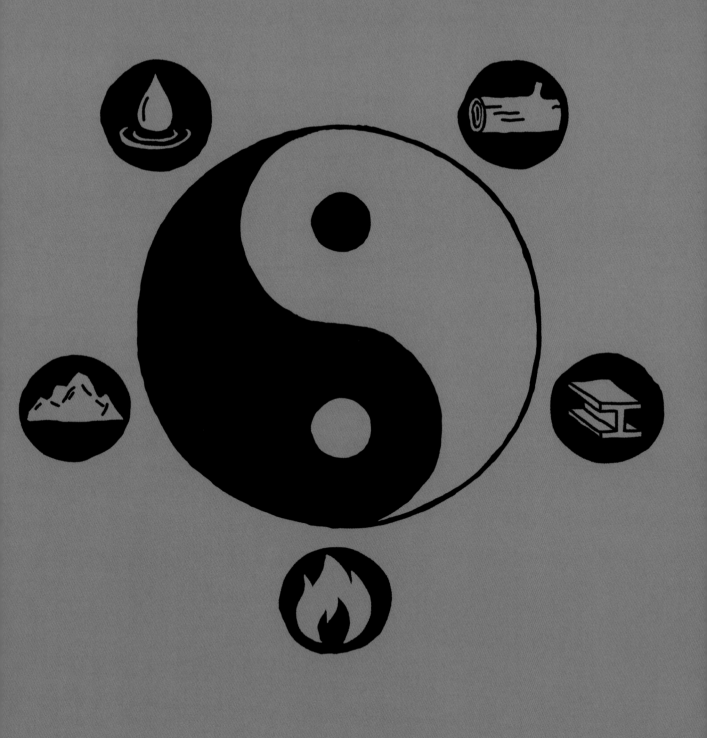

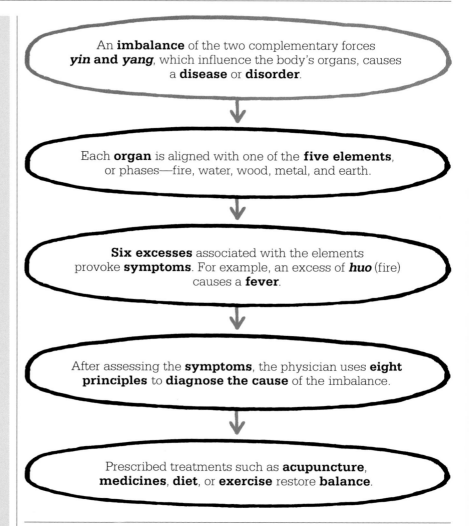

An **imbalance** of the two complementary forces **yin** and **yang**, which influence the body's organs, causes a **disease** or **disorder**.

Each **organ** is aligned with one of the **five elements**, or phases—fire, water, wood, metal, and earth.

Six excesses associated with the elements provoke **symptoms**. For example, an excess of **huo** (fire) causes a **fever**.

After assessing the **symptoms**, the physician uses **eight principles** to **diagnose the cause** of the imbalance.

Prescribed treatments such as **acupuncture**, **medicines**, **diet**, or **exercise** restore **balance**.

The foundational text of traditional Chinese medicine is the *Huangdi Neijing* (*The Yellow Emperor's Classic of Internal Medicine*). It was written around 300 BCE, during the Warring States period before China was unified under a single emperor, but it includes earlier ideas, such as the diagnostic methods of legendary physician Bian Qiao, described in his *Nanjing* (*Classic of Difficulties*).

The core principles of traditional Chinese medicine are far older. They are attributed to three mythical emperors. Emperor Fuxi created the *bagua*, eight symbols that represent the fundamental components of reality (Heaven, Earth, Water, Fire, Wind, Thunder, Mountain, and Lake). Each symbol is made up of three lines that are either broken (*yin*) or unbroken (*yang*). Shennong, the Red Emperor, discovered which plants had medicinal uses and which were toxic. Huangdi, the Yellow Emperor, invented acupuncture and was taught by the gods how to mix magical healing powders and use the pulse for diagnosis.

Whatever their origins, *yin* and *yang* (the universal concept on which Chinese medical philosophy is based), examination and diagnosis

See also: Ayurvedic medicine 22–25 ▪ Roman medicine 38–43 ▪ Islamic medicine 44–49 ▪ Medieval medical schools and surgery 50–51 ▪ Pharmacy 54–59 ▪ Anesthesia 112–117 ▪ Vitamins and diet 200–203

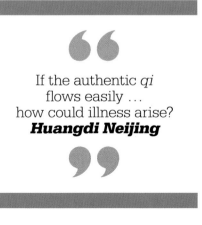

If the authentic *qi* flows easily … how could illness arise?
Huangdi Neijing

(the procedure for healing), and acupuncture and herbs (the means of healing), are the essence of traditional Chinese medicine, brought together in the *Huangdi Neijing*. Its text takes the form of discussions between the Yellow Emperor and his ministers. Huangdi asks questions about medical problems, and his advisers reply, setting out the core tenets of Chinese medical knowledge.

The key principles

The *Huangdi Neijing* describes the oppositions of *yin* and *yang*, the five elements (fire, water, wood, metal, and earth), and *qi*—the energy that flows along channels (meridians) of the body, sustaining life. The text also sets out diagnostic procedures, such as taking the pulse or looking at the patient's tongue, as well as treatments, including acupuncture, the prescription of herbs, massage, diets, and physical exercise.

The concept of balance between *yin* and *yang* is key; they are seen as opposed yet complementary forces that govern different aspects of the body and manifest their influences in different ways. *Yin* is cool, dark, passive, feminine, and most akin to water, while *yang* is hot, bright, active, and masculine, with a kinship to fire. An imbalance between them causes disease.

Each of the major internal organs is influenced either by *yin* or *yang*. The *yin* organs—the heart, spleen, lungs, kidney, liver, and pericardium (a thin sac around the heart)—are seen as solid, with functions that include regulating and storing key substances such as blood and *qi*. The *yang* organs—the small intestine, large intestine, gallbladder, stomach, and urinary bladder—are considered hollow; their function is to digest nutrients and eliminate waste.

The five elements, interacting in a system called *wu-xing*, each correspond to a *yin* and *yang* organ—fire to the heart/small intestine, water to the kidney/bladder, wood to the liver/gallbladder, metal to the lungs/large intestine, and earth to the spleen/stomach. Interactions between the elements create a dynamic, self-adjusting cycle of sheng (generating or nurturing), *ke* (controlling), *cheng* (overacting), and *wu* (rebelling). The vital force *qi* passes through the meridians, animating the organs. Taking in food and air replenishes *qi*. Without it, the body will die, and where it is deficient, the body will sicken.

Diagnosing disease

Traditional Chinese medicine aims to identify and correct imbalances in the body's *yin* and *yang*, *wu-xing*, and *qi*. A deficit of *yin*, for example, might appear as insomnia, night sweats, or a rapid pulse, while a lack of *yang* could cause cold limbs, a pale tongue, or a sluggish pulse. At a basic level, eight diagnostic principles help identify the complex patterns of disharmony. The first two principles are *yin* and *yang*, which help define the six other principles—deficiency, cold, interior, excess, heat, and exterior.

A physician can further diagnose the cause of external disorders according to six excesses (wind, »

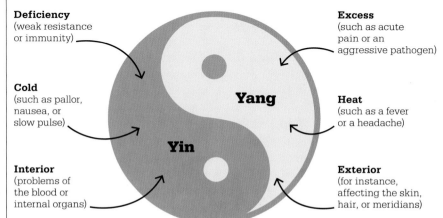

Deficiency (weak resistance or immunity)

Cold (such as pallor, nausea, or slow pulse)

Interior (problems of the blood or internal organs)

Excess (such as acute pain or an aggressive pathogen)

Heat (such as a fever or a headache)

Exterior (for instance, affecting the skin, hair, or meridians)

Yang

Yin

Traditional Chinese medicine uses eight principles to define disorders during diagnosis. They are *yin* and *yang* and the six principles they govern: the *yin* principles are deficiency, cold, and interior; the opposite *yang* principles are excess, heat, and exterior.

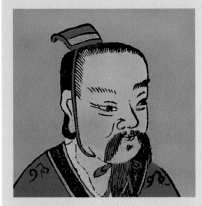

Bian Qiao

Born in the 5th century BCE, Bian Qiao is the first Chinese physician of whom anything is known—largely thanks to a biography written some 300 years after his death by historian Sima Qian. The story goes that a mysterious figure gave the young Qiao a book of medical secrets and a bunch of herbs, then disappeared. After taking the herbs in a solution for 30 days, Bian Qiao could see through the human body to diagnose disease.

As Bian Qiao traveled across the country, treating disorders and performing surgery, his fame as a gifted healer grew. Among the many near-miraculous cures was that of Zhao Jianzi, chief minister of the kingdom of Jin, whom Ban Qiao revived by using acupuncture after he had fallen into a coma and was believed dead.

In 310 CE, Bian Qiao was assassinated by a rival—Li Mi, a royal medical officer.

Key works

Nanjing (*Classic of Difficulties*)
Bian Qiao Neijing (*Bian Qiao's Classic of Internal Medicine*)

coldness, summer heat, dampness, dryness, and fire) that are allied to the elements. Internal problems are related to seven emotions: anger, happiness, thoughtfulness, sadness, fear, surprise, and anxiety.

In the 4th century BCE, Bian Qiao's *Nanjing* set out four key stages of diagnosis: observing a patient (especially the face and tongue); listening to the voice and internal sounds (and smelling the breath and body odors); asking the patient about symptoms; and taking the pulse. In the late 3rd century CE, Wang Shuhe wrote the *Maijing* (*Pulse Classic*), explaining where the pulse should be taken on the wrist—at the *cun* (close to the hand), the *guan* (slightly higher on the arm), or the *chi* (farthest up the arm). Taking a reading on the right wrist, he advised, was best for measuring *yin*, and on the left for *yang*. To gauge the health of different organs, he recommended taking two pulse measurements—first by pressing lightly, then more heavily—at each pulse point.

In traditional Chinese medicine, every diagnosis is tailored to the individual patient, as reflected in the saying *yin bing tong zhi; tong bin yi zhi*, or "different diseases, the same treatment; the same disease, different treatments." In other words,

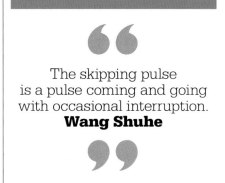

> The skipping pulse is a pulse coming and going with occasional interruption.
> **Wang Shuhe**

people with different symptoms may require the same treatment, while treatments for those with similar symptoms may differ.

A cure by needles

The aim of acupuncture is to correct the body's imbalances by inserting needles into the skin at key points to redirect the flow of *qi* along the body's 12 principal meridians and a host of minor ones. These points may be at some distance from the area where the problem appears; to remedy pain

Chinese physicians prescribed many exercises to help restore the body's balance. This image is part of a silk manuscript from the 2nd century BCE, found in a tomb in south central China.

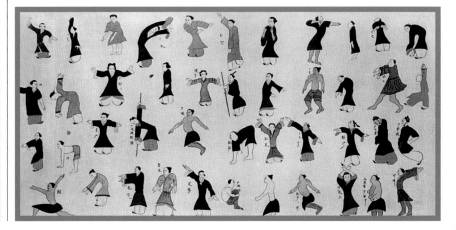

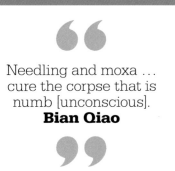

Needling and moxa …
cure the corpse that is
numb [unconscious].
Bian Qiao

in the lower back, for instance, the acupuncture points are located on the hand. The first key text, listing 349 points, was the *Systematic Classic of Acupuncture and Moxibustion*, written around 260 CE by Huangfu Mi and revised around 630 CE by Zhen Quan. By 1030, there were 657 points, as set out by Wang Weiyi, a renowned acupuncturist who made life-sized bronze models to illustrate the location of the points.

Moxibustion and more

A further key component of Chinese medicine is moxibustion—burning the herb mugwort (moxa) on or very near the surface of the skin to stimulate *qi*. As with acupuncture, herbal medicine, dietary rules, and other treatments were all refined during the 1st millennium CE. Leading Han dynasty physician Zhang Zhongjing (150–219 CE) wrote about diet and typhoid but is best known for *Shang han za bing lun* (*Treatise on Fevers and Other Diseases*). His contemporary Hua Tuo is considered to be China's first anesthetist; he used a powder called *mafeisan* (thought to have contained opium, cannabis, and small quantities of toxic herbs), which was dissolved in water and given to patients before surgery.

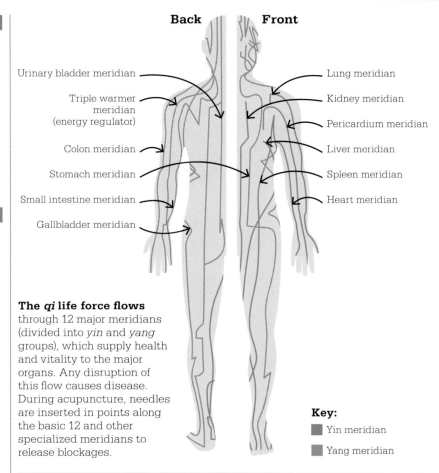

Back Front

Urinary bladder meridian
Triple warmer meridian (energy regulator)
Colon meridian
Stomach meridian
Small intestine meridian
Gallbladder meridian

Lung meridian
Kidney meridian
Pericardium meridian
Liver meridian
Spleen meridian
Heart meridian

The *qi* life force flows through 12 major meridians (divided into *yin* and *yang* groups), which supply health and vitality to the major organs. Any disruption of this flow causes disease. During acupuncture, needles are inserted in points along the basic 12 and other specialized meridians to release blockages.

Key:
■ Yin meridian
■ Yang meridian

With the advent of European medicine, introduced by Jesuit missionaries in the late 16th century, imperial China increasingly viewed acupuncture as mere superstition, and herbal treatments became the chief therapeutic tool of Chinese doctors. Physician Li Shizhen's 53-volume *Bencao Gengmu* (*Compendium of Materia Medica*) of 1576 lists 1,892 herbs and more than 11,000 combinations of herbs to prescribe for specific diseases.

Walking on two legs

As Western influence increased from the mid-19th century, traditional Chinese medicine was criticized for its perceived lack of scientific basis. It underwent a revival after the establishment of the People's Republic in 1949, partly because the new Communist government pledged to provide wider healthcare to a population of over 500 million, for whom there were only 15,000 physicians trained in Western medicine. The combination of modern and traditional medicine became known as the "walking-on-two-legs policy."

While scientists still point out the lack of clinical evidence for its efficacy, traditional Chinese medicine (TCM) is thriving today. Acupuncture is widely used to treat pain, and the inclusion of TCM in a 2018 World Health Organization diagnostic compendium looks set to further boost its influence. ■

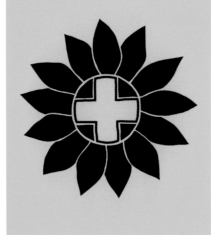

NATURE ITSELF IS THE BEST PHYSICIAN

HERBAL MEDICINE

IN CONTEXT

BEFORE

c. 2400 BCE A Sumerian cuneiform tablet records 12 recipes for drugs, including plant sources.

c. 1550 BCE The Ebers papyrus includes more than 700 plant species used by the ancient Egyptians to create medicines.

c. 300 BCE In ancient Greece, Theophrastus's *Historia Plantarum* classifies over 500 medicinal plants.

AFTER

512 CE The oldest surviving copy of *De Materia Medica* is produced for the daughter of the Roman emperor Olybrius.

c. 1012 *The Canon of Medicine* by Islamic physician Ibn Sina compiles material from many sources, including Dioscorides.

1554 Italian botanist and physician Pier Andrea Mattioli writes a lengthy commentary on *De Materia Medica*.

Many ancient societies employed herbs in medicinal treatment and recorded their uses. The Egyptian Ebers papyrus, a collection of medical texts compiled around 1550 BCE, cites 700 plant species to be used as herbal remedies and applications. In ancient Greek culture, Homer's epic poems the *Iliad* and *Odyssey*, both composed around 800 BCE, mention more than 60 plants with medicinal uses. However, it was only with the advent of a more scientific approach to medicine, initiated by the work of Hippocrates in the 5th century BCE, that a more consistent method of classifying plants according to their therapeutic action was taken.

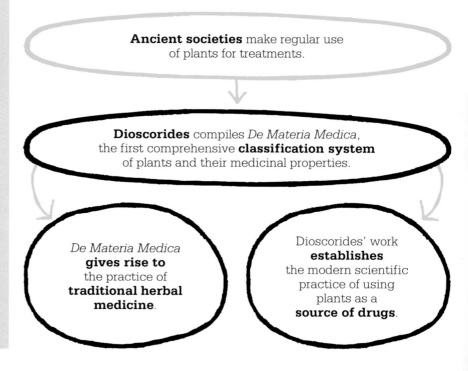

Ancient societies make regular use of plants for treatments.

Dioscorides compiles *De Materia Medica*, the first comprehensive **classification system** of plants and their medicinal properties.

De Materia Medica **gives rise to** the practice of **traditional herbal medicine**.

Dioscorides' work **establishes** the modern scientific practice of using plants as a **source of drugs**.

See also: Greek medicine 28–29 ▪ Roman medicine 38–43 ▪ Islamic medicine 44–49 ▪ Medieval medical schools and surgery 50–51 ▪ Pharmacy 54–59 ▪ Aspirin 86–87 ▪ Homeopathy 102

Pedanius Dioscorides

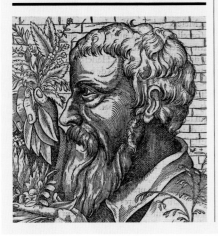

Born in Anazarbus (modern-day Turkey) around 40 CE, Dioscorides served as a surgeon in the Roman army during the reign of Emperor Nero. This enabled him to travel extensively throughout the eastern Mediterranean and to collect information on medically useful plants that grew in the region. By about 70 CE, he had used this knowledge to produce his *De Materia Medica*, a comprehensive five-volume textbook on herbal medicine. Written in his native Greek, it was organized according to the therapeutic properties of the plants, as well as the other substances he included. When it was later translated into Latin and Arabic, its neat organization was obscured by the editors' habit of alphabetizing his original lists of drugs. In illustrated form, it became a favorite of medieval manuscript copyists and of publishers of early printed books during the late Renaissance. Dioscorides died around 90 CE.

Key work

c. 70 CE *De Materia Medica* (*On Medicinal Substances*)

Pioneering botanist Theophrastus of Lesbos (a pupil of Aristotle) refined classification systems in the late 4th century BCE. In his *Historia Plantarum* (*Enquiry into Plants*), he devised a method for categorizing 500 medicinal plants according to detailed groupings such as physical features, habitats, and practical use.

De Materia Medica

The full development of herbal medicine came with the work of the Roman soldier–physician Dioscorides in the 1st century CE. His seminal text, *De Materia Medica* (*On Medicinal Substances*), assimilated his knowledge of plants based on years of observing their medicinal uses. Dioscorides' key insight was to arrange the work according to the physiological effect each drug had on the body, such as a diuretic effect (increased production of urine) or an emetic effect (causing vomiting). He recorded 944 drugs, of which more than 650 have a plant origin, and detailed their physical properties, as well as how they should be prepared, their medicinal effect, and the diseases against which they were effective. Many of these plants, such as willow and camomile, treated a range of conditions and became the mainstays of medieval herbals.

The rise of herbals

De Materia Medica was influential during Roman times, and even after the fall of the Roman Empire in the 5th century, it remained a key text. When Rome fell and its libraries were destroyed, many other medical works were lost, yet *De Materia Medica* survived thanks

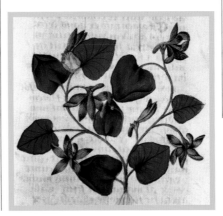

to copies that were made by scholars in the Byzantine and then Islamic empires. Dioscorides' work was widely translated and became the prime means by which classical medical knowledge was transmitted.

During the medieval period, *De Materia Medica* inspired a new genre of herbals—extensive compilations of medically useful plants. In the Renaissance, it had a further revival with the publication of lavish printed editions, including commentaries by scholars.

De Materia Medica established the modern scientific appreciation of plants as a crucial source of new drugs (leading, for example, to the extraction of medicinal quinine in 1820). It also bolstered the continuing practice of traditional herbal medicine, using plants and plant preparations directly for their therapeutic value. ∎

De Materia Medica became the foundation text for herbal medicine and pharmacology for 16 centuries. These hand-drawn sweet violets are from a 15th-century illustrated edition.

TO DIAGNOSE, ONE MUST OBSERVE AND REASON

ROMAN MEDICINE

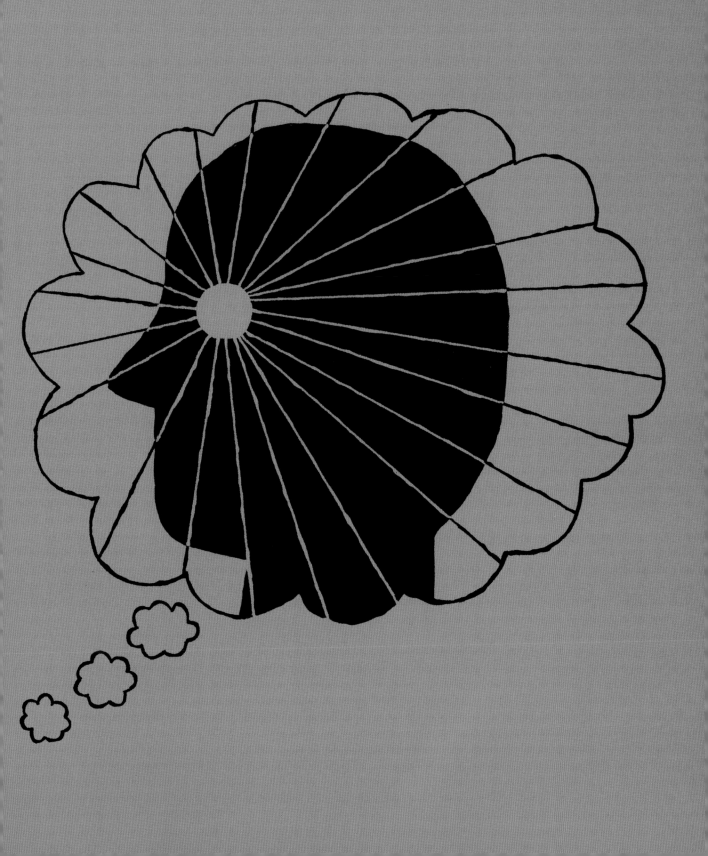

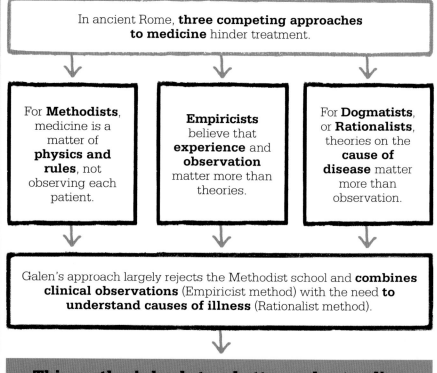

In ancient Rome, **three competing approaches to medicine** hinder treatment.

For **Methodists**, medicine is a matter of **physics and rules**, not observing each patient.

Empiricists believe that **experience and observation** matter more than theories.

For **Dogmatists**, or **Rationalists**, theories on the **cause of disease** matter more than observation.

Galen's approach largely rejects the Methodist school and **combines clinical observations** (Empiricist method) with the need **to understand causes of illness** (Rationalist method).

This synthesis leads to a better understanding of disease and to new medical theories.

T he Roman Empire, at its peak under the emperor Trajan in the 2nd century CE, stretched 1.9 million sq miles (5 million sq km) across Europe, North Africa, the Middle East, and western Asia. Its citizens took pride in their bath houses and aqueducts, but in reality, streets were insanitary and disease common. Yet Rome made strides in hygiene, and its contributions to medicine have had a lasting impact.

Greek roots

Roman medicine arose out of a synthesis of traditional practices, such as herbal healing, and the more theoretical and scientific approaches that had evolved in Greece since the 5th century BCE. At first, the principal borrowings from the Greek medical world were religious, in particular the adoption of the Greek deity Asclepios as the Roman god of healing. Then in 219 BCE, the Spartan doctor Archagathus arrived in Rome, marking the start of a change in the Roman attitude toward medicine. Archagathus was renowned for his ability to cure skin ailments and to heal wounds received in battle—a valuable skill at a time when the Romans knew little of surgery but were becoming embroiled in the Second Punic War against Carthage.

Although some in Rome called Archagathus "the Butcher," his treatment centers for soldiers paved the way for Rome's *valetudinaria*, or military hospitals, and he popularized Greek medical theories. The most important of these was the theory of the humors, developed by the Greek physician Hippocrates in the 5th century BCE. It proposed that the body was composed of four vital fluids—blood, yellow bile, black bile, and phlegm—and that an excess or lack of any of these was a sign of illness. The physician's role was to identify an imbalance and restore the patient to balance, which would ensure their continued health.

Schools of thought

As Greek medical tradition became accepted into Roman culture, Greek doctors came to Rome in increasing numbers. However, they met with varying levels of hostility. Historian and senator Cato the Elder, writing in the 2nd century BCE, rejected Greek innovations in favor of more traditional remedies, such as the use of cabbage: he recommended it for ailments ranging from stomach disorders to deafness.

Despite its opponents, Greek medicine became well established in Rome. Its results were clearly too effective to ignore. Over time, however, its followers fractured into a number of competing schools.

The Methodists, founded by the Greek physician Asclepiades in 50 BCE, applied a philosophical approach. This was based on the work of the philosopher Democritus, who had theorized that the Universe was made of atoms. Methodists believed the body was simply a physical construct and that with good hygiene, diet, and drugs, it could be easily put back into order. They decried the medical profession, believing that the basics of medicine could be learned in a few months.

By contrast, the Empiricists— founded by the Greek physician Philinus of Cos in c. 250 BCE— believed medical knowledge could be advanced by observing patients and identifying the visible signs of disease. However, they also believed that nature was fundamentally incomprehensible and that speculation on the causes of illness was pointless, so they had little interest in exploring the internal human anatomy.

A third medical school, the Rationalists or Dogmatists, placed greatest importance in physicians devising an underlying theory to guide their treatment of a disease. This was valued above examining the patient's particular symptoms. The Rationalists were more able than the Empiricists to devise general principles in dealing with diseases but did not promote any close clinical observation of specific cases. If a theory proved incorrect, it could lead to disastrous results.

Combined theories

It took a physician of rare ability to create a synthesis from these competing schools of thought. Claudius Galen, a Roman physician from Pergamum (in modern-day

> It is impossible for anyone to find the correct function of a part unless he is perfectly acquainted with the action of the whole instrument.
> **Claudius Galen**
> *De Usu Partium Corporis Humani,* c. 165–175 CE

Turkey), was such a man. By drawing on specific aspects of each school that aligned with his own theories, he created a medical approach that would remain common practice for over a thousand years.

Galen absorbed Greek philosophy and medical theories in his native Pergamum, but after he had moved to Rome in 162 CE, he developed them further. Like Hippocrates, he saw the human body as one complete system that should not be treated as a collection of isolated organs that yielded disparate sets of symptoms. To understand disease and to treat patients, Galen believed the physician must closely observe both inside and outside the human body. Only then could he apply a theoretical framework, based on »

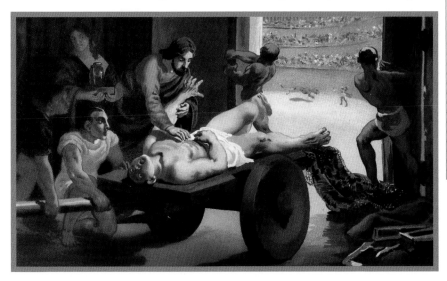

When serving as physician for a gladiatorial school, Galen gained first-hand experience of the internal human anatomy through treating the wounded and examining the dead.

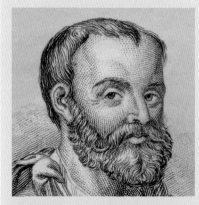

Claudius Galen

Born in Pergamum (in modern-day Turkey) in 129 CE, Galen decided to become a doctor after the healing god Asclepios appeared to his father in a dream. He studied at Pergamum, Smyrna, and then Alexandria, where he had access to medical texts in the Great Library.

After five years as chief physician to the gladiatorial school in Pergamum, Galen moved to Rome in 162 CE. There, his growing medical reputation and abrasive personality won him enemies. Forced to leave in 166, he was brought back by Emperor Marcus Aurelius in 169 to serve as imperial physician—a post he also held under Commodus and Septimius Severus. Galen died in c. 216. A prolific writer, he left around 300 works, including books on linguistics, logic, and philosophy, as well as medicine, but only about half of these have survived.

Key work

c. 165–175 CE *De Usu Partium Corporis Humani* (*On the Usefulness of the Parts of the Human Body*)

the humors of Hippocrates, when proposing cures. With this approach, Galen combined Rationalist and Empiricist thought—but he remained skeptical of the Methodist school.

Clinical observation

Galen believed an understanding of anatomy together with direct observation and experiment were fundamental medical requirements. During his time as chief physician to a Pergamum gladiatorial school, he had observed elements of the musculature and internal organs exposed by wounds. Yet human dissection was forbidden by Roman law, so he was confined to the dissection of animals. Galen's experiments on barbary apes, cattle, and pigs enabled him to make certain advances, such as understanding that the arteries

contained blood. During one experiment, he severed the laryngeal nerve of a live pig, which continued to struggle but was no longer able to squeal. This confirmed Galen's own hypothesis concerning the nerve's role in vocalization.

Galen's emphasis on observation extended to the clinical examination of patients' external symptoms as a means to diagnose and to prescribe correct cures. During the Antonine Plague, which erupted in 165 CE, Galen recorded symptoms of patients he examined. In all cases, he saw vomiting, upset stomachs, and foul breath, but the patients whose bodies became covered in black scabs that fell off after a few days tended to survive. In contrast, patients who excreted dark black stools would usually die. Galen did not understand the cause of this

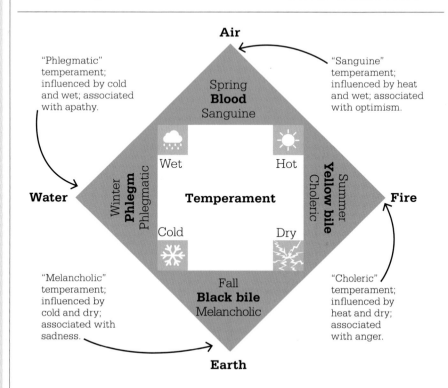

Galen linked each of the four humors to a season, an element (such as air), and a temperament (such as sanguine). Ideally, humors remained balanced; an excess or lack of one could result in illness.

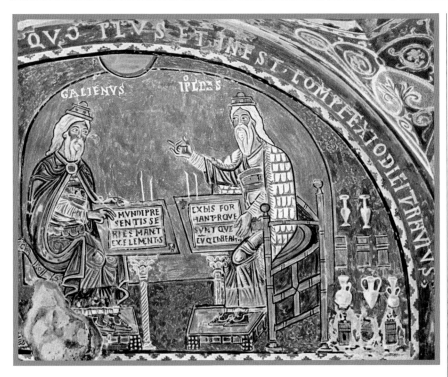

Although separated by centuries, Galen and Hippocrates are portrayed together in this 13th-century Byzantine fresco in Italy as the most significant physicians of the ancient world.

disease, which may have been smallpox, and little could be done other than to make the patients comfortable. However, his detailed recording of the symptoms is a testament to his commitment to understanding the signs of disease.

Galen's medical ideas were rooted in his development of Hippocrates' theory of humors. He expanded Hippocrates' idea on the variables of hot and cold, and wet and dry—each of which played a role in the equilibrium of the body. A person who has a tendency to coldness and dryness, Galen believed, would have a soft constitution and be slim. He also considered that the relative combinations of these factors affected temperament. The person

with high levels of cold and dry, for example, would most likely be melancholic. Galen also claimed that high levels of yellow bile would contribute to intelligence.

Lasting fame

Although Galen was Rome's most famous physician, there were others who carried out groundbreaking work. The mid-1st century CE saw Aulus Celsus, who dealt with diet and surgery, and identified many skin disorders. Soranus of Ephesus in the early 2nd century was a pioneer of obstetrics and gynecology. Yet it was Galen's work that survived the fall of Rome in 476, in books that were translated and transmitted via Islamic physicians from the 7th century, to become the basis of medieval European medicine.

Ironically, despite his emphasis on practical experimentation and clinical observation, it was Galen's elevation to the status of ultimate

medical authority that impeded progress in both areas. He had carried out most of his anatomical research on animals, and many of his results were invalid for humans. Yet Galen's authority meant later practitioners were so certain of his work that for centuries those performing dissections simply rejected any contradictory evidence before them. As more physicians attempted to replicate Galen's experiments, the flaws in his theories appeared. With the work of Flemish physician Andreas Vesalius in 1543, Galen's authority as an anatomist collapsed.

Despite this fall from grace, Galen's contribution to medicine was immense. The Islamic physician al-Razi (854–925), who wrote *Doubts about Galen*, was still supportive of his methods rather than his findings. Modern physicians work on the basis that an accurate knowledge of human anatomy combined with close clinical observation of symptoms is essential to treating disease. As such, Galen continues to be a towering influence on the practice of medicine. ∎

> In the course of a single dissection … Galen has departed on two hundred or more occasions from the true description of the harmony, function, and action of the human parts.
> **Andreas Vesalius**
> *De Humani Corporis Fabrica*, 1543

KNOW THE CAUSES OF SICKNESS AND HEALTH

ISLAMIC MEDICINE

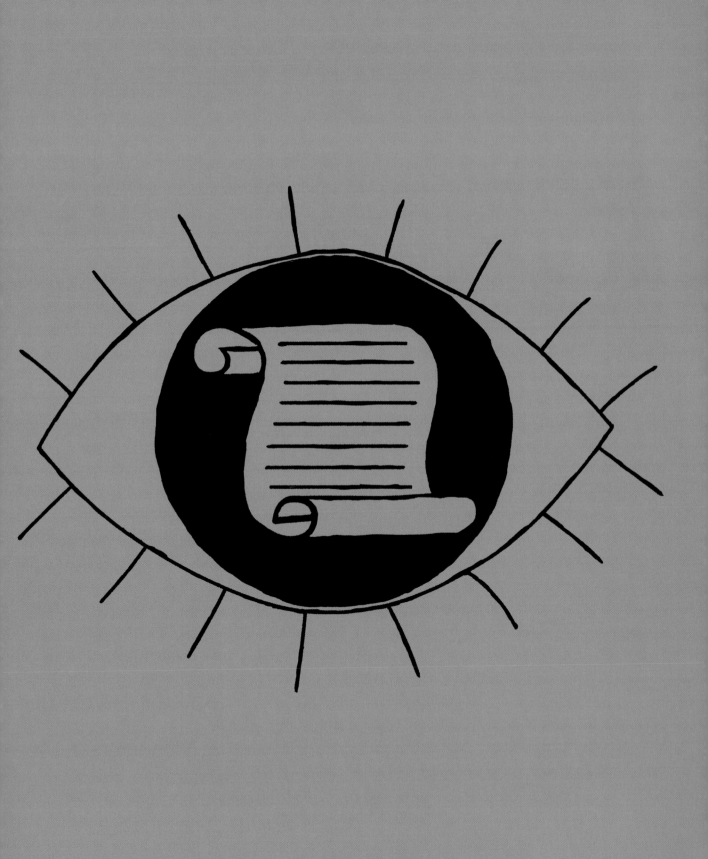

IN CONTEXT

BEFORE

4th–6th century CE The world's first medical center develops at Gondeshapur under the patronage of Sassanian kings from Shapur I.

627 The first mobile hospital is a tent for the Muslim wounded, set up during the *Ghazwah Khandaq* (Battle of the Ditch).

c. 770 Caliph al-Mansur founds the *Bayt-al Hikma* (House of Wisdom), where many ancient medical texts are translated into Arabic.

AFTER

12th–13th century In Spain, the first Latin translation of Ibn Sina's *Al-Qanun fi al-Tibb* (*The Canon of Medicine*) appears.

1362 After the Black Death ravages Europe, Ibn al-Khatib of Granada writes a treatise on contagious infections.

1697 Ibn Sina's *Qanun* is still on the curriculum at the medical school in Padua, Italy.

> Truth in medicine is an unattainable goal, and the art as described in books is far beneath the knowledge of an experienced and thoughtful physician.
> **Al-Razi**

The fall of the western Roman Empire in the late 5th century CE led to a steep decline in the level of medical knowledge and practice in Europe, but Hellenistic (Greek) culture had survived in the empire's eastern provinces, conquered by the armies of a new religion—Islam—in the 7th century. There, the medical theories from ancient Greece and ancient Rome were transmitted to early Islamic physicians by Nestorian (Eastern) Christians who worked in the medical center at Gondeshapur in Iran under the Persian Sasanian emperors.

This interest continued under the Islamic caliphs, particularly the Abbasids, whose capital Baghdad (founded in 762) became a vibrant economic, cultural, and scientific center. In the late 8th century, caliph al-Mansur established the *Bayt al-Hikma*, or House of Wisdom, which became a base for the translation of ancient texts into Arabic. Men such as Ibn Ishaq (808–873), the court physician who translated the works of Hippocrates and Galen, ensured that Islamic physicians had access to the medical theories of the Greek and Roman world. A new era of Islamic medicine developed, fueled by luminaries such as al-Razi (854–925) and Ibn Sina (980–1037), known in the West as Rhazes and Avicenna respectively.

Early Islamic hospitals

From the start, Islamic medicine embraced the practicalities of treatment, as well as medical theory. In the 7th century, Islam's first mobile hospital had treated battlefield injuries, and the academy at Gondeshapur had become a renowned center of medical treatment and learning. Islam's first documented general hospital—or *bimaristan* (Persian for "place of the sick")—was founded around 805 by caliph al-Rashid in Baghdad and quickly achieved fame. Within a century, another five had been built, and more were later established around the Middle East.

Medical schools had close links to such hospitals, and students could observe patients being treated by qualified doctors. Some hospitals had separate wards for infectious diseases, gastrointestinal problems, eye ailments, and mental illnesses. As a result of such first-hand clinical experience, early Islamic physicians made important advances in identifying disorders and devising effective cures.

Clinical expertise

In the 9th century, al-Razi, the chief physician to the caliph in Baghdad, wrote more than 200 texts and commentaries developing the principles of earlier Greek, Roman, Syrian, Islamic, and Indian medical

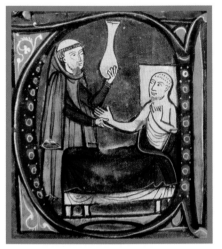

Al-Razi examines a patient and holds up a matula, a vessel for collecting urine, in a French image from the 13th century. Al-Razi pioneered a scientific approach to uroscopy, the study of urine.

> The physician … must always make the patient believe that he will recover, for the state of the body is linked to the state of the mind.
> **Kitab al-Hawi fi al-Tibb, c. 900**

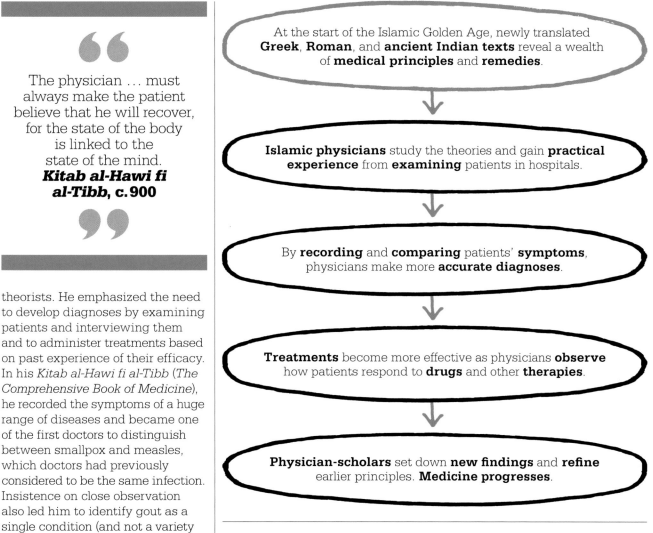

At the start of the Islamic Golden Age, newly translated **Greek**, **Roman**, and **ancient Indian texts** reveal a wealth of **medical principles** and **remedies**.

Islamic physicians study the theories and gain **practical experience** from **examining** patients in hospitals.

By **recording** and **comparing** patients' **symptoms**, physicians make more **accurate diagnoses**.

Treatments become more effective as physicians **observe** how patients respond to **drugs** and other **therapies**.

Physician-scholars set down **new findings** and **refine** earlier principles. **Medicine progresses**.

theorists. He emphasized the need to develop diagnoses by examining patients and interviewing them and to administer treatments based on past experience of their efficacy. In his *Kitab al-Hawi fi al-Tibb* (*The Comprehensive Book of Medicine*), he recorded the symptoms of a huge range of diseases and became one of the first doctors to distinguish between smallpox and measles, which doctors had previously considered to be the same infection. Insistence on close observation also led him to identify gout as a single condition (and not a variety of conditions, as the Greeks had supposed), and he concluded from his clinical experience that many diseases did not follow the course that Galen, the great Roman physician, had suggested.

Among al-Razi's many insights were his views on mental illness and the connection between mind and body. He championed the idea that mental disorders should be treated in the same way as physical diseases and prescribed

therapies involving diet, medicines, and even music and aromatherapy. He also urged that patients should be encouraged to believe in the possibility of improvement and the efficacy of a treatment, as this was likely to produce better outcomes.

Licensed to practice

Al-Razi was revered as not only a model practitioner but also as a teacher. Not everyone matched his high standards, however, and in

931, caliph al-Muqtadir ordered the licensing of all physicians when he heard that an error had caused a patient's death. When medical students passed their examinations, they took the Hippocratic Oath and received a license from a *muhtasib* (inspector general).

A great medical manual

The idea that medicine should be based on a comprehensive system of observation, experimentation, »

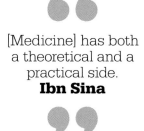

> [Medicine] has both a theoretical and a practical side.
> **Ibn Sina**

and testing in order to establish diagnoses and devise the best treatment reached its most developed form in the work of Ibn Sina. His *Al-Qanun fi al-Tibb* (*The Canon of Medicine*), published around 1012, gathered knowledge from Greek, Roman, Persian, and Arabic works and combined it with his own clinical observations to create the most comprehensive medical manual of the medieval era. In the 12th century, it was translated into Latin and became an essential part of the training for medical students in Europe for around 400 years.

The *Qanun* ran to more than a million words in five volumes. The first book dealt with the origins of diseases. Drawing much from the Hippocratic and Galenic theory of humors, Ibn Sina classified the possible causes of disease, both extrinsic (such as the climate of the region) and intrinsic (such as whether the patient has excessive sleep/rest or excessive movement/ activity), alongside other causes (such as the habits and constitution of the person). Ibn Sina believed that the four humors interacted with the "elements" (earth, air, fire, and water) and the patient's anatomy to cause disease. An excess of moisture, for example, might cause tiredness or digestive disorders, while elevated heat could induce thirst or a racing pulse. Like Galen and Hippocrates, he considered that direct observation of a patient could determine which factor was out of balance.

Drugs, diseases, and cures

The second book of the *Qanun* catalogued about 800 remedies and medicines from plant, animal, and mineral sources, together with the diseases they could treat most effectively. Ibn Sina drew from Indian and Greek authorities, then offered his own opinions of the efficacy of remedies, their differing strengths, and certain variations in recipes from different sources.

With advice partly taken from Galen, Ibn Sina also set down seven rules for experimenting with new drugs. He cautioned that medicines should not be exposed to excessive heat or cold, and that a drug should be tested on a patient who suffered from one rather than multiple conditions and given only in small doses at first to observe the effect. In the third and fourth books, Ibn Sina covers disorders of specific parts of the body, from head to toe, including tuberculosis affecting the lungs (correctly identified as contagious) and cataracts of the eye, and those that affect the whole body or several different parts, such as fevers, ulcers, fractures, and skin conditions. The fifth and final book describes a number of complex preparations and treatments and a collection of preventive measures, including diet and exercise. Ibn Sina's recognition that prevention is better than cure set him several centuries ahead of medieval European physicians.

Built on earlier advances

Before Ibn Sina, a constellation of Islamic physicians had contributed to the advancement of medical science. In the late 8th century, Jabir Ibn Hayyan (known in Europe as Geber), who was the court physician to caliph al-Rashid, formalized the study of pharmacology. Although many of the 500 works attributed to him were probably written by his later followers, Jabir himself brought experimental rigor to the traditional practice of alchemy, which sought

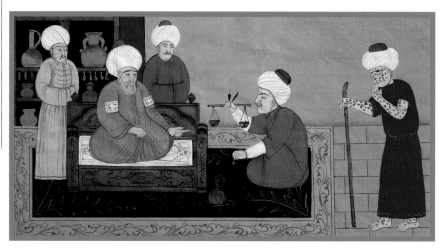

A pharmacist weighs out a medicine for a patient suffering from smallpox in this illustration from Ibn Sina's *Canon of Medicine*. Islamic pharmacists—like doctors—were trained and licensed.

Ibn Sina

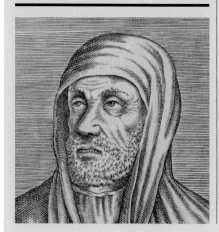

Born in 980 CE near Bukhara (in present-day Uzbekistan), Ibn Sina, the son of a government official, studied Islamic philosophy, law, and medicine. At the age of 18, he successfully treated Nuh Ibn Mansur, the Samanid sultan of Bukhara, which gained him a position at court and access to the extensive royal library.

The collapse of the Samanids in 999 forced Ibn Sina to flee, and he spent several years in Khorasan, a region covering parts of northeast Iran, Afghanistan, and Central Asia, before moving to Hamadan, a city in west central Iran. There, he was court physician and vizier to the Buyid ruler Shams ad-Dawla. In 1022, Ibn Sina moved to Isfahan, under the patronage of Persian prince Ala al-Dawlah, and completed his major works. He died in 1037 from the aftereffects of a slave adding excessive opium to one of his remedies.

Key works

c. 1012 *Al-Qanun fi al-Tibb* (*The Canon of Medicine*)
c. 1027 *Kitab al-Shifa* (*Book of Healing*)

to transform one substance into another (notably base metals into gold). A brilliant chemist, he catalogued key processes, such as crystallization and evaporation, and invented the alembic, a jar used for distillation. Jabir's work gave pharmacists of his time the tools to develop new drugs.

Other notable precursors to Ibn Sina include al-Tabari, a 9th-century Persian physician who taught al-Razi and wrote the seven-part *Firdous al-Hikmah* (*Paradise of Wisdom*)— one of the earliest encyclopedias of Islamic medicine. Al-Tamimi, a 10th-century physician in Cairo,

If the physician is able to treat with nutrients, not medication, then he has succeeded.
Kitab al-Hawi fi al-Tibb, c. 900

Egypt, was renowned for his extensive knowledge of medicinal herbs; for his guide to nutrition, plants, and minerals (*al-Murshid*); and for an antidote for snakebite so successful that he called it *tiryaq al-faruq* ("the cure of salvation").

In Cordoba, Spain, Andalusian court physician and the medieval era's greatest surgeon al-Zahrawi compiled the 30-part *Kitab al-Tasrif* (*The Methods of Medicine*) in the late 10th century. It included a surgical treatise outlining many sophisticated techniques, such as the removal of bladder stones, the excision of cancerous tumors from breasts, as well as gynecological operations and an early form of plastic surgery to mitigate damage caused by wounds.

Lasting influence

A product of the Islamic Golden Age, Islamic medicine had a significant impact on Western Europe from the medieval era until the 17th century, when new scientific ideas emerged during the Age of Enlightenment. Islamic medicine was advanced in many ways, with its emphasis on well-being, its insistence on observation of the patient as the basis for diagnosis, the keeping of detailed patient records, the inclusive nature of its hospitals that treated all members of society, the training of doctors, and the employment of female physicians and nurses. Its teaching lives on, especially in the Unani system of medicine practiced in Iran, Pakistan, and India. ∎

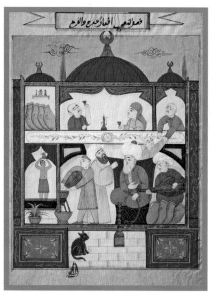

Ibn Sina teaches his students the principles of hygiene in this image from a 17th-century Ottoman manuscript. Ibn Sina taught daily at a local medical school during his later life in Isfahan.

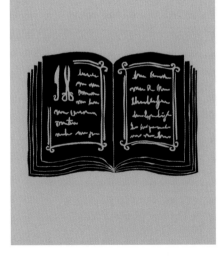

LEARNED, EXPERT, INGENIOUS, AND ABLE TO ADAPT
MEDIEVAL MEDICAL SCHOOLS AND SURGERY

After the fall of the Roman Empire, what remained of Greco-Roman medical knowledge in Western Europe retreated into monasteries. The Benedictine monastic order of the Catholic Church, founded in the 6th century CE, insisted that each of its monasteries had an infirmary with a monk in charge. One of the first of these was Montecassino, in southern Italy. In the early 800s, the Holy Roman Emperor Charlemagne decreed that every cathedral and monastery in his kingdom should have a hospital attached. Monks provided palliative care and treated a wide range of ailments. Many

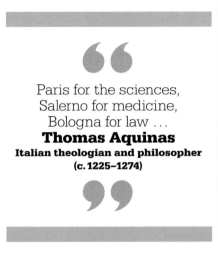

> Paris for the sciences, Salerno for medicine, Bologna for law ...
> **Thomas Aquinas**
> **Italian theologian and philosopher**
> **(c. 1225–1274)**

monasteries had their own medicinal garden for herbal remedies. Some had qualified apothecaries, and their in-depth knowledge of plants enabled them to prescribe a range of herbal or mineral remedies, as they carried out basic procedures such as bloodletting. Beyond the monasteries, medical schools advanced new ideas and skills, epitomized in the late 12th century by the master surgeon Roger of Salerno, or Rogerius.

Schola Medica Salernitana
The first formal medical teaching school emerged from the European Dark Ages in the 9th century CE in Salerno, southern Italy. It drew on influences from Islamic, Jewish, Greek, and Roman medicine. For four centuries, the reputation of this school, Schola Medica Salernitana, as a center of teaching excellence was probably unrivaled in medieval Europe. Students, teachers, and those seeking medical treatment traveled long distances to reach Salerno. In 1099, for example, Robert II of Normandy traveled from northern France to receive medical attention. Salerno had the world's most extensive medical library, with

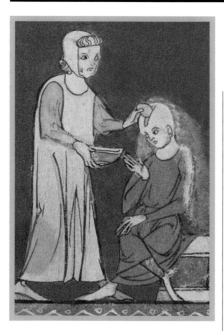

texts by Islamic physicians al-Razi (854–925) and Ibn Sina (980–1037), and other texts from Montecassino reflecting the teachings of ancient Greece and Rome. The school provided thorough curriculum-based teaching, typically with three years of study followed by four years of hands-on training.

An illustration showing a cranial operation, taken from Rogerius's *Practica Chirurgiae*. His work brought academic respect to the discipline of surgery.

Women were welcomed as students and teachers at Salerno. In the early or mid-12th century, the most prominent of these was Trota (or Trocta), a physician, educator, and writer. Her specialties were gynecology and midwifery, but she gave students a grounding in a range of diagnostic tools, including how to analyze urine, check pulse rates, and examine skin tone.

Roger of Salerno

Salerno's reputation peaked in the late 12th century, when Rogerius (c. 1140–1195) became its most famous teacher and surgeon. His *Practica Chirurgiae* (*Practice of Surgery*) was considered a standard text for at least 300 years. Written in 1180, it was the first work to deal with treatments arranged anatomically, describing diagnoses and treatments for diseases and disorders of the head, neck, arms, chest, abdomen, and legs. Rogerius's pioneering work included methods for detecting tears in the cerebral membrane (the Valsalva maneuver) and realigning damaged tissues (reanastomosis).

Medical schools spread

By the 12th century, other medical schools had been set up in Europe, including those at Montpellier in France, Bologna and Padua in Italy, Combria in Portugal, Vienna in Austria, and Heidelberg in Germany—all modeled on Salerno.

French surgeon Guy de Chauliac (c. 1300–1368) studied at Montpellier and Bologna and was appointed to the most prestigious position in Europe—personal physician to Pope Clement VI. Chauliac's *Chirurgia Magna* (*Great [work on] Surgery*) covered an array of subjects, including anatomy, anesthetics, bloodletting, drugs, fractures, and wounds. The seven-volume text was translated from Latin into many languages and became a new authority for surgeons until the 17th century, when new medical theories began to emerge. ∎

The Black Death

One of the deadliest pandemics in human history, the Black Death was a devastating outbreak of bubonic plague that killed 25 to 200 million people in Asia, Europe, and North Africa in the mid-14th century. It probably originated in Central or East Asia and spread west, peaking in Europe between 1347 and 1351. Up to half of Europe's population perished, with cities faring particularly badly. For instance, the population of Florence, Italy, fell from 110,000 to 50,000 during this period. Most people who contracted the disease died within days.

At the time, the cause of the plague was not understood, but some physicians blamed "a great pestilence in the air" (the miasma theory). It is now known that the bacteria responsible for it were carried by rat fleas. Rats were commonplace in overcrowded, unhygienic cities, and they were also transported from port to port on boats. The idea of quarantine first emerged in the city-state of Ragusa (modern Dubrovnik, Croatia) in 1377.

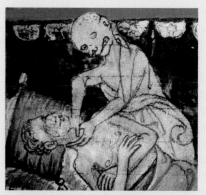

A 14th-century depiction of Death strangling a victim of bubonic plague. Guy de Chauliac distinguished between this and pneumonic plague.

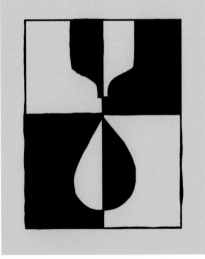

THE VAMPIRE OF MEDICINE
BLOODLETTING AND LEECHES

IN CONTEXT

BEFORE

c. 400 BCE Hippocrates promotes his theory of the four humors, which becomes the basis for bloodletting.

c. 1000 CE Al-Zahrawi describes surgical instruments for use in bloodletting.

AFTER

1411 French healer Peretta Peronne is prosecuted for carrying out bloodletting, a practice forbidden to women.

1719 Austrian surgeon Lorenz Heister develops the spring lancet.

1799 First US president George Washington dies from shock and loss of blood after being bled excessively by his doctors.

1828 Research by French doctor Pierre Louis suggests the medicinal use of leeches is of little value, leading to a reduction in the procedure.

The practice of medicinal bloodletting—the removal of blood to cure disease—is thought to have originated in ancient Egypt around 3000 BCE. It passed into ancient Greek culture during the 5th century BCE, and was formalized as a procedure after the physician Hippocrates declared blood to be one of the four bodily humors that must remain in balance to preserve health.

Bloodletting was widespread in Europe by the medieval era. In 1163, the Church forbade clerics carrying out the procedure, so barbers performed bloodletting and other surgery, using instruments such as fleams (blades with handles), lancets (needles), or the medicinal leech (*Hirudo medicinalis*) to suck blood and anesthetize the wound.

Bridging the gap

The divide between physicians, who dispensed cures, and barber-surgeons, who operated directly on the body, only began to close in the 1250s, when doctors such as Italy's Bruno da Longobucco argued that bloodletting should not be left to barber-surgeons alone. Bloodletting then became a central medical tool until the 19th century: one French doctor, François Broussais (1772–1838), was branded the "Vampire of Medicine" for his leech-mania.

Today, leeches are still used to remove congested blood in some operations, and bloodletting plays a role in treating conditions such as hemochromatosis (a disorder causing an accumulation of excess iron in the blood). ∎

> Bloodletting frequently strangles fever … it imparts strength to the body.
> **Benjamin Rush**
> American physician (1746–1813)

See also: Greek medicine 28–29 ▪ Roman medicine 38–43 ▪ Medieval medical schools and surgery 50–51 ▪ Blood circulation 68–73

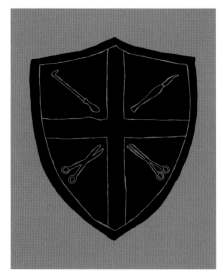

WARS HAVE FURTHERED THE PROGRESS OF THE HEALING ART
BATTLEFIELD MEDICINE

IN CONTEXT

BEFORE
c. 500 BCE Sushruta describes a form of tourniquet that can prevent arterial bleeding during amputations.

c. 150 BCE Galen advises against tourniquets, claiming that they increase bleeding.

c. 1380 CE The use of a wicker stretcher to carry a casualty from the battlefield to safety is recorded in France.

AFTER
1847 Russian surgeon Nikolai Pirogov introduces ether to be used as an anesthetic in the Crimean War.

1916 In World War I, British chemist Henry Dakin designs a disinfectant to kill bacteria without damaging the flesh.

1937 In the Spanish Civil War, Canadian surgeon Norman Bethune's refrigerated trucks, the first mobile blood banks, allow blood transfusions to take place near the front line.

Wounds inflicted in battle have engaged doctors since ancient times. The Edwin Smith papyrus, an Egyptian surgical text from c. 17th century BCE, details treatments for injuries sustained in battle. The Roman army gained significant expertise in battlefield medicine. Yet by the medieval era, techniques had barely progressed, and most serious wounds resulted in death either from shock or bacterial infection.

Pioneering techniques
During a battle in 1537, French army barber-surgeon Ambroise Paré ran out of the boiling oil traditionally used to treat gunshot wounds. (It was believed to purge the body of poisonous gunpowder.) Resorting to a folk remedy of egg yolk, rose oil, and turpentine, he found that the wounds healed more rapidly and with much less pain. Paré later pioneered the use of ligatures rather than cauterization to seal amputations and developed the *Bec de corbin* ("crow's beak"), a clamp to secure the ligature

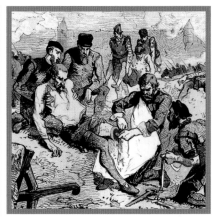

Ambroise Paré's ligature technique (tying arteries during amputations to stop hemorrhaging) represented a significant surgical breakthrough.

during the procedure. His many other advances include long forceps to extract bullets from wounds and the use of pain relief in surgery.

Paré's work inspired others such as Dominique-Jean Larrey, a French surgeon in the Napoleonic Wars, who introduced military ambulances to transport casualties to safety and pioneered the concept of "triage" to assess the urgency of cases. ∎

See also: Plastic surgery 26–27 ▪ Roman medicine 38–43 ▪ Scientific surgery 88–89 ▪ Triage 90 ▪ Blood transfusion and blood groups 108–111

THE ART OF PRESCRIBING LIES IN NATURE

PHARMACY

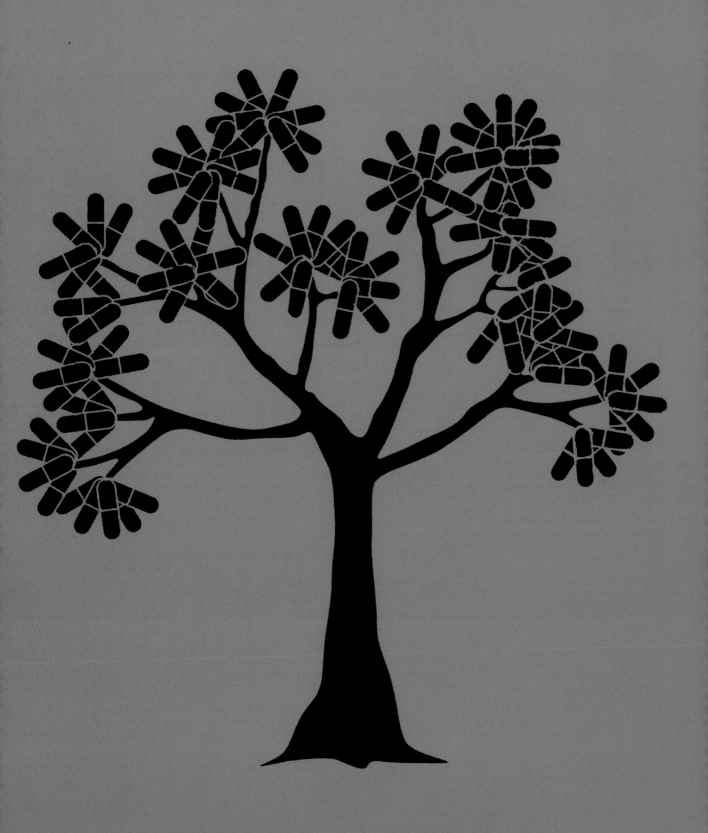

IN CONTEXT

BEFORE

c. 70 CE Dioscorides writes *De Materia Medica*.

c. 780 Jabir ibn Hayyan develops ways of purifying and mixing drugs.

1498 The first official pharmacopeia, *Ricettario Fiorentino*, is issued in Italy.

AFTER

1785 British physician William Withering conducts one of the first clinical drug trials, proving the efficacy of digitalin.

1803 The first known alkaloid, morphine, is isolated by Louis Derosne.

1828 Friedrich Wöhler synthesizes urea from nonorganic compounds.

1860s Claude Bernard proves drugs have specific sites of action in the body.

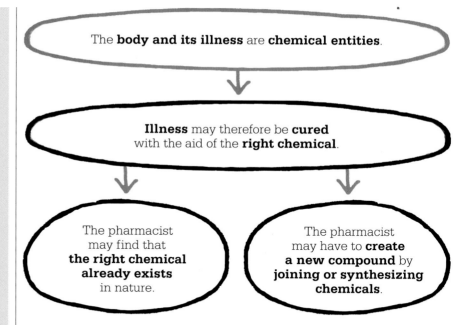

The **body and its illness** are **chemical entities**.

↓

Illness may therefore be **cured** with the aid of the **right chemical**.

↓ ↓

The pharmacist may find that **the right chemical already exists** in nature.

The pharmacist may have to **create a new compound** by **joining or synthesizing chemicals**.

Pharmacy is the idea that certain substances can be used to treat or prevent disease or to correct bodily functions. Today, people take it for granted that if they are ill, a doctor will prescribe drugs to make them better. Such demand has made the production of pharmaceuticals one of the world's biggest industries, with an estimated worth of around $1.5 trillion.

One of the first major proponents of pharmacy was the 16th-century Swiss physician Philippus von Hohenheim, who went by the name of Paracelsus. Paracelsus was an alchemist, not a modern scientist, and his theories involved occult concepts, but in placing chemistry at the heart of treatment for disease, he characterized the new focus of Renaissance science and initiated the field of pharmacology.

Ancient origins

The idea of using particular substances to heal ailments goes back to prehistoric times, and even animals often know instinctively to home in on certain plants or minerals when sick. Surviving papyri tell us that ancient Egyptian physicians wrote healing recipes for their patients and recognized the purgative qualities of plant materials such as senna and castor oil. Folk healers also passed down knowledge about the curative properties of herbs, and in Greek and Roman times, physicians began writing these down. Around 70 CE, the Greek military surgeon Dioscorides produced *De Materia Medica*—a compendium of known medical treatments, mostly plant-based—which remained the go-to book for medicaments until the 18th century.

Knowledge like this depended on finding naturally occurring substances, especially herbs. The idea of creating chemical drugs emerged in the Muslim world around the 8th century CE. Persian polymath Jabir ibn Hayyan (known as Geber in Europe) began to experiment with

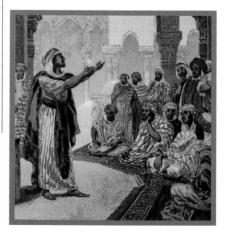

Jabir ibn Hayyan, known as the "father of early chemistry," promoted greater understanding of chemical processes through his teaching, texts, and experiments in the 8th century CE.

processes such as crystallization and distillation in his laboratory, creating concoctions which, as a physician, he tested on his patients. He was chiefly interested in the chemistry of poisons and how they react in the body. Among the hundreds of texts attributed to him is the oldest known systematic classification of chemical substances.

The first pharmacopeias

Most physicians in medieval Europe had little interest in drugs and still adhered to the ancient teachings of Galen on rebalancing the body's humors in order to treat illness. It was left to apothecaries to dispense chemical remedies, many of which were ineffective and some even harmful. In 1478, however, the printing of Dioscorides's *De Materia Medica,* previously only circulated as hand-copied manuscripts, sparked new interest in the concept of using formulations for healing.

In 1498, eager to regulate the apothecary trade and banish quack remedies, the medical authorities in Florence, Italy, published the *Ricettario Fiorentino (Florentine Book of Prescriptions)*—the first pharmacopeia. Still utilized by

> 66
> The patients are your textbook, the sickbed is your study.
> **Motto of Paracelsus**
> 99

physicians today, pharmacopeias are official lists of medicinal drugs, giving their effects and directions for their use.

The "Luther of medicine"

During the 16th century, Paracelsus revolutionized the preparation and prescription of chemical compounds. A contemporary of Martin Luther, the iconoclastic German priest who challenged the prevailing orthodoxy of the Church, Paracelsus was labeled the "Luther of medicine" for his attempts to reform orthodox medical opinion. He challenged its reliance on the traditional teachings of Galen and Ibn Sina (Avicenna) and rejected the concept of the four humors.

Instead of an imbalance in bodily fluids, Paracelsus regarded disease as an intrusion into the body—in some ways anticipating germ theory. He also argued that book learning is of little use when treating patients: what matters is learning from observation and »

Alchemists prepared cures that often included tiny amounts of toxic ingredients and used processes such as distillation, which foreshadowed modern drug production.

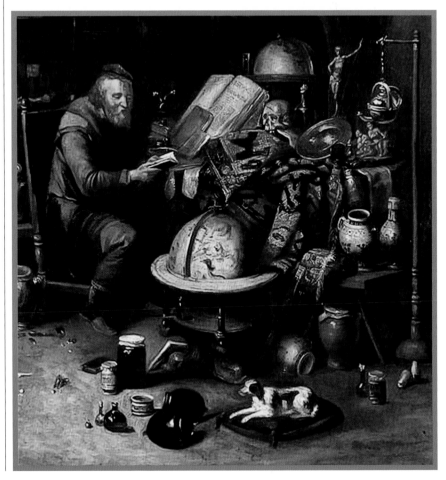

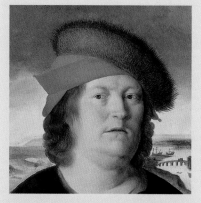

Paracelsus

Born in Einsiedeln, Switzerland, in 1493, Philippus Aureolus Theophrastus Bombastus von Hohenheim took the name Paracelsus (meaning "beyond Celsus," the Roman physician) to show his rejection of ancient Roman teaching after studying medicine at universities in Austria, Switzerland, and Italy.

Paracelsus found university learning so out of touch that he spent years traveling widely, learning from folk healers and alchemists. By the time he returned to Austria in 1524, he was famous for his miraculous cures. He opened his lectures to all, burned ancient medical texts, and stressed the value of practical learning. He looked to chemistry and metals for cures, but his iconoclastic style and interest in the occult made him enemies. He redeemed his reputation with his book *Der grossen Wundartzney* (*The Great Surgery Book*) in 1536, and became sought after and wealthy, but died in the White Horse Inn in Salzburg in 1541 in mysterious circumstances.

Key works

1536 *The Great Surgery Book*
1538 *Third Defense*

experimentation. Foreshadowing modern pharmaceutical methods, he conducted experiments to make medicinal compounds, heating and distilling metals to transform them into substances that might defeat disease. Among his discoveries was laudanum, derived from powdered opium and alcohol, which became the prime relief for people in severe pain until the discovery of morphine in the 19th century. He was also one of the first physicians to treat syphilis with mercury, which remained almost the only treatment for the disease until the 20th century despite its terrible side effects.

The active principle

After his death, Paracelsus's ideas continued to circulate through his written works. For two centuries, his followers developed the field of iatrochemistry, a form of medicinal chemistry. Regarding the body as a chemical system and disease as a disturbance in this framework, they used chemical processes to extract the "active principle" from natural substances, which was then administered to rebalance the body.

Resistance to iatrochemistry persisted in some medical circles (not least because of the high toxicity of some of the substances used), but in late 17th-century France, scientists began to follow up on Paracelsus's assertion that there is an active principle or key chemical in plants that gives them medicinal qualities. They hypothesized that if they could extract or harvest this, as Paracelsus suggested, they might be able to reproduce it in large amounts.

In 1803, French pharmacist Louis Charles Derosne found that morphine was the active ingredient in opium. In 1809, Louis Vauquelin isolated nicotine in tobacco. Soon after, Pierre-Joseph Pelletier and Joseph-Beinamé Caventou identified quinine in cinchona, caffeine in coffee, and strychnine in the seeds of the "poison nut" tree, *Strychnos nux-vomica*.

The isolation of these organic compounds led to the realization that they all contained nitrogen and behaved as bases, which form salts when combined with acids. In 1819, German pharmacist Wilhelm Meissner dubbed them "alkaloids." Soon another class of active organic compounds was identified: glycosides. These included digitalin, a heart stimulant extracted from foxgloves, and salicin, the painkiller

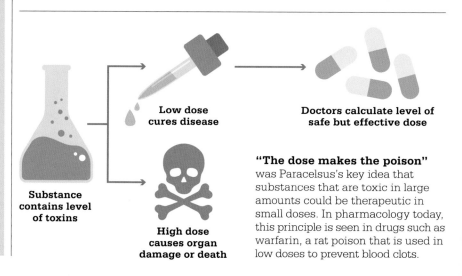

Substance contains level of toxins

Low dose cures disease

High dose causes organ damage or death

Doctors calculate level of safe but effective dose

"The dose makes the poison" was Paracelsus's key idea that substances that are toxic in large amounts could be therapeutic in small doses. In pharmacology today, this principle is seen in drugs such as warfarin, a rat poison that is used in low doses to prevent blood clots.

The pharmaceutical industry today uses new technologies to mass produce drugs, but the research, testing, and development of formulations still reflect the processes developed by Paracelsus.

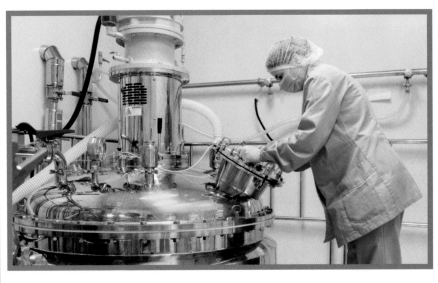

discovered in willow bark by British cleric Edward Stone in the 1760s and later manufactured as aspirin, the first mass-market painkiller.

Drug action

While chemists isolated organic compounds in the early 19th century, physiologists began to pin down their effects in the body. In France, François Magendie showed the painkilling effect of morphine in 1818, and the spasms caused by strychnine in 1819. Drugs at that time were presumed to have a general action throughout the body, but in 1856, Magendie's assistant Claude Bernard found that curare, a poison used by South American Indigenous peoples, had a specific local effect. Although it is carried through the body in the bloodstream, curare acts only at the point where nerves contact muscles, preventing them from moving. In this way, the poison causes paralysis and, when it hits the chest muscles, inhibits breathing, resulting in death.

> "
> Poisons and medicines
> are oftentimes
> the same substances
> given with different intents.
> **Peter Mere Latham**
> **British physician**
> **(1789–1875)**
> "

Bernard's research demonstrated that drugs interact with chemical structures in or on cells (later called receptors). Understanding this chemical action forms the basis of drug development and testing today.

Big business

As the 19th century progressed, advances in chemical and industrial processes enabled the manufacture of drugs to treat the ailments of the large populations crowding into new urban centers. In 1828, German chemist Friedrich Wöhler synthesized an organic substance, urea, from inorganic elements. This refuted the prevailing belief that organic substances could only be produced from living organisms. It also suggested that medicines based on organic compounds could be synthesized from inorganic materials.

A breakthrough moment came in 1856, when 18-year-old British chemistry student William Henry Perkin, tasked with finding a way to synthesize quinine, accidentally made the first synthetic dye, a deep purple which he called mauveine. Other synthetic dyes soon followed, fueling a major new dyestuff and fashion industry.

By the mid-19th century, it was clear that many of these dyes had medical applications, and large dye-making companies—such as CIBA and Geigy in Switzerland and Hoechst and Bayer in Germany—began to market them as pharmaceuticals, redirecting their chemical capabilities toward the production of synthesized drugs.

Bayer began producing aspirin in 1899, and Hoechst launched Salvarsan, the first effective drug for syphilis, in 1910. Salvarsan marked the development of a new range of "magic bullet" targeted chemical drugs. Designed to lock on to specific disease-causing pathogens, these drugs left the rest of the body unharmed.

During the 20th century, the development of synthetic insulin formulas to manage diabetes, the production of vaccines, and the manufacture of antibiotics such as penicillin turned pharmaceuticals into a lucrative global industry. Yet the use of drugs as a core treatment for ailments, the methods of their production, and the essence of their action still draw on the basic approach and principles outlined by Paracelsus. ∎

TEACH NOT FROM BOOKS BUT FROM DISSECTIONS

ANATOMY

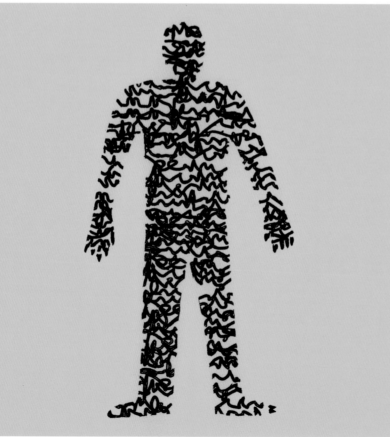

IN CONTEXT

BEFORE

c. 1600 BCE In ancient Egypt, the Edwin Smith papyrus, the oldest known medical treatise, lists traumas to the organs.

2nd century CE Galen publishes works on anatomy that are largely based on his dissections of animals.

c. 1012 Persian physician Ibn Sina completes *The Canon of Medicine*, which includes a classification of organs.

1490s Leonardo da Vinci begins his anatomical studies based on direct observation of the human form.

AFTER

1832 The Anatomy Act is passed in Britain, enabling doctors and students to dissect donated bodies.

1858 Henry Gray publishes his influential work *Anatomy: Descriptive and Surgical.*

Until the discovery of X-rays in 1895 ushered in medical imaging, the only way to see inside the whole human body was by dissecting the dead. As cultural taboos hindered this, physicians based their knowledge of bones and organs on animal dissection. Flemish anatomist Andreas Vesalius revolutionized anatomical study in the 16th century, when he proved through his own dissections of the human body that many earlier theories were wrong. Using corpses from public hangings, he established the importance of accurate anatomical knowledge gained from first-hand observation.

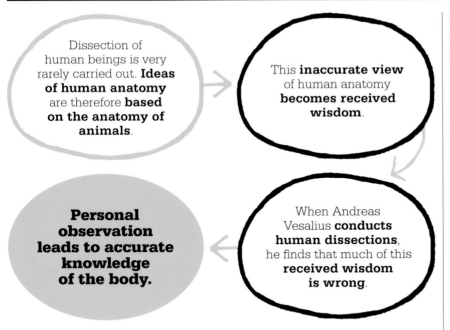

Dissection of human beings is very rarely carried out. **Ideas of human anatomy** are therefore **based on the anatomy of animals**.

This **inaccurate view** of human anatomy **becomes received wisdom**.

When Andreas Vesalius **conducts human dissections**, he finds that much of this **received wisdom is wrong**.

Personal observation leads to accurate knowledge of the body.

Physicians had long known that they needed to understand the structure and placement of organs in order to treat disease. Ancient Egyptian texts display knowledge of human organs, probably gained from mummification. The word anatomy (from the Greek *ana-tome*, meaning "a cutting up") was coined in the 4th century BCE by Aristotle, who dissected animals and made generalizations from his findings. The Greek physician Herophilus took this a stage further around 275 BCE by dissecting hundreds of human corpses. Allegations that he had dissected live bodies led to public revulsion for anatomy, and the practice largely stopped.

Galen's legacy

Until Vesalius, the most influential early anatomist was the Roman doctor Galen, in the 2nd century CE. Galen derived his knowledge from the dissection of dogs, apes, and other animals and from examining wounded gladiators when he was chief physician to the gladiator school in Pergamum. Galen's texts became established orthodoxy for more than 1,300 years. The work of Islamic physician Ibn al-Nafis, who carried out dissections in Egypt in the 13th century, and contradicted Galen with his correct description of pulmonary circulation, was not translated into Latin until 1547.

New interest

As new universities sprang up in Europe, interest in anatomy revived, beginning at the medical school in Salerno, Italy, founded in the 9th century. A Church ban on clergy performing surgery did not extend to human dissection, and in 1231, Holy Roman Emperor Frederick II ruled that a human dissection should take place every five years. In 1240, he also decreed that all surgeons had to study anatomy for at least a year.

Dissection became a regular part of university courses. In general, assistant barber-surgeons rather than professors performed human dissections, while junior academic staff read out relevant sections from Galen. In 1315, Mondino de Luzzi, professor of anatomy at the University of Bologna, presided over his first public dissection of a human body. He published *Anathomia* in 1316, but, like other anatomy texts of the time, it espoused the hallowed anatomical texts of Galen.

The study of anatomy began to change in the late 15th century, after Renaissance artists introduced a more realistic style of portraiture involving a closer study of the human form. From around 1490, Italy's famous artist, scientist, and engineer Leonardo da Vinci performed dissections in Florence, Milan, Rome, and Pavia and made detailed anatomical sketches of the human skeleton, muscles, and organs. It was Leonardo who provided the first clinical description of cirrhosis of the liver.

In Bologna, Giacomo Berengario da Carpi produced a book in 1521 that amended Mondino's work. Venetian anatomist Niccolò »

> Through dissection of the dead, we gain accurate knowledge.
> **Andreas Vesalius**
> *De Humani Corporis Fabrica*

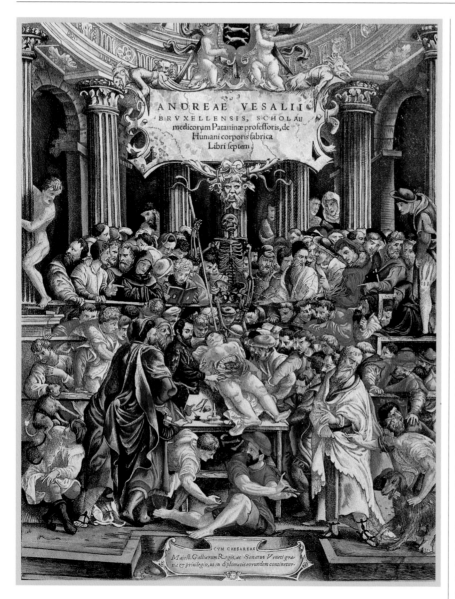

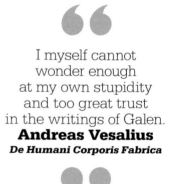

about human anatomy were wrong on several important points. For example, Vesalius found that the human breastbone is made up of three segments, not seven as Galen had said; the human liver has four lobes, not five; and the mandible (lower jaw) is made up of a single bone, not two. Vesalius also established that the humerus (the upper arm's bone) was not the second-longest bone in the body, as Galen had maintained—the tibia and fibula are longer.

Trailblazing masterpiece

In 1543, Vesalius published *De Humani Corporis Fabrica Libri Septem* (*Seven Books on the Structure of the Human Body*), the first comprehensive illustrated work on anatomy. Printed to exacting standards in Basel, Switzerland, the seven sections on the skeleton, musculature, vascular system, nerves, gastrointestinal system, heart and lungs, and brain were illustrated with 82 plates and around 400 separate drawings. The artists are unnamed, but may have come from the studio of the great Venetian painter Titian. Vesalius's book provoked a storm

Massa included his own observations in *Liber Introductorius Anatomiae* (*Introductory Book of Anatomy*), published in 1536. Generally, however, conclusions drawn from dissections were still made to fit the theories of Galen.

Anatomical revolution

Andreas Vesalius established the principle that proper understanding of the human body can only come from direct observation. Working in

Dissections were part tutorial, part public spectacle, as the title page of *De Humani Corporis Fabrica Libri Septem* shows. Audiences included dignitaries, members of the public, and students.

Italy at the University of Padua, which had a longstanding tradition of practical anatomy, Vesalius carried out the dissections himself and produced charts to illustrate his lessons for students. He discovered that Galen's theories

of criticism for contradicting Galen, not least from his own professor, Jacobus Sylvius, who had taught Vesalius dissection in Paris. Some critics attacked the book for its scandalous nudity, but most of Vesalius's peers soon accepted his ideas. In 1561, however, Gabriele Fallopio, professor of anatomy at Padua, who may have been taught by Vesalius, published his own book, *Observationes Anatomicae* (*Anatomical Observations*), in which he corrected some of Vesalius's errors. Vesalius replied by criticizing Fallopio, who is now largely forgotten save for the tubes connecting each ovary to the uterus, which he identified in the book and which bear his name to this day.

In the 1550s, a professor of anatomy at Rome, Bartolomeo Eustachi, prepared plates with 47 anatomical drawings—intended for a book called *De Dissensionibus ac Controversiis Anatomicus*—that were just as detailed as those in *De Humani Corporis Fabrica*. If Eustachi had not died before the book was published, he might have shared the title of Father of Anatomy with Vesalius. Instead, his fame is largely confined to the eustachian

The lavish illustration in *De Humani Corporis Fabrica* was designed to entertain and amaze, as well as instruct readers. Its lively figures are often set against imaginary landscapes.

tube, connecting the middle ear and the upper throat, which he identified and described.

New tool, new texts

The invention of the microscope in the early 17th century enabled scientists to examine aspects of the human anatomy that are invisible to the naked eye. By the 18th century, the study of anatomy had revolutionized medical and surgical education. William Hunter, a Scottish anatomist, obstetrician, and physician to Queen Charlotte from 1764, used his observations of childbirth to understand the structure of the uterus. In 1768, Hunter established an influential private school of medicine at his home in London.

The publication of *Anatomy: Descriptive and Surgical* by British surgeon Henry Gray in 1858 marked the moment when the study of anatomy became mainstream. Later retitled *Gray's Anatomy*, this

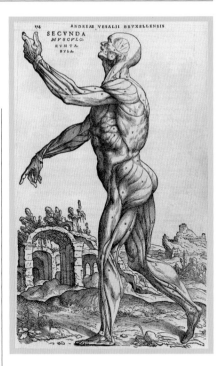

comprehensive manual with annotated illustrations has been an essential handbook for medical students ever since.

Vesalius's legacy to anatomy was not just *De Humani Corporis Fabrica* itself, but the principle behind it—that true knowledge of the human body can only be gained from direct and careful examination. ∎

Andreas Vesalius

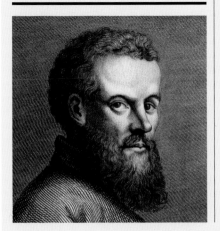

Born in Brussels, Belgium (which was then part of the Habsburg Netherlands), in 1514, Vesalius was the son of the apothecary to Holy Roman emperors Charles V and Maximilian I. He studied medicine at Louvain, Paris, and Padua. The day after graduating in 1538, he became professor of surgery at Padua.

Vesalius's presentation of *De Humani Corporis Fabrica* to Charles V earned him a post as imperial physician in 1544. He secured the same position with Philip II in 1559. This took him to Spain, but he left five years later,

possibly to avoid a charge of heresy. While on a pilgrimage to the Holy Land, Vesalius heard he had been reappointed to his Padua post, but on the voyage to Italy, he was shipwrecked on the Greek island of Zakynthos. Short on funds, he died there in 1564.

Key works

1538 *Six Anatomical Plates*
1543 *De Humani Corporis Fabrica Libri Septem* (*Seven Books on the Structure of the Human Body*)

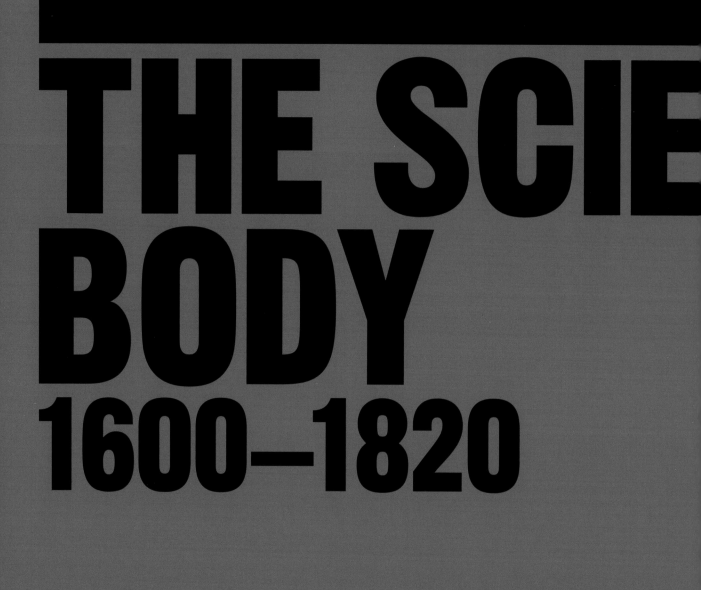

THE SCIE
BODY
1600–1820

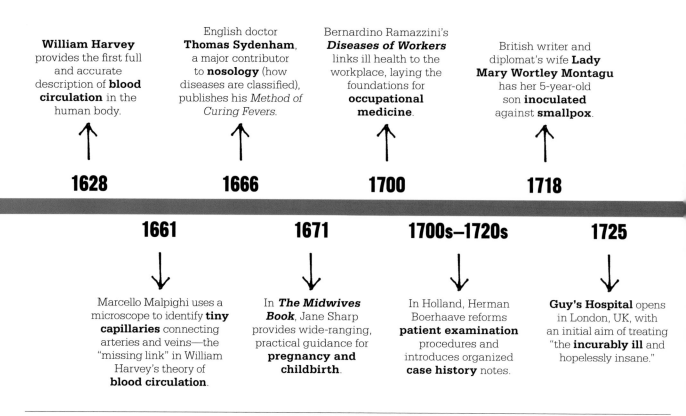

William Harvey provides the first full and accurate description of **blood circulation** in the human body.

1628

English doctor **Thomas Sydenham**, a major contributor to **nosology** (how diseases are classified), publishes his *Method of Curing Fevers*.

1666

Bernardino Ramazzini's *Diseases of Workers* links ill health to the workplace, laying the foundations for **occupational medicine**.

1700

British writer and diplomat's wife **Lady Mary Wortley Montagu** has her 5-year-old son **inoculated** against **smallpox**.

1718

1661

Marcello Malpighi uses a microscope to identify **tiny capillaries** connecting arteries and veins—the "missing link" in William Harvey's theory of **blood circulation**.

1671

In *The Midwives Book*, Jane Sharp provides wide-ranging, practical guidance for **pregnancy and childbirth**.

1700s–1720s

In Holland, Herman Boerhaave reforms **patient examination** procedures and introduces organized **case history** notes.

1725

Guy's Hospital opens in London, UK, with an initial aim of treating "the **incurably ill** and hopelessly insane."

As the Scientific Revolution gathered pace during the 17th century, major medical advances arrived with increasing rapidity, fueled by ingenious inventions, innovative procedures, and new philosophies from other scientific fields. The new scientific approach also influenced the Enlightenment, or the Age of Reason, which advocated the application of rational thought and observation to every aspect of society and incited political revolution in 18th-century North America, France, and beyond.

Scientific approach

The doctrines of the 2nd-century Roman physician Claudius Galen that had ruled European medicine for some 1,500 years would now be steadily eroded. Under the influence of leading European scientists, the concept of scientific method began to take shape: the idea of formulating a hypothesis, designing a trial or experiment to test it, analyzing the results, and drawing conclusions. Medical practitioners began to adopt this approach to assess diagnoses, treatments, and outcomes.

In 1628, after almost 20 years of personal research and scientific experiments, English physician William Harvey published *De Motu Cordis et Sanguinis* (*On the Motion of the Heart and Blood*), which described for the first time how the heart pumps blood around the whole body. In 1661, Italian biologist Marcello Malpighi supplied the one missing link in Harvey's account—how blood in the arteries passes into the veins. Using a microscope, the instrument that revolutionized scientific research, Malpighi identified capillaries that are 10 times thinner than human hairs and link arteries and veins.

Many physicians had resisted Harvey's conclusions at first because they contradicted Galen's theory that blood was produced by the liver, but the evidence was now irrefutable. Harvey's approach also encouraged more physicians to use their own observations rather than remain bound to ancient texts.

Benefits across society

English midwife Jane Sharp used her decades of observation and hands-on experience to inform *The Midwives Book* (1671), which advanced understanding of the birth process, breastfeeding, and infant care. Italian professor of medicine Bernadino Ramazzini carefully

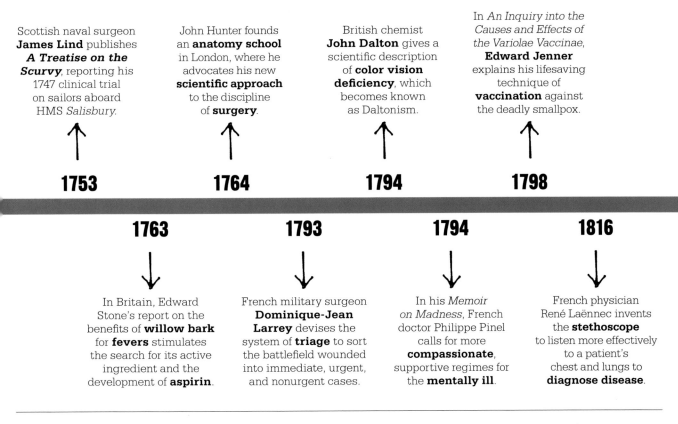

Scottish naval surgeon **James Lind** publishes ***A Treatise on the Scurvy***, reporting his 1747 clinical trial on sailors aboard HMS *Salisbury*.

John Hunter founds an **anatomy school** in London, where he advocates his new **scientific approach** to the discipline of **surgery**.

British chemist **John Dalton** gives a scientific description of **color vision deficiency**, which becomes known as Daltonism.

In *An Inquiry into the Causes and Effects of the Variolae Vaccinae*, **Edward Jenner** explains his lifesaving technique of **vaccination** against the deadly smallpox.

1753   **1764**   **1794**   **1798**

1763   **1793**   **1794**   **1816**

In Britain, Edward Stone's report on the benefits of **willow bark** for **fevers** stimulates the search for its active ingredient and the development of **aspirin**.

French military surgeon **Dominique-Jean Larrey** devises the system of **triage** to sort the battlefield wounded into immediate, urgent, and nonurgent cases.

In his *Memoir on Madness*, French doctor Philippe Pinel calls for more **compassionate**, supportive regimes for the **mentally ill**.

French physician René Laënnec invents the **stethoscope** to listen more effectively to a patient's chest and lungs to **diagnose disease**.

researched disorders encountered in 54 different types of work, in the first major study of occupational diseases, published in 1700.

Scottish doctor James Lind carried out the earliest controlled clinical experiment in 1747, when he methodically administered different remedies to sailors with scurvy; his experiment established that what we now know as vitamin C could cure the disease, which is fatal if untreated. Clergyman Edward Stone reasoned that willow bark, the precursor of aspirin, might help reduce fevers and similarly proved his hypothesis by observing its beneficial effects on patients.

At a time when surgeons were often barbers and not medically qualified, Scottish surgeon John Hunter took a rigorous approach to the study of anatomy to inform his work. At his school of anatomy, he refined the practice of surgery, which he would perform only after detailed observation of his patients' conditions, often practicing on animals before he operated to test the efficacy of an intervention.

Hunter had honed his skills as a military surgeon in the Seven Years' War of the 1760s. In France, at the end of the century, another military surgeon—Dominique-Jean Larrey—conceived the idea of triaging the battlefield wounded to ensure those most seriously injured were treated first. Triage became widely used during wars and was then more generally adopted in hospitals from around 1900.

Unlike scientific discoveries, which take time to trickle down, practical advances such as triage have an immediate benefit. Early in the 18th century, the emergence of hospitals that treated all who were sick, regardless of wealth or religion, improved the lives of many ordinary people. By the end of the century, kinder health care had also been extended to the mentally ill, spurred by the work of Philippe Pinel in France and William Tuke in Britain.

The birth of vaccination
Perhaps the greatest medical advance of this era was vaccination. British physician Edward Jenner's experiments in 1796, using cowpox inoculation to protect against smallpox, laid the basis for the procedure, since used to prevent killer diseases such as polio or diphtheria. Vaccination currently prevents between 2 and 3 million deaths globally each year. ∎

THE BLOOD IS DRIVEN INTO A ROUND

BLOOD CIRCULATION

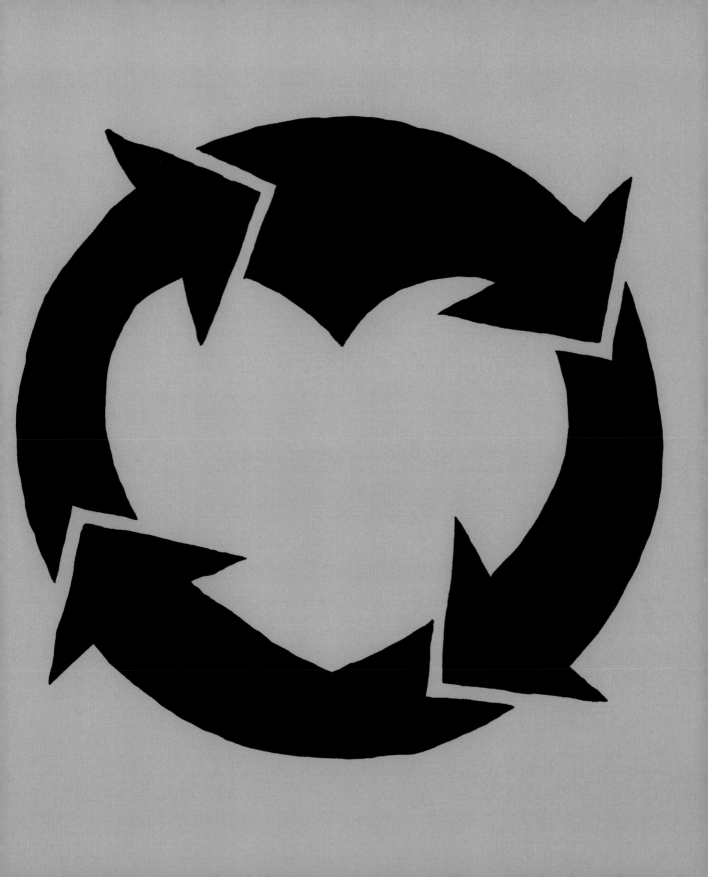

IN CONTEXT

BEFORE

2nd century CE Claudius Galen asserts that blood is produced in the liver and then consumed by the organs.

c. 1275 Ibn al-Nafis describes pulmonary circulation of blood.

1553 The idea of pulmonary circulation is put forward by Michael Servetus in his book *Christianismi Restitutio* (*Christianity Restored*).

AFTER

1661 Marcello Malpighi discovers capillaries, the missing link in the double circulatory system.

1733 Stephen Hales describes and measures blood pressure (the pressure of arterial blood).

1953 American surgeon John Gibbon performs the first successful operation on a human using the heart-lung machine (the first heart bypass machine).

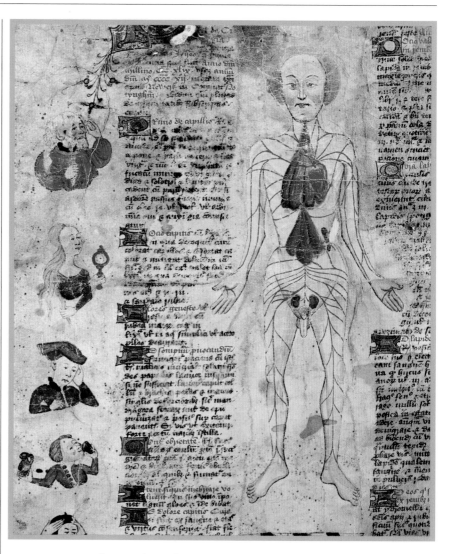

I n 1628, English physician William Harvey published a new theory about the circulation of the blood. Through rigorous experiments over 10 years, he had discovered the source and route of blood in the body. His ideas challenged theories that had prevailed for almost 1,500 years.

Early theories

Ancient doctors understood that blood was essential for human life, that it moved around the body in some way, and that the heart played an essential role in this, but the

process was unclear to them. In ancient China, the *Huangdi Neijing* (*The Yellow Emperor's Classic of Medicine*) hypothesized that blood became mixed with *qi* (life force) and spread energy around the body. In Greece, Hippocrates believed that the arteries carried air from the lungs and that the heart had three chambers, or ventricles.

The most influential theories were those of the 2nd-century-CE Roman doctor Claudius Galen. He understood that the body had both arteries and veins but thought, incorrectly, that blood was produced

Galen's theory that blood came from the liver is illustrated in *De Arte Phisicali et de Cirugia* (*On the Art of Medicine and Surgery*) by English master surgeon John Arderne (1307–c. 1390).

in the liver and was then carried through the body by the veins. Crucially, Galen argued that blood was absorbed by body tissues and had to be constantly replenished; he did not believe that it returned to the liver or the heart or that it circulated around the body. Even so, he did surmise that the right side of the heart nourished the lungs

See also: Greek medicine 28–29 ▪ Traditional Chinese medicine 30–35 ▪ Roman medicine 38–43
▪ Islamic medicine 44–49 ▪ Bloodletting and leeches 52 ▪ Anatomy 60–63 ▪ Blood transfusion and blood groups 108–111

> The penetration of the blood into the left ventricle is from the lung, after it has been heated within the right ventricle.
> **Ibn al-Nafis**
> *Commentary on Anatomy in Ibn Sina's Canon, c. 1275*

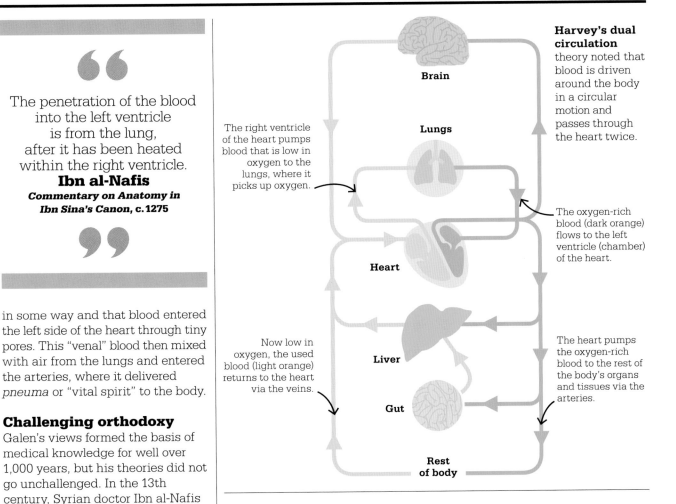

Harvey's dual circulation theory noted that blood is driven around the body in a circular motion and passes through the heart twice.

Brain

Lungs

The right ventricle of the heart pumps blood that is low in oxygen to the lungs, where it picks up oxygen.

The oxygen-rich blood (dark orange) flows to the left ventricle (chamber) of the heart.

Heart

Liver

Now low in oxygen, the used blood (light orange) returns to the heart via the veins.

The heart pumps the oxygen-rich blood to the rest of the body's organs and tissues via the arteries.

Gut

Rest of body

in some way and that blood entered the left side of the heart through tiny pores. This "venal" blood then mixed with air from the lungs and entered the arteries, where it delivered *pneuma* or "vital spirit" to the body.

Challenging orthodoxy

Galen's views formed the basis of medical knowledge for well over 1,000 years, but his theories did not go unchallenged. In the 13th century, Syrian doctor Ibn al-Nafis established that there are no pores between the right and left ventricles of the heart, as Galen had supposed, and that blood must travel between the two sides of the heart by some other means. He suggested that this must be the lungs, establishing the principle of pulmonary circulation and solving one of the biggest mysteries of blood circulation.

Al-Nafis's theory was a major step forward, but the manuscript in which he explained his theory was not known to European scholars until it was translated into Latin in 1547, nor did it solve the

problem of how blood circulated through the body as a whole. In 1553, Spanish anatomist and theologian Michael Servetus restated the concept of pulmonary circulation, but he was burned as a heretic at the age of 42 and his books were suppressed, so his theories were not widely known.

At around the same time, Italian anatomist Realdo Colombo rediscovered the principle of pulmonary circulation. Colombo published his observations, based on dissections of human and animal cadavers, in *De Re Anatomica* (*On

Things Anatomical*) in 1559. In the 16th century, human dissection became more popular in Europe. However, acquiring corpses for this purpose was limited, and it was not sanctioned by the Catholic Church.

Dual system

William Harvey may have known of Colombo's work, since he studied at Padua University in Italy. He also had access to the anatomical drawings of Flemish physician and artist Andreas Vesalius. Harvey expanded on Colombo's ideas by considering the wider matter of » blood's circulation beyond the lungs. In 1628, he came up with the theory that the body has a dual circulatory system and that the blood passes through the heart twice. He realized that blood passed between the heart and the lungs and from the heart to the rest of the body. This discovery was crucial, facilitating many future medical advances.

Practical experiments

Harvey came to his conclusions through a series of experiments. First, he concentrated on Galen's assertion that blood was produced in the liver. He drained the blood from sheep and pigs and measured their left ventricles. He calculated that if each heartbeat emptied the ventricle of blood—and if Galen was right in saying that blood was constantly being created rather than circulated through the body—then the amount of blood pumped daily would be around 10 times the volume of the entire animal. The body of a dog, for example, would

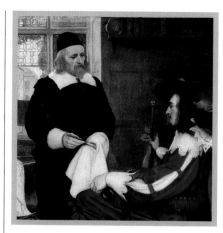

Harvey explains his theories to his patron, King Charles I. After Charles I's execution in 1649, Harvey lost his position as chief physician at St. Bartholomew's Hospital.

have to produce and consume about 414 pints (235 liters) of blood each day. This seemed impossible.

In another experiment, Harvey opened up a live snake and compressed the vein entering the heart, which then emptied of blood, proving that he had stopped the circulation of the snake's blood. Harvey also demonstrated that when a tourniquet is applied to the arm of a human and the veins become engorged, the blood can be

pushed through the blockage in the direction of the heart, but it is impossible to push it backward.

Harvey's experiments proved that blood not only circulates throughout the body, but does so in a one-way direction. He calculated that blood must circulate outward from the left ventricle through the arteries, inward to the right ventricle through the heart, and back to the left ventricle by means of the lungs. He realized there must be small connections between the arteries and veins to allow this to happen, but he could not observe any himself.

Hostile reception

In 1628, Harvey published his theories in *De Motu Cordis et Sanguinis* (*On the Motion of the*

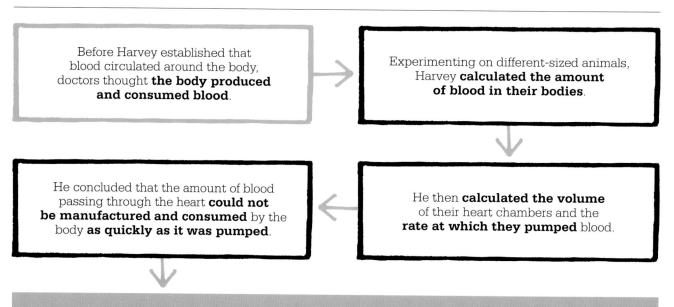

Before Harvey established that blood circulated around the body, doctors thought **the body produced and consumed blood**.

Experimenting on different-sized animals, Harvey **calculated the amount of blood in their bodies**.

He then **calculated the volume** of their heart chambers and the **rate at which they pumped** blood.

He concluded that the amount of blood passing through the heart **could not be manufactured and consumed** by the body **as quickly as it was pumped**.

Harvey established that the same blood circulates.

> The animal's heart is the basis of its life, its chief member, the sun of its microcosm; on the heart all its activity depends, from the heart all its liveliness and strength arise.
> **William Harvey**
> *De Motu Cordis et Sanguinis*

Heart and Blood). They were not very well received to begin with. Physicians were so steeped in Galen's doctrines that they resisted the idea of double circulation, and many mocked Harvey's practical approach through experimentation.

Harvey's failure to find the means by which blood passed from the arterial to the venous system provided his critics with a specific loophole, which they used to undermine his theory. In 1648, French physician Jean Riolan pointed out that the animal anatomy, on which Harvey had based many of his findings, might not operate in the same way as the human body and questioned "how such a circulation takes place without causing upset and mixing of the body's humors."

New understandings

It was not until 1661, after the recently invented microscope had been sufficiently improved, that Italian biologist Marcello Malpighi observed the network of tiny capillaries that connect the arterial and venous systems. This missing piece in the dual circulation theory vindicated Harvey, albeit four years after his death. By the late 17th century, the double circulation of the blood in the cardiovascular system had itself become medical orthodoxy, entirely replacing the long-held Galenic view.

Harvey's discovery led to a long series of medical advances, starting with the rejection of the age-old theory that bloodletting and the application of blood-sucking leeches were helpful in removing "excess" blood from the system. The importance of blood pressure, as first described by British clergyman and scientist Stephen Hales in the 1730s, and of hypertension (high blood pressure), outlined by Thomas Young in 1808, were breakthroughs in knowledge of the cardiovascular system. In the 1890s, the new cuff sphygmomanometer (an inflatable arm band for measuring blood pressure) gave doctors a powerful diagnostic tool when assessing the health of the heart.

In finding the solution to an enduring medical mystery and replacing outmoded theories with firm evidence-based ideas about the circulation of the blood, William Harvey ranks among the most important medical pioneers. ∎

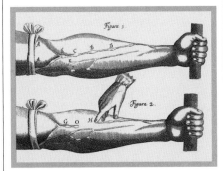

To prove that venal blood flowed toward the heart, Harvey ligatured an arm to make the veins obvious. He then tried to push the blood in the vein away from the heart, to no avail.

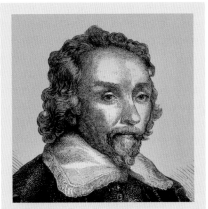

William Harvey

Born in 1578, William Harvey was the son of a Kent farmer. After studying medicine at Cambridge University, he enrolled at the University of Padua, where he studied under celebrated anatomist Hieronymus Fabricius.

Returning to London in 1602, Harvey became chief physician at St. Bartholomew's Hospital in 1609 and Lumleian lecturer of the Royal College of Physicians in 1615. His appointment as chief physician to James I in 1618 (and to his successor Charles I in 1625) gave him considerable prestige and partly shielded him from critics when he published his theory of double circulation in 1628. His other important work concerned the development of animal embryos, in which Harvey disproved the long-held theory of spontaneous generation of life. He died in 1657.

Key works

1628 *De Motu Cordis et Sanguinis (On the Motion of the Heart and Blood)*
1651 *Exercitationes de Generatione Animalium (On Animal Generation)*

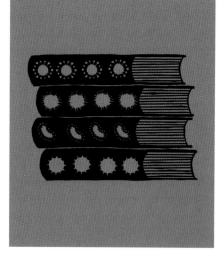

A DISEASE KNOWN IS HALF CURED

NOSOLOGY

IN CONTEXT

BEFORE

c. 175 CE Galen develops Hippocrates' idea of the four humors, which becomes the basis for diagnosing disease.

1532 In England, the City of London begins to issue Bills of Mortality.

1554 Jean Fernel outlines an early scientific approach to nosology in *Universa Medicina*.

AFTER

1853 In Brussels, Belgium, the first International Statistical Congress calls for a uniform, international classification of causes of death.

1883 German psychiatrist Emil Kraepelin publishes an influential classification system for mental disorders.

1949 American scientist Linus Pauling suggests that some diseases can be classified according to the molecular structure of the microorganism causing them.

From the time of Hippocrates in ancient Greece until the mid-17th century, when English doctor Thomas Sydenham began his work, physicians in Europe had based diagnoses on the erroneous theory of the four humors. The theory attributed disease to excesses of phlegm, blood, yellow bile, or black bile and grouped disorders accordingly.

When diagnosing his patients' complaints, Sydenham, by contrast, based his conclusions on careful, objective observation of symptoms and signs and used the same approach to classify disorders. The classification of diseases was later termed nosology.

Sydenham's endeavors were timely in an era when infectious diseases and epidemics, such as the Great Plague of 1665, had decimated urban populations. The ability to distinguish between different types of illness in order to treat them effectively was urgently required.

Objective observation

One practical effort to monitor disease was the City of London's Bills of Mortality, which listed generic causes of death (such as "pox"), but these were not based on detailed medical examinations. French physician Jean Fernel had included a section on types of disease in his *Universa Medicina* (1554), but Sydenham's work marked the true start of modern nosology.

Sydenham was among the first to describe scarlet fever, which he distinguished from measles. He

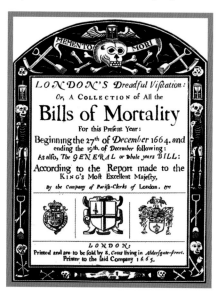

The Bills of Mortality, published weekly, listed who had died, what they had (allegedly) died of, and where outbreaks of diseases had occurred to help people avoid areas of infection.

See also: Greek medicine 28–29 ▪ Roman medicine 38–43 ▪ Medieval medical schools and surgery 50–51 ▪ Pharmacy 54–59 ▪ Histology 122–123 ▪ The World Health Organization 232–233 ▪ Pandemics 306–313

also identified chronic and acute forms of gout and separated them from other rheumatic disorders. His recognition that symptoms, such as fever, were not the disease itself but the body's reaction to disease was also a significant contribution to medicine. His *Medical Observations* of 1676 became a standard textbook for the next 200 years.

Nosology after Sydenham

The concept of classifying diseases gained momentum. In 1763, French physician François Boissier de Sauvages published *Nosologia Methodica*, which grouped 2,400 physical and mental disorders in 10 major classes, with more than 200 genera. Six years later, Scottish physician William Cullen published *Synopsis Nosologiae Methodicae*, which became widely used.

By 1869, when the Royal College of Physicians in London published its monumental *The Nomenclature of Diseases*, more countries were recognizing the need for a uniform system for classifying disease.

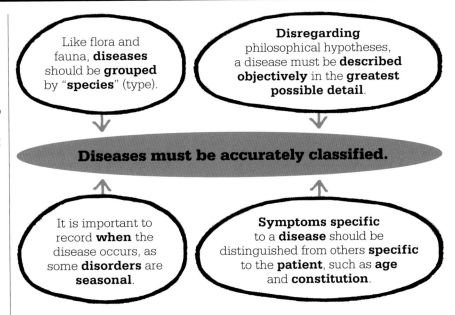

Like flora and fauna, **diseases** should be **grouped** by "**species**" (type).

Disregarding philosophical hypotheses, a disease must be **described objectively** in the **greatest possible detail**.

Diseases must be accurately classified.

It is important to record **when** the disease occurs, as some **disorders** are **seasonal**.

Symptoms specific to a **disease** should be distinguished from others **specific** to the **patient**, such as **age** and **constitution**.

At a meeting in Chicago, Illinois, in 1893, the International Statistical Institute adopted the *International List of Causes of Death*, compiled by French statistician Jacques Bertillon. It was later renamed the *International Classification of Diseases* (ICD), which the WHO now updates and manages. The ICD classifies all known diseases, disorders, and injuries; establishes universally comparable statistics on cause of death; categorizes newly identified diseases; and, crucially, allows health information to be shared and compared worldwide. ▪

Thomas Sydenham

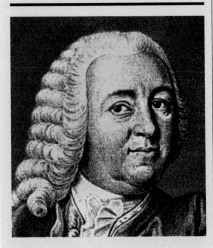

Born in 1624, Sydenham served in the army of Oliver Cromwell in the English Civil War before and after completing medical studies at Oxford University. In 1663, he passed the College of Physician examinations, allowing him to practice as a doctor in London.

In his 1666 treatise on fevers and later works, Sydenham began to develop his nosological system, which reflected his belief that close examination of patients and the course of an illness were crucial for classifying disease. He also championed effective herbal treatments, such as willow bark (the source of aspirin) for fevers and cinchona bark (which contains quinine) for malaria. Many physicians opposed his ideas, but prominent supporters included philosopher John Locke and scientist Robert Boyle.

Long after his death in 1689, Sydenham's innovative work on nosology won him recognition as the "English Hippocrates."

Key works

1666 *The Method of Curing Fevers*
1676 *Medical Observations*
1683 *The Management of Arthritis and Dropsy*

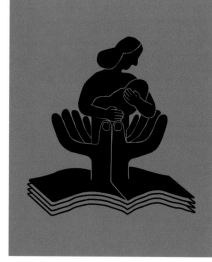

HOPE OF A GOOD, SPEEDY DELIVERANCE

MIDWIFERY

IN CONTEXT

BEFORE
1540 The first midwifery manual printed in England is *The Byrth of Mankynd*, a translation of German physician Eucharius Rösslin's *Der Rosengarten*.

1651 Nicholas Culpeper publishes his practical and wide-ranging *Directory for Midwives*.

AFTER
1902 In Britain, the Midwives Act establishes the Central Midwives Board to train and license midwives.

1920s Mary Breckinridge founds the Frontier Nursing Service (FNS) in Kentucky. She demonstrates that midwives can achieve safer births than doctors.

1956 The Natural Childbirth Trust (later the National Childbirth Trust) is founded in the UK to promote natural childbirth led by midwives.

Women learn to be midwives from other women. They are **not formally trained or educated**.

⬇

Early books on midwifery are **written by men**, and books on medicine and human biology are in **Greek or Latin**. Few women can read in these languages.

⬇

Jane Sharp writes *The Midwives Book* in English to educate women in "**the conception, breeding, bearing, and nursing of children**."

Jane Sharp's 1671 *The Midwives Book* is a comprehensive manual on pregnancy and childbirth that provided a badly needed female voice of experience. Previously, every British book on childbirth had been written by men. They included *A Directory for Midwives*, a popular text by English herbalist Nicholas Culpeper, later known as the father of midwifery, despite Culpeper's own admission that he had never attended a birth. Sharp, by comparison, had been a "practitioner in the art of midwifery" for more than 30 years. Although little else is known about her, the knowledge and understanding of medicine and human biology that is evident in her book indicate that she had been formally educated.

Invaluable advice

Sharp's book is divided into sections. They include: male and female anatomy; conceiving and the problems doing so; the different

See also: Women in medicine 120–121 ▪ Nursing and sanitation 128–133 ▪ Birth control 214–215 ▪ Hormonal contraception 258 ▪ In vitro fertilization 284–285

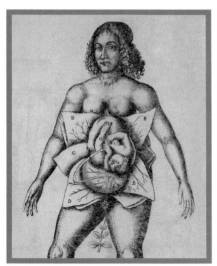

The Midwives Book contains illustrations of the womb. This one shows how "the child lies therein near the time of its birth" and the role of the placenta.

stages of fetal development; and childbirth and the complications that can arise during labor. In the childbirth section, Sharp refutes the common advice that women should lie in one position during labor and suggests that they move around, choosing whatever position feels best. Sharp also puts to bed the then-popular notion that any physical deformities in offspring were God's retribution or punishment for the sins of their parents, and instead explains the biological causes of some of these conditions.

A final section in the book provides practical advice on life after childbirth, including guidance on breastfeeding and the correct way to handle infants, who are described as "tender twigs." There is also advice, perhaps aimed at fathers, for the comfort and care of a new mother, who should be "put to as little trouble as you can, for she has endured enough pain already."

Women only

The Midwives Book clearly states that midwifery should be an exclusively female occupation. When Sharp refers to the books of male rivals, including Culpeper's *Directory for Midwives*, she is quick to point out any errors. She also gives female midwives career advice, urging them to seek out a formal education in order to understand the many texts in Greek and Latin that could further their knowledge of biology and medicine, and recommends that they learn basic surgical procedures, so that a physician may not need to be called in when complications arise in childbirth.

Ahead of its time

The Midwives Book had run to four separate editions by 1725, and remained the go-to text for midwives and doctors for many decades afterward. It was visionary in its

Midwifery is doubtless one of the most useful and necessary of all arts for the being and well-being of mankind.
Jane Sharp
The Midwives Book

content and approach. Sharp used science to dismiss unfounded religious and paternalistic beliefs while offering practical advice and arguing for the betterment of women. The text is testament to a woman who broke into the male-dominated field of printed knowledge on the subjects of science and medicine. Remarkably, *The Midwives Book* is still in print today. ▪

Sharp and sexuality

Jane Sharp's writing is clear, witty, and often ironic in tone, not least when it discusses male and female sexuality. Sharp dismisses the common notion that the female reproductive organs are responsible for sexual dissatisfaction and places the blame on men instead, explaining: "True it is that … motion [an erection] is always necessary, but the Yard moves only at some times, and riseth sometimes to small purpose."

Sharp celebrates the female reproductive organs, marveling at the vagina and cervix's ability to expand, open, and close as "the works of the Lord." She also emphasizes the importance of clitoral stimulation and female orgasm in conception—ideas that were virtually unheard of in the 17th century. Sharp's candid views represent an important, progressive voice at a time when gender roles and notions of women's sexuality were extremely limited.

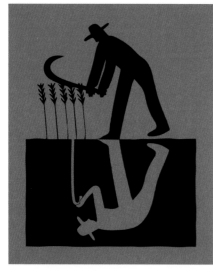

THE HARVEST OF DISEASES REAPED BY WORKERS
OCCUPATIONAL MEDICINE

IN CONTEXT

BEFORE
4th century BCE Hippocrates comments on occupational health after discovering the link between poisoning and mining.

1st century CE Roman author Pliny the Elder recommends workers wear masks to protect against dust.

1533 The Swiss physician Paracelsus publishes his findings on the diseases of miners.

AFTER
1842 British social reformer Edwin Chadwick publishes guidance on sanitary conditions for workers.

1910 American physician Alice Hamilton is appointed as a state investigator of occupational diseases and compiles a report on the effects of industrial poisons on workers in Illinois.

I n 1700, while professor of medicine at Modena University, Italian physician Bernardino Ramazzini published his pioneering book *Diseases of Workers*. It detailed the disorders encountered in 54 different occupations and warned against the factors that could cause them, including the hazards of poor posture; repetitive and strenuous movements; and the dangers of abrasive and irritating substances, such as dust, mercury, and sulfur. *Diseases of Workers* represented a breakthrough in the treatment and prevention of workplace disease

and injuries, and, for his work in this area, Ramazzini is often referred to as the father of occupational medicine.

Ramazzini's research took place during a time of economic recession in Italy and, in particular, a crisis in the agricultural sector in northern Italy where he was based. He believed that workers' disorders had a significant socioeconomic impact and began to investigate ways to minimize their risk and improve workers' health. To do this, Ramazzini visited workplaces, investigated conditions, and talked

Occupational cancer

Bernardino Ramazzini observed the potential link between certain occupations and cancer while investigating job-related risks among women, including midwives, wet nurses, and nuns. He found that nuns were more likely to develop breast cancer than other women but less likely to get cervical cancer, which he attributed to the nuns' celibacy.

Published in 1713, this study was an early example of epidemiology, which compares the risks of illnesses in different

populations. The theory of occupational cancer was later confirmed in 1775 by British surgeon Percivall Pott, who found that exposure to soot was causing scrotal cancer among chimney sweeps. In 1788, an Act of Parliament forbade the use of young boys as sweeps, but – unlike countries where sweeps wore protective clothing – death rates remained high in Britain until the mid-20th century, when new heating and cooking technology became the norm.

See also: Greek medicine 28–29 ▪ Roman medicine 38–43 ▪ Pharmacy 54–59 ▪ Case history 80–81
▪ Epidemiology 124–127 ▪ Evidence-based medicine 276–277

*… in this curious branch
of medicine …
the clear waters of truth
are so often muddied by
mutual antagonisms, quarrels
over wages and hours,
and over unionization.*
Alice Hamilton
American physician (1869–1970)

to the workers about what they did
and the health problems afflicting
them. This approach was unusual
at a time when medical attention
was almost exclusively the domain
of the rich and powerful, but
Ramazzini considered talking to
workers essential to the scientific
success of his studies. He famously
recommended that all physicians
add a new diagnostic question to
those suggested by Hippocrates:
"What is your occupation?"

Prevent and protect

In his book, Ramazzini highlighted
the dangerous and often exploitative
conditions workers were subjected
to and recommended a range of
protective measures. Starch makers,
for example, should limit their
exposure to dust by working

Reports on industrial poisoning in
the early 20th century highlighted the
plight of workers such as these pottery
manufacturers, whose exposure to lead
glazes resulted in chronic illness.

outdoors; cleaners of cesspits
should wear protective masks;
and blacksmiths should not stare
too long at molten substances.

In the science we now call
ergonomics, Ramazzini suggested
that workers should not sit or stand
for too long, that those performing
repetitive or strenuous tasks take
regular breaks, and that those
performing "activities requiring
an intense effort of the eyes …
now and again drop their work and
turn their eyes elsewhere." Where
preventive measures were not
possible, or poor occupational
health had caused a lasting problem,
Ramazzini also recommended the
worker be found alternative forms
of employment.

Published during the Age
of Reason, *Diseases of Workers*
signaled the slow emergence
of a wider focus on public health
issues. Translated into several
languages, its advice soon gained
further relevance when the
Industrial Revolution radically
affected the way people lived
and worked. ▪

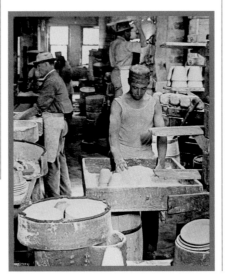

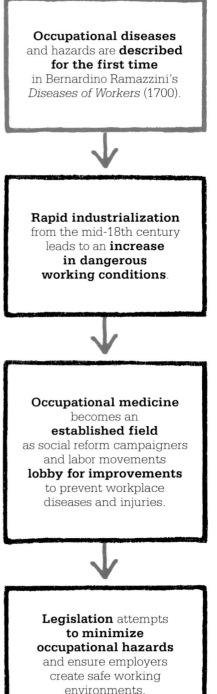

Occupational diseases
and hazards are **described
for the first time**
in Bernardino Ramazzini's
Diseases of Workers (1700).

Rapid industrialization
from the mid-18th century
leads to an **increase
in dangerous
working conditions**.

Occupational medicine
becomes an
established field
as social reform campaigners
and labor movements
lobby for improvements
to prevent workplace
diseases and injuries.

Legislation attempts
**to minimize
occupational hazards**
and ensure employers
create safe working
environments.

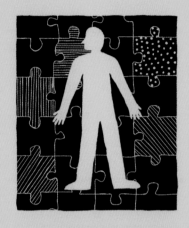

THE PECULIAR CIRCUMSTANCES OF THE PATIENT
CASE HISTORY

The classical medical tradition that began with Hippocrates in the 5th century BCE emphasized the key importance of examining patients, with both questions and the careful noting of symptoms. In the 2nd century CE, the Roman physician Rufus of Ephesus championed interrogating patients and taking a pulse as a diagnostic measure.

During the medieval era, doctors further refined their assessments of patients by introducing techniques such as examining the urine. Yet a general lack of consistency in approach meant that one patient's symptoms could not be measured against another's; differences or common characteristics between cases could not be compared, and there was no attempt to keep records for future reference.

The birth of case notes

A shift in attitude was established by the work of Herman Boerhaave, a Dutch physician who lectured and was a professor at the University of Leiden, the Netherlands, from 1701 to 1729.

As part of Boerhaave's reform of the university's medical faculty, he insisted that students observe their instructors examining the patients and making records of their diagnoses. Boerhaave made daily rounds with his students; he performed new examinations, including examinations of patients' urine, and reviewed and amended the notes that had previously been recorded. Boerhaave emphasized in particular the usefulness of

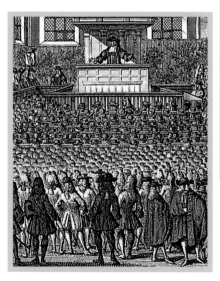

Boerhaave was a gifted lecturer and taught the importance of clinical examination and patient records to a wide audience, disseminating his knowledge throughout Europe.

See also: Greek medicine 28–29 ▪ Roman medicine 38–43 ▪ Islamic medicine 44–49 ▪ Nosology 74–75
▪ Hospitals 82–83 ▪ The stethoscope 103 ▪ Cancer screening 226–227

postmortems as a means of a final diagnosis. He used the technique to find the cause of death of Baron van Wassenaer, a Dutch admiral who had torn his esophagus while overeating (an affliction that was later named Boerhaave syndrome).

New techniques
The new discipline of taking case histories (known as anamnesis) to diagnose patients spread from the Netherlands throughout Europe, thanks to the many foreign students who studied under Boerhaave. Yet he and his successors found their examinations were hampered by the lack of diagnostic tools—even thermometers, for example, were still not advanced enough to take accurate readings.

In 1761, Austrian physician Leopold Auenbrugger invented the technique of percussion—tapping on the surface of the body as a means of diagnosis. Then in the early 19th century, instruments such as the reflex hammer, stethoscope, and pleximeter were developed, enabling physicians to refine their diagnoses.

> A patient provides their **personal details** and **main concerns or symptoms**, details of **medical and surgical history**, and any **current medications**.

> A physician **compiles** all these details into a **formalized case history** and **updates them** as treatment progresses.

> The patient's **case history notes** are **made available to other physicians** in case further treatment is required.

In the mid-19th century, French physician Pierre Charles Alexandre Louis furthered Boerhaave's work. In a Paris hospital, Louis carried out detailed clinical research into patients, and by comparing the data he collected, he was able to make informed assessments of their conditions. Louis insisted that physicians discover the previous health of a patient, their occupation and family history, and the details of their present symptoms—all this was recorded and updated during the patient's treatment and referred to in the case of a postmortem.

The routine taking of patients' clinical histories today shows that Boerhaave's insight still lies at the heart of modern medical practice. ∎

Herman Boerhaave

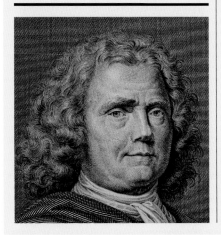

Sometimes known as the "Dutch Hippocrates," Herman Boerhaave was born in the Netherlands in 1668. He studied philosophy and medicine and spent his career at the University of Leiden, serving as lecturer; professor of botany, medicine, and chemistry; and rector of the university.

Boerhaave's teaching and innovative diagnostic practices attracted students from all over Europe and enhanced Leiden's reputation. Aiming to systematize the medical developments that had occurred over the previous two centuries, he produced new editions of works such as *De Humani Corporis Fabrica* by Andreas Vesalius. Boerhaave believed that fluids circulated in the body via elastic vessels and that disease occurred when this flow was disturbed, and he frequently diagnosed purging to remove excess blood. Boerhaave died in 1738.

Key works

1708 *Institutes of Medicine*
1709 *Aphorisms on the Recognition and Treatment of Diseases*

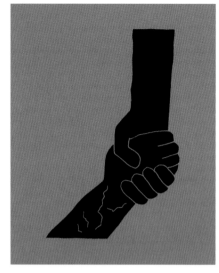

TO RESTORE THE SICK TO HEALTH AS SPEEDILY AS POSSIBLE
HOSPITALS

Throughout much of human history, the sick have been cared for at home. Temple-based healing, practiced in ancient Greece, is the earliest evidence of some form of community healthcare provision. However, nothing like the modern idea of a hospital—a dedicated building staffed with medical personnel—emerged until the 1st century CE, when the Roman army began building *valetudinaria*, medical establishments to treat sick and wounded legionnaires.

Hospitals, complete with wards, appeared in the Islamic world from the 9th century, some also offering care for the elderly and for those with mental illness. In Christian Europe, care for the sick in the medieval period was associated with spiritual care and poor relief.

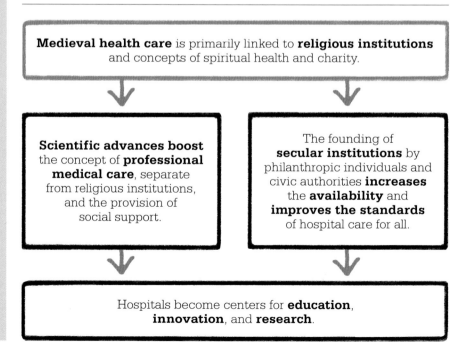

Medieval health care is primarily linked to **religious institutions** and concepts of spiritual health and charity.

Scientific advances boost the concept of **professional medical care**, separate from religious institutions, and the provision of social support.

The founding of **secular institutions** by philanthropic individuals and civic authorities **increases** the **availability** and **improves the standards** of hospital care for all.

Hospitals become centers for **education**, **innovation**, and **research**.

See also: Islamic medicine 44–49 ▪ Medieval medical schools and surgery 50–51 ▪ Case history 80–81 ▪ Scientific surgery 88–89 ▪ Triage 90 ▪ Hygiene 118–119 ▪ Nursing and sanitation 128–133 ▪ Palliative care 268–271

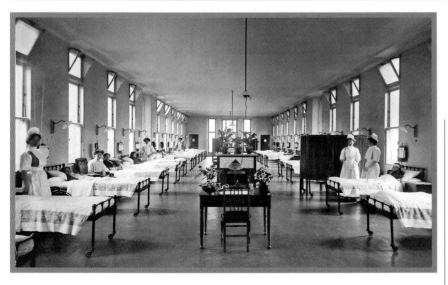

Advances in understanding about sanitation transformed the design and organization of many hospitals, including King's College, London, which moved from cramped conditions to modern, hygienic premises in 1913.

Monasteries became centers for healing and the nucleus for proto-hospitals such as St. Bartholomew's, London, which was founded in 1123.

A new secular model

The 16th-century Reformation of the Church weakened the link between religion and health care in the West, and many monasteries and their hospitals disappeared. While some were taken over by civic authorities, a lingering notion that hospitals were just hospices for the poor meant that surviving institutions became places to shut away the destitute and those with infectious diseases.

During the 17th and 18th centuries, the emergence of a merchant class with funds and a belief in philanthropic giving, the growth of cities, and the dawn of scientific medicine led to the birth of hospitals in their modern form. One of the first, Guy's Hospital in London, UK, was founded in 1721 by Thomas Guy. A wealthy publisher and businessman, he had made his fortune through shares in the South Sea Company, which profited from the slave trade. Aiming to provide a hospital for the "incurably ill and hopelessly insane," Guy's state-of-the-art establishment opened to patients in 1725 with 100 beds and 50 staff, including a bed-bug killer.

Similar hospitals founded by wealthy individuals, charitable or civic trusts, and universities created places where, for the first time, the general public were admitted without consideration of religion or wealth. The first general hospital in the US was founded in Philadelphia in 1751. New York's Bellevue Hospital, while originally attached to a poorhouse, was by 1816 one of a range of American medical establishments that offered care and trained physicians. In Germany, Berlin's Charité, originally founded as a quarantine hospital for plague victims, became a military hospital, and then a teaching hospital in 1828.

Today, we take for granted that hospitals are places dedicated to excellence in the healing of the sick using the most advanced techniques possible. Yet without the establishment of progressive institutions such as Guy's Hospital, the marriage of patient care and science they initiated might have occurred far more slowly, if at all. ▪

Centers for education and innovation

In the 18th century, the founding of new secular institutions such as Guy's Hospital, London, and the boost to scientific research provided by Enlightenment thinkers began to alter the focus of hospital medicine.

Prussia's Medical Edict of 1725, which set standards for the training of doctors, was a first sign that hospitals would, as well as caring for the sick, become centers for education. By 1750, Edinburgh's Royal Infirmary had a clinical ward for instructing students, and by the 1770s, trainee doctors in Vienna were also learning on the wards.

By the 19th century, hospitals had developed into centers for innovation, as well as education. Advances such as handwashing to reduce disease transmission, introduced by Hungarian doctor Ignaz Semmelweis in 1847, and the recommendations proposed by Florence Nightingale in the 1860s, effected changes in medical practice that still underpin modern hospital care.

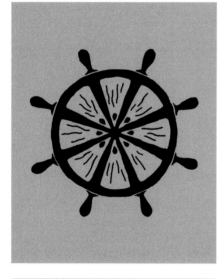

GREAT AND UNKNOWN VIRTUE IN THIS FRUIT
PREVENTING SCURVY

While working as a surgeon on the British naval vessel HMS *Salisbury* in 1747, Scottish physician James Lind reportedly performed a controlled clinical experiment on 12 sailors who were suffering from scurvy. The disease, which was ravaging the navy, was not yet understood. Lind divided his patients, whose symptoms were allegedly similarly advanced, into six pairs. Each pair was given a different dietary supplement that had been suggested as a cure: vinegar, sea water, cider, oranges and lemons, diluted sulfuric acid, or a mixture of garlic and mustard seeds. He found that those given citrus fruit recovered from the illness most quickly, and one sailor was fit for duty after only six days. Those given the other "cures" recovered slowly or not at all.

Scurvy is now known to result from a lack of vitamin C (ascorbic acid) in the body, and symptoms begin to develop after about a month of deprivation. Early signs include extreme lethargy and aching joints. If untreated, bleeding gums, loose teeth, and hemorrhaging of the skin follow, then death.

The disease was endemic among sailors, who were often at sea for months at a time and had to subsist on an appalling diet lacking in fruit and vegetables. Portuguese explorer Ferdinand Magellan lost most of his crew to scurvy on an expedition across the Pacific Ocean in 1520. By the mid-18th century, with increases in shipping, naval activity, and the length of voyages, the scale of the problem was immense. This "plague of the sea"

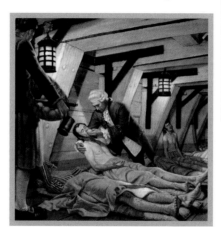

James Lind's experiment in 1747 was one of the first controlled medical trials. Participants shared the same diet, environment, and symptoms, so Lind could accurately compare the effects of his prescribed supplements on scurvy.

See also: Greek medicine 28–29 ▪ Roman medicine 38–43 ▪ Vitamins and diet 200–203 ▪ Evidence-based medicine 276–277

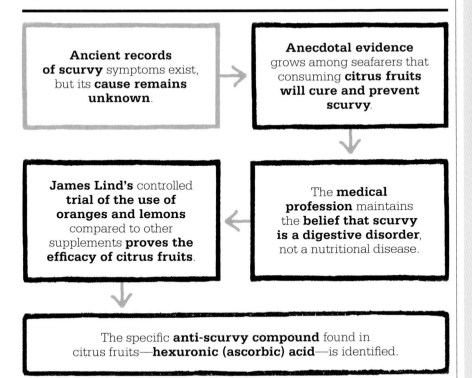

Ancient records of scurvy symptoms exist, but its **cause remains unknown**.

Anecdotal evidence grows among seafarers that consuming **citrus fruits will cure and prevent scurvy**.

The **medical profession** maintains the **belief that scurvy is a digestive disorder**, not a nutritional disease.

James Lind's controlled **trial of the use of oranges and lemons** compared to other supplements **proves the efficacy of citrus fruits**.

The specific **anti-scurvy compound** found in citrus fruits—**hexuronic (ascorbic) acid**—is identified.

probably killed more than 2 million sailors between the 15th and the 19th centuries—more than died from storms, combat, and every other disease combined.

Long-known disease

The symptoms of scurvy had been described by the ancient Egyptians, Hippocrates was aware of the disease, and several seafarers had suggested that citrus fruit might be preventative before Lind's trial. One of these was Portuguese explorer Vasco da Gama, who successfully treated his crew with oranges after they succumbed to scurvy in 1497.

Despite similar reports, the medical establishment remained wedded to the idea that scurvy was a digestive complaint caused by a lack of "fixed air" in the tissues and, with no way of keeping fruit fresh for long periods, citrus was not adopted as an antiscorbutic. Shortly after Lind's death, however, the British navy succumbed to pressure from naval physicians to supply all sailors with lemon juice. A similar policy was adopted by other maritime nations in the early 19th century. ▪

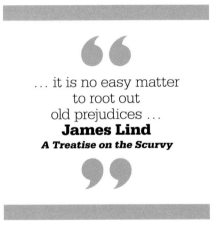

… it is no easy matter to root out old prejudices …
James Lind
A Treatise on the Scurvy

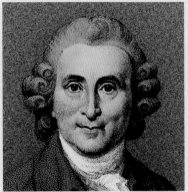

James Lind

Born in Edinburgh, Scotland, in 1716, James Lind was apprenticed to a surgeon at the age of 15 and joined the Royal Navy in 1739. After conducting experiments with a group of sailors on HMS *Salisbury* who were suffering from scurvy, he published his findings in *A Treatise on the Scurvy* in 1753. Lind's recommendation that sailors be given juice from citrus fruits to prevent scurvy led to British sailors being called "limeys."

Lind returned to his native Edinburgh to practice medicine, but in 1758, he was persuaded to become the chief physician at the newly opened Haslar Royal Naval Hospital in Gosport, Hampshire. From then until his retirement 25 years later, he proposed many measures to improve health and hygiene on naval vessels, though he was often frustrated that these were slow to be implemented. Many historians regard him as one of the first clinical investigators of the modern era. Lind died in Gosport in 1794.

Key work

1753 *A Treatise on the Scurvy*

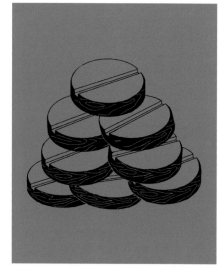

THE BARK OF A TREE IS VERY EFFICACIOUS
ASPIRIN

spirin is one of the most widely used drugs in the world. It has a spectrum of applications, from relieving pain and reducing inflammation to preventing strokes and treating cardiovascular conditions. Its active ingredient is acetylsalicylic acid, a compound originally derived from the willow tree.

A cure for agues

The medicinal properties of willow have been known for thousands of years. In the 5th century BCE, the Greek physician Hippocrates prescribed willow leaf tea for fever and pain, in particular for women in childbirth.

The analgesic (pain-relieving) properties of willow bark were rediscovered in the 18th century by British clergyman Edward Stone. Nibbling on a piece of willow bark while out walking, he was struck by its bitterness. It reminded him of cinchona bark, the source of quinine used to treat malaria. Aware of the folk belief that harmful agents and their panaceas are often found side by side, Stone reasoned that willow might be a cure for fevers.

Edward Stone

The son of a gentleman farmer, Edward Stone was born in the English town of Princes Risborough, Buckinghamshire, in 1702. At the age of 18, he attended Wadham College, Oxford, and was ordained a deacon and priest in 1728. He became a fellow of the college two years later.

In 1745, Stone moved to Chipping Norton, Oxfordshire, as chaplain at Bruern Abbey, where he also served as priest in several parish churches.

In addition to his duties as a cleric and his interest in medicine and science, Stone was appointed a justice of the peace for Oxfordshire in 1755.

A fire at Bruern Abbey ended Stone's chaplaincy in 1764. He died in Chipping Norton in 1768 and was buried in the churchyard at Horsenden.

Key work

1763 "An account of the success of the bark of the willow in the cure of agues"

See also: Greek medicine 28–29 ▪ Herbal medicine 36–37 ▪ Pharmacy 54–59 ▪ Cancer therapy 168–175 ▪ Electrocardiography 188–189 ▪ Antibiotics 216–223

The creation of aspirin

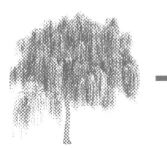 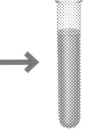 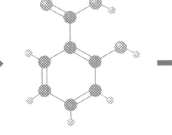 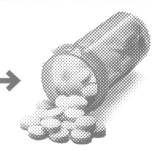

The analgesic and anti-inflammatory effect of willow (*Salix* spp.) is discovered by accident when its bark is chewed.

Chemists isolate the active ingredient— salicylic acid, a natural compound—that produces the analgesic effect.

The chemical structure of salicylic acid can now be determined. This allows chemists to synthesize it—create it artificially.

Salicylic acid is modified to create acetylsalicylic acid—a safer form of the compound, better known as aspirin.

Fevers (or "agues") were associated with damp, marshy environments, such as those in which willow trees typically grow.

Over the next few years, Stone treated 50 patients with fevers or suspected malaria with small doses of powdered willow bark in water delivered every four hours. He found the infusion to be very effective, and in 1763, he wrote to the president of the Royal Society about his remedy, in a landmark paper entitled "An account of the success of the bark of the willow in the cure of agues."

Active ingredient

After the publication of Stone's findings, more pharmacists began using willow bark. In 1827, German chemist Johann Buchner succeeded in isolating the bitter substance. He called it salicin, and it contained the active ingredient salicylic acid. Two years later, French pharmacist Henri Leroux managed to extract 1 oz (30 grams) of purified salicin from 3.3 lb (1.5 kg) of willow bark. The drawback of salicylic acid was that it caused gastrointestinal irritation, which some patients could not tolerate.

In 1897, at the pharmaceutical company Bayer based in Germany, chemist Felix Hoffmann created a safe form of the drug by altering the structure of salicylic acid. This new chemical, acetylsalicylic acid, was given the name aspirin. Frenchman Charles Gerhardt had treated acetyl chloride with sodium salicylate in 1853, but Hoffmann's version, which was instigated by his supervisor Arthur Eichengrün, was the first to be suitable for medical use.

Bayer marketed aspirin in 1899, originally as a powder that reduced temperature and inflammation, and sales of the first analgesic took off across the world. ■

That many … remedies lie not far from their causes was so very apposite to this particular case that I could not help applying it.
Edward Stone
Letter to the Royal Society, 1763

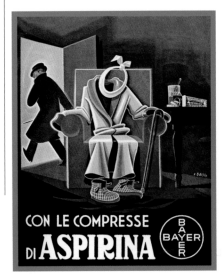

An Italian advertisement from 1935 illustrates the transforming effects of taking aspirin tablets to treat different types of pain.

CON LE COMPRESSE DI ASPIRINA BAYER

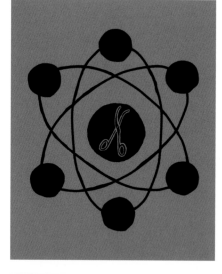

SURGERY HAS BECOME A SCIENCE

SCIENTIFIC SURGERY

IN CONTEXT

BEFORE

c. 17th century BCE The Egyptian Edwin Smith papyrus describes operations for the treatment of wounds.

c. 1150 CE The Arab surgeon Ibn Zuhr (Avenzoar) performs a tracheotomy on a goat to prove the safety of the procedure on humans.

1543 Andreas Vesalius publishes his *De Humani Corporis Fabrica*, showing depictions of internal human anatomy in previously unparalleled detail.

AFTER

1817 John Hunter's pupil Astley Cooper carries out the first operation to ligate the abdominal aorta.

1846 American dentist Henry Morton first uses ether as an anesthetic in an operation.

2001 The first-ever remote operation using robotic surgery is carried out in the US.

One of the first medical disciplines to make real advances was the practice of surgery. In ancient Egypt, c. 17th century BCE, the Edwin Smith papyrus outlined different surgical procedures. Later, Roman military surgeons refined surgical practice around the 1st century BCE, and key anatomical advances were made during the Renaissance. However, internal surgery was hampered by a lack of anesthesia or pain relief. There was also little understanding when it came to the long-term effects of an operation. The success or failure of a particular procedure might be apparent to the surgeon, but rarely did anyone examine the impact of surgery in detail.

Surgical discipline

In the 18th century, Scottish surgeon John Hunter established a scientific and methodical basis for surgery. He honed his skills as a military surgeon during the Seven Years' War in the 1760s. From his studies of gunshot

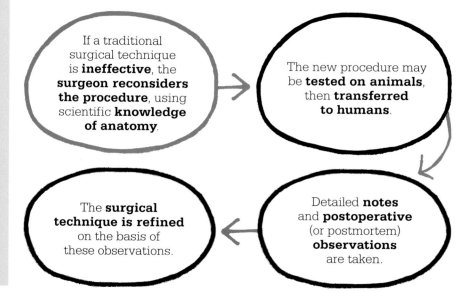

If a traditional surgical technique is **ineffective**, the **surgeon reconsiders the procedure**, using scientific **knowledge of anatomy**.

The new procedure may be **tested on animals**, then **transferred to humans**.

Detailed **notes** and **postoperative** (or postmortem) **observations** are taken.

The **surgical technique is refined** on the basis of these observations.

See also: Plastic surgery 26–27 ▪ Battlefield medicine 53 ▪ Anesthesia 112–117
▪ Antiseptics in surgery 148–151 ▪ Robotics and telesurgery 305

wounds, Hunter concluded that the opening of damaged tissue in order to extract bullet fragments (which was common practice at the time) in fact aggravated infections rather than diminished them.

On returning to London, Hunter aligned his surgical procedures to an understanding of anatomy and physiology. He made detailed observations of disease in living patients, and also conducted postmortem dissections. Hunter would devise an operation on the basis of his observations and practice on animals before conducting it on a human patient. This rigorous and inductive approach made him the founder of scientific surgery.

In 1785, Hunter carried out his most famous operation on the knee of a 45-year-old coachman, who had a popliteal aneurysm that swelled to fill the entire back of his knee. Instead of opening up the wound and scooping out the aneurysm, Hunter opened up the muscles and inserted ligatures (bindings)—these pressed against the blood vessels to steady the blood flow. The patient was able to walk again and, when

later he died of a fever, Hunter's postmortem revealed the aneurysm had gone, leaving no sign of infection.

In 1786, Hunter became one of the first physicians to recognize the process of metastasis in cancer. He noted the presence of tumors in a male patient's lungs that were similar to those on the man's thigh, and in doing so foreshadowed the clinical discipline of oncology.

Enduring influence

Hunter's focus on direct scientific observation refined the practice of surgery, earning him great acclaim. Many of his contemporaries and pupils, such as Joseph Lister, emulated Hunter's methods and carried forward his insistence that surgery (and the development of new operations) must have a basis in science, not tradition. This discipline continues to inform core surgical developments in the 21st century. ▪

The Hunter brothers, William and John, are depicted mid-dissection at William's school of anatomy. It was open to anyone who could pay to observe and learn surgical techniques.

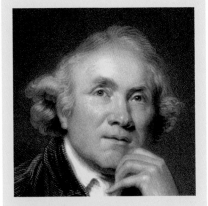

John Hunter

Born in Scotland, in 1728, John Hunter moved to London at age 21 to join his brother William, an anatomist. Hunter studied surgery at St. Bartholomew's Hospital and gained practical experience when he was then commissioned as an army surgeon in 1760.

Hunter later set up his own anatomy school in London in 1764, and used it as the base for his wide-ranging interests, such as comparative anatomy, the circulatory system of blood in pregnant women and the fetus, venereal disease, and the transplantation of teeth. He also taught Edward Jenner, the pioneer of vaccination.

Hunter became a fellow of the Royal Society in 1767, and later personal surgeon to King George III in 1776. He died in 1793, leaving his collection of more than 10,000 anatomical specimens to the Royal College of Surgeons.

Key works

1771 *The Natural History of the Human Teeth*
1786 *A Treatise on the Venereal Disease*
1794 *A Treatise on the Blood, Inflammation, and Gunshot Wounds*

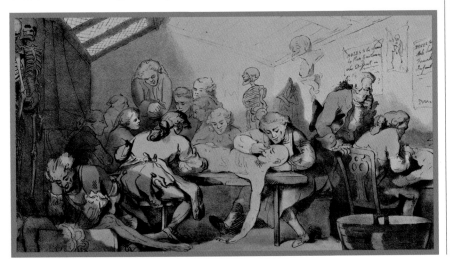

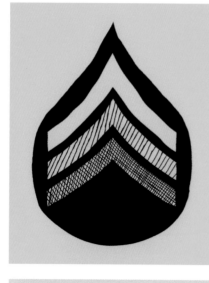

THE DANGEROUSLY WOUNDED MUST BE TENDED FIRST
TRIAGE

IN CONTEXT

BEFORE
c. 1000–600 BCE Assyrian "asu" are the first recorded military physicians to tend the wounded during battles.

c. 300 BCE–400 CE Roman armies develop systems to evacuate and treat the wounded.

16th century Barber-surgeons work on the battlefield; their increasingly skilled treatment raises the status of surgeons.

AFTER
1861–1865 Union surgeon Jonathan Letterman creates a new system of battlefield care during the Civil War.

1914–1918 The *Ordre de Triage*, devised by Belgian doctor Antoine Depage, sets out guidelines for the treatment of soldiers during World War I.

1939–1945 In World War II, army medics triage injuries in mobile aid stations close to battlefield front lines.

I n 1793, while on campaign with Napoleon, French military surgeon Dominique-Jean, Baron Larrey first used a system termed "triage" ("sorting") to manage the treatment of soldiers wounded on the battlefield, separating them into immediate, urgent, and nonurgent cases. Regardless of rank, the most seriously wounded, who in earlier campaigns had often been left to die, were taken to nearby medical tents on another of Larrey's innovations—*ambulances volantes* ("flying ambulances"), which were horse-drawn gun carriages specially adapted to carry the wounded from the battlefield.

Larrey's triage system, together with the first teams of medical attendants who stretchered the wounded, greatly reduced the total fatalities among Napoleon's men.

Triage in civilian settings
The triage concept further evolved in battlefield settings throughout the 19th and 20th centuries. As hospitals in Western nations

> The triage nurse makes quick decisions that can be the difference between life and death.
> **Lynn Sayre Visser**
> **American triage nurse and educator**

became more efficiently managed in the early 1900s, their emergency departments developed triage systems—both to decide the order for treating incoming patients and, in the field, to prioritize those needing very urgent medical care after a major accident or disaster.

Today, triage is widely used in civilian settings, and, depending on the country, may have three to five levels, ranging from immediate and resuscitation to nonurgent. ∎

See also: Battlefield medicine 53 ▪ Hospitals 82–83 ▪ Scientific surgery 88–89 ▪ Nursing and sanitation 128–133

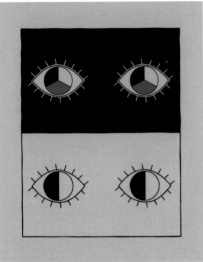

A PECULIARITY IN MY VISION
COLOR VISION DEFICIENCY

John Dalton was a British meteorologist and chemist, but he is also known for his 1794 description of the eye disorder that affected him and his brother. He found it difficult to detect the color red, while orange, yellow, and green appeared to merge into shades of yellow to beige. Later dubbed Daltonism, his was a red-green form of the defect better known as color blindness, or (more accurately) color vision deficiency.

Dalton's account interested the scientific community. Within a decade, British physicist Thomas Young proposed that the eye has three types of cone (photoreceptors responsible for color vision)—one each for blue, green, and red—to provide the full color spectrum. If one type is defective (in Dalton's case, the green receptor), color vision deficiency results.

Limited color range
In 1995, DNA from Dalton's eye, preserved after his death, showed he had deuteranopia, one of three types of red-green color vision deficiency. Lacking M-cones that react to medium-wave light, he could only distinguish between two or three colors rather than the full spectrum visible with normal vision. Rarer blue-yellow color deficiencies (tritanomaly and tritanopia) make it hard to distinguish between blue and green, and yellow and red.

While screening tests now help eye experts identify color vision deficiency, there is still no remedy. ∎

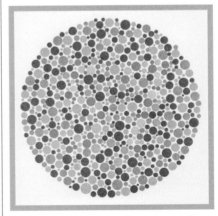

This color dot test plate, devised by Shinobu Ishihara, helps detect red-green color vision deficiency in those unable to see the figure 57.

See also: Islamic medicine 44–49 ▪ Anatomy 60–63 ▪ Inheritance and hereditary conditions 146–147 ▪ Physiology 152–153

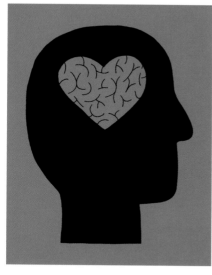

NO LONGER FEARED, BUT UNDERSTOOD
HUMANE MENTAL HEALTH CARE

IN CONTEXT

BEFORE
c. 8000 BCE A skull unearthed at Taforalt, a cave in Morocco, bears evidence of trepanning (drilling into the skull), possibly to cure a mental disorder.

1406 The first mental hospital opens in Valencia, Spain.

AFTER
1927 Austrian psychiatrist Manfred Sakel introduces insulin coma therapy. Schizophrenics are injected with insulin to put them into a low blood sugar coma.

1949 Portuguese neurologist Egas Moniz receives the Nobel Prize for introducing lobotomy (severing connections in parts of the brain) to treat serious mental illness. The procedure is later discredited for causing personality changes.

1950s French scientists develop antipsychotic drugs to treat schizophrenia and bipolar disorder.

Before the 18th century, people with **mental illness** are **feared** and **removed from society**.

↓

Their **humanity is denied** and their **condition becomes worse**.

↓

The Enlightenment fosters notions of **common humanity**, **individual liberty**, and **universal rights**.

↓

The **humane treatment of mental illness**, known as *traitement moral*, is introduced.

The diagnosis and treatment of mental illness raises a unique set of problems, in particular the judgment of what "normal" means in terms of behavior. Throughout the medieval period, the belief that people could be possessed by demons that had to be driven out was common. The world was dominated by fear of plague, famine, and war, and superstition was rife. At best, the mentally ill experienced social stigma; at worst, they were accused of witchcraft.

Asylums to house the mentally ill increased in number during the 16th century. Most of their patients were confined against their will and were often chained. They were likened to animals, without the capacity to reason or experience pain. Asylums made no pretense at helping the mentally ill recover, and patients were expected to tolerate their miserable existence without complaint.

Traitement moral
Scientific understanding of mental illness barely changed during the 17th century, but in the 18th century, social reformers in Europe began to turn their attention to

See also: Lithium and bipolar disorder 240 ▪ Chlorpromazine and antipsychotics 241 ▪ Behavioral and cognitive therapy 242–243

> The managers of these institutions … are frequently men of little knowledge and less humanity …
> **Philippe Pinel**
> *Treatise on Insanity*, **1801**

the mentally ill. Italian physician Vincenzo Chiarugi removed the chains from his psychiatric patients in the 1780s and encouraged good hygiene, recreation, and some occupational training. In Paris in the 1790s, Philippe Pinel sought to prove his hypothesis that mentally ill patients would improve if treated with compassion. He introduced his *traitement moral* (moral treatment), a regime of improved nutrition and living conditions.

In Britain, Quaker philanthropist William Tuke established the York Retreat along similar lines in 1796. Tuke also believed in the therapeutic and moral value of physical work for patients.

The moral treatment advocated by Pinel and Tuke reached the US in the early 19th century. Again, the focus was on spiritual and moral development, as well as the

The York Retreat, shown here in 1887, was founded on "moral treatment" of the mentally ill. Patients were viewed with compassion and treated as guests rather than prisoners.

rehabilitation of patients, who were encouraged to engage in manual labor and recreational pastimes. By the end of the century, however, moral treatment had largely been abandoned. Asylums had become overcrowded and individual care could no longer be provided.

Mental hygiene

By the late 19th century, the mental hygiene movement promoted by reformer Clifford Beers in the US was replacing moral treatment. Beers was motivated by the poor treatment he had received for his own depression and anxiety. He recommended an approach to mental health that focused on the patient's total well-being. Beers' book *A Mind That Found Itself* (1908), and the National Committee for Mental Hygiene that he founded in 1909, influenced mental health services across the world. Beers' ethos is at the heart of mental health provision today. ∎

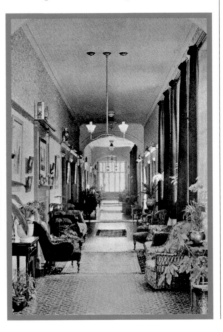

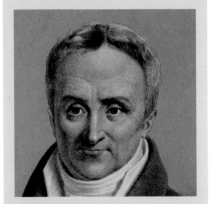

Philippe Pinel

Born in Jonquières, France, in 1745, Philippe Pinel was the son of a master surgeon. Abandoning his studies in theology in 1770, Pinel attended France's leading medical school at the University of Montpellier, supporting himself during his training by translating medical and scientific texts and teaching mathematics.

In 1778, Pinel moved to Paris, where he edited the medical journal *Gazette de santé*, regularly including articles on mental illness. In 1793, he was appointed superintendent of the Bicêtre hospice, and two years later, became chief physician of the Salpêtrière hospital, which had 600 beds for the mentally ill. It was at Bicêtre and Salpêtrière that he devised his *traitement moral*, and chains were removed from patients who had been restrained for decades. Pinel worked at Salpêtrière for the rest of his life and died in 1826.

Key works

1794 *Memoir on Madness*
1801 *Treatise on Insanity*

TRAINING THE IMMUNE SYSTEM

VACCINATION

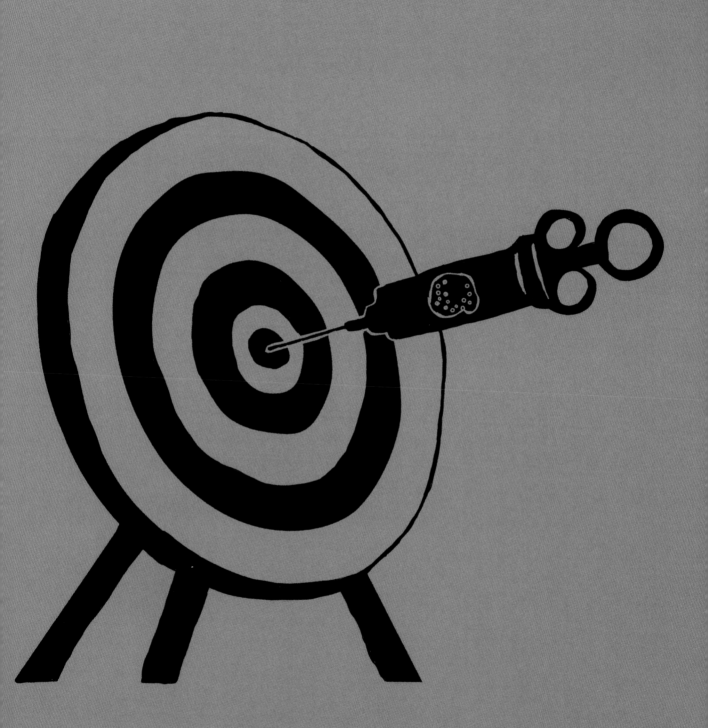

IN CONTEXT

BEFORE

c. 590 CE Chinese healers begin to practice inoculation.

1713 Emmanuel Timoni describes mass inoculation in Constantinople.

1718 Lady Mary Wortley Montagu has her young son inoculated in Constantinople.

1721 In the American colonies, pastor Cotton Mather urges variolation to protect against a smallpox epidemic.

AFTER

1921 French scientists Albert Calmette and Camille Guérin create BCG, the first vaccine against tuberculosis.

1953 Jonas Salk, an American virologist, discovers a vaccine for polio.

1980 The World Health Organization declares that "Smallpox is dead!"

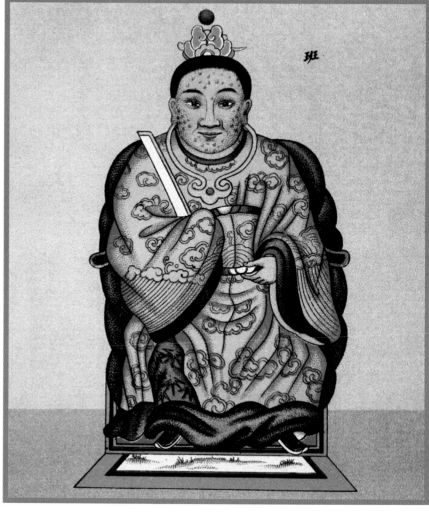

Vaccines are one of the greatest medical success stories of all time. In the developed world, they have been so effective at containing many infectious diseases that it is easy to forget just how terrible diseases such as smallpox, diphtheria, polio, and tetanus once were.

Vaccination, or immunization, works by priming the body's defenses with a safe version of the germ (or part of the germ) that causes the disease. This enables the immune system to build up resistance, or immunity, to the disease—and the more people

who are immune to the disease, the less it can spread. The key to vaccination's success is the idea of the "safe version," and this was the great breakthrough made by British physician Edward Jenner in 1796 with his smallpox vaccine.

The deadly pox

Smallpox is a highly contagious disease that is caused by two forms of the variola virus. It has now been completely eradicated from the world, but until Jenner's vaccine, its effects were devastating. In the 18th century, nearly half a million people in Europe alone died from

Yu Hoa Long was the Chinese god of recovery from smallpox, a disease that was seen by many cultures as a divine punishment for sins committed.

the disease each year. And as European explorers, traders, and settlers spread across the globe, they took with them smallpox and other diseases, which decimated native populations that had never before been exposed to these germs.

Those who were lucky enough to survive smallpox were often scarred for life with pockmarked faces, the effect of the terrible pustules or "pox" that erupt. One

See also: Germ theory 138–145 ▪ The immune system 154–161 ▪ Virology 177 ▪ Attenuated vaccines 206–209 ▪ Global eradication of disease 286–287 ▪ HIV and autoimmune diseases 294–297 ▪ Pandemics 306–313

> The small-pox, so fatal,
> and so general amongst us,
> is here entirely harmless
> by the invention of
> ingrafting [variolation] …
> **Lady Mary
> Wortley Montagu**
> Letter to a friend, April 1717

third of survivors went blind. In 18th-century England, largely due to smallpox, just one child in three survived beyond the age of 5.

It had been known at least as far back as Roman times that those who survived smallpox somehow gained immunity. In fact, former smallpox victims were often called upon to nurse the sick. Healers across Asia (especially China), Africa, and Europe had long tried to replicate this natural immunity through the practice of variolation (inoculation), in which healthy people were deliberately infected with matter from someone with an apparently mild version of the disease.

Variolation usually involved rubbing crushed smallpox scabs into cuts on the hand, or blowing them in pellets into the nostrils. In a practice known as "buying the pox," parents would purchase scabs or contaminated clothing with which to infect their children.

With luck, people who had been inoculated would fall moderately ill for a few days, then recover with full immunity. It was a high-risk strategy, as a significant number of those inoculated would die. Also, children who survived variolation could become carriers of the disease. But smallpox was so devastating that many people were prepared to risk it. Some, such as girls raised in the Caucasus for the Ottoman sultan's harems in Constantinople (now Istanbul), had no choice.

The royal experiment

The idea of inoculation began to catch the attention of European physicians around 1700. In 1713, Greek doctor Emmanuel Timoni described how he had seen Greek female inoculators successfully inoculating thousands of children in Constantinople during a smallpox epidemic. Venetian physician Jacob Pylarini, who practiced variolation in the city, wrote a book about it in 1715. Then, British writer Lady Mary Wortley Montagu, who had been left severely disfigured by the disease, observed the practice.

Impressed by the apparent success of "ingrafting," Lady Mary asked embassy surgeon Charles

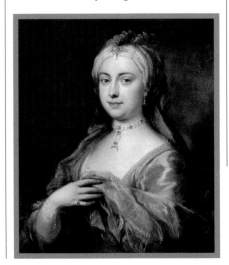

> In 1736, I lost
> one of my sons …
> by the small-pox.
> I long regretted bitterly …
> that I had not given it to him
> by inoculation.
> **Benjamin Franklin**
> American statesman (1706–1790)

Maitland to oversee the inoculation of her 5-year-old son Edward by one of the Greek female inoculators in 1718. She became a prominent advocate of the technique, and on their return to Britain, she asked Maitland to inoculate her daughter.

Soon after, in 1721, Maitland received a Royal Commission to conduct what may have been the world's first clinical trial. The aim was to prove to the British royal family that inoculation worked. Under the watchful eye of the country's leading physician, Hans Sloane, Maitland inoculated six condemned prisoners in Newgate Prison, who were persuaded to cooperate in return for then being released. They survived and, a few months later, Maitland repeated the trial with orphaned children, who also survived. **»**

Smallpox survivor Lady Mary Wortley Montagu was instrumental in bringing the practice of inoculation to the notice of British physicians. She had lost her brother to the disease when he was 20.

News of Maitland's achievements spread quickly, and the practice of inoculation was adopted across Europe and in the American colonies. In 1721, Massachusetts pastor Cotton Mather and doctor Zabdiel Boylston became forceful advocates. In 1738, with a serious smallpox epidemic threatening the state of Carolina, around 1,000 people were treated. In Britain that year, nearly 2,000 people were inoculated in Middlesex.

Variolation was a hazardous procedure, with at least one in 30 dying from the disease as a direct result, but the introduction of inoculation on a large scale soon demonstrated that the risk was considerably lower than from dying in an epidemic. In 1757, an 8-year-old boy was inoculated with smallpox, one of thousands to be treated that year. His name was Edward Jenner.

The safe version

Jenner went on to be dubbed the "father of immunology," with an assured place in the history of medicine. But back in the 1770s, he was a country physician who, like other doctors of the period,

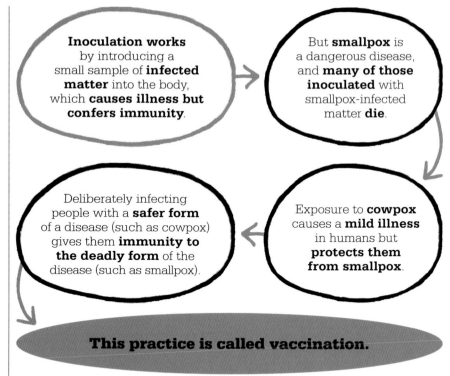

Inoculation works by introducing a small sample of **infected matter** into the body, which **causes illness but confers immunity**.

But **smallpox** is a dangerous disease, and **many of those inoculated** with smallpox-infected matter **die**.

Deliberately infecting people with a **safer form** of a disease (such as cowpox) gives them **immunity to the deadly form** of the disease (such as smallpox).

Exposure to **cowpox** causes a **mild illness** in humans but **protects them from smallpox**.

This practice is called vaccination.

I hope that someday the practice of producing cow pox in human beings will spread over the world—when that day comes, there will be no more small pox.
Edward Jenner, 1798

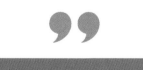

inoculated many of his patients to protect them from smallpox. He was intrigued by stories that people—typically milkmaids—who had contracted a mild infection, cowpox, from their cows had acquired an immunity to the much deadlier smallpox, and he wondered whether cowpox could provide a safer method of inoculation.

One day, Jenner is said to have overheard a dairymaid boasting, "I shall never have smallpox for I have had cowpox. I shall never have an ugly pockmarked face." He began to gather data in earnest. In nearly 30 cases, he found examples of previous exposure to cowpox appearing to give immunity to smallpox. Although Jenner did not know it, cowpox is caused by the vaccinia virus, which can be transmitted to humans and is closely related to the variola virus responsible for smallpox.

In 1796, Sarah Nelmes, a dairymaid, went to see Jenner about a rash on her right hand. He diagnosed her with cowpox and decided to test his theory, using James Phipps, the 8-year-old son of his gardener, as his guinea pig. Jenner made a few scratches on one of the boy's arms and rubbed in some of the cowpox material he had taken from pockmarks on the infected dairymaid's hand. Within a few days, the boy became mildly ill with cowpox but soon recovered.

Having established that cowpox could be transferred from person to person, Jenner proceeded to the next step in his experiment. This was to test whether the cowpox would in fact protect James from smallpox. Jenner inoculated the boy with material from a fresh smallpox lesion. James did not develop smallpox symptoms either then or in the future.

Jenner continued to collect further case histories and also followed up his initial experiment with others, which confirmed his original theory that cowpox did in fact protect against smallpox. In 1798, he published his findings in a book entitled *An Inquiry into the Causes and Effects of the Variolae Vaccinae, a Disease Discovered in some of the Western Counties of England, Particularly Gloucestershire, and Known by the Name of the Cow Pox*. The technique of introducing material under the skin to confer protection against disease became universally known as vaccination, a word derived from the Latin name for the cow (*vacca*), in recognition of Jenner's discovery.

Spreading the word

Jenner sent a vaccine to anyone who requested it and, with the support of other doctors, vaccination spread rapidly throughout Britain. By 1800, it was being practiced in most European countries and in the United States. The following year, Jenner published an article, "On the Origin of the Vaccine Inoculation," summarizing his discoveries and expressing his hope that "the annihilation of the smallpox, the most dreadful scourge of the human species, must be the final result of this practice."

Although Jenner was the first person to carry out a scientific investigation into vaccination and its effects, he may not have been the first to discover the technique. When a smallpox epidemic hit the English county of Dorset in 1774, local farmer Benjamin Jesty was determined to protect his family. He took material from the udder of an infected cow and used a small needle to introduce it into the arms of his wife and two sons. (Jesty had had cowpox already, so he did not vaccinate himself.) The experiment worked, and the family remained free of smallpox. But it would be a further 25 years before Jenner's experiments and dogged promotion of vaccination changed the way medicine was practiced forever.

A mixed reception

Jenner's findings did not meet with universal acceptance. Some of the most vocal objections came from the clergy, who reasoned that smallpox was a God-given fact of life and death and any attempt to

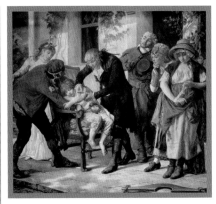

This painting by Gaston Melingue shows Jenner vaccinating James Phipps in 1796. Jenner was so grateful to the boy that he later built a house for him in his home town of Berkeley.

interfere with divine intention was blasphemy. There were also those who were fearful of having material from diseased cows introduced into their bodies, an objection readily satirized by the caricaturists of the day. When vaccination with cowpox was made compulsory in 1853, it led to protest marches and impassioned demands for freedom of choice from anti-vaccination campaigners.

For decades after Jenner's breakthrough discovery, the source of the vaccine continued to be **»**

Edward Jenner

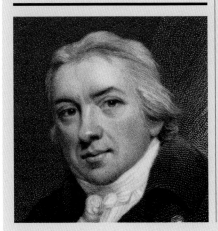

Born in Berkeley, Gloucestershire, UK, in 1749, Edward Jenner was orphaned at age 5 and went to live with his older brother. In 1764, he began an apprenticeship with a local surgeon, after which, at 21, he became a student of the famous surgeon John Hunter in London.

Jenner's interests were wide: he helped classify new species brought back from the South Pacific by botanist Joseph Banks; built his own hydrogen balloon; and studied the life cycle of the cuckoo. He also played the violin and wrote poetry. Jenner married in 1788 and had four children. In a hut in the garden of his family home, dubbed the "Temple of Vaccinia," he vaccinated the poor for free. Having won widespread recognition, he died in 1823.

Key works

1798 *An Inquiry into the Causes and Effects of the Variolae Vaccinae*
1799 *Further Observations on the Variolæ Vaccinæ, or Cow Pox*
1801 "On the Origin of the Vaccine Inoculation"

Vaccination was feared by many people. This 1802 cartoon by James Gillray depicts Jenner vaccinating a nervous woman, while around her cows sprout from other people's bodies.

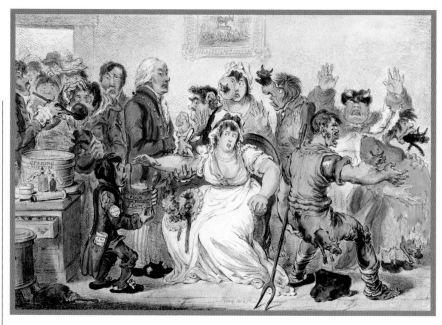

the cowpox sores on the arms of infected dairymaids. Few efforts were made to use cowpox material taken directly from cattle. In the 1840s, Italian physician Giuseppe Negri was one of the first to use bovine material to vaccinate people directly, but it was not until 1864 that French medics Gustave Lanoix and Ernest Chambon transported a calf infected with cowpox from Naples in Italy to Paris and set up an "animal vaccine" service.

There were obvious advantages to animal vaccination. Over the course of a few weeks, one heifer could provide enough vaccine for thousands of doses. A small herd could vaccinate a city. Another benefit was that patients no longer risked cross-infection with other diseases from a human donor. Chambon took his ideas to the United States, where "virus farms" became established toward the end of the century. By 1902, around a quarter of the population of New York, about 800,000 people, had been vaccinated.

> Medicine has
> never before produced
> any single improvement
> of such utility.
> **Thomas Jefferson**
> **3rd US president (1801–1809)**

Until the 1870s, smallpox was the only disease for which there was a vaccine. But that all changed when microbiologists Louis Pasteur in France and Robert Koch in Germany showed that diseases are caused by tiny microbes, or germs. In 1877, Pasteur began to argue that if a vaccine could be found for smallpox, then it could for all diseases.

Weakened germs

Eager to prove his theory, Pasteur tried inoculating chickens with cholera bacteria, but most of the chickens died. In 1879, he made a startling discovery. Just before he went away on vacation, he instructed his assistant to inoculate the birds using a fresh bacteria culture. The assistant forgot, and on his return, Pasteur inoculated the chickens with the old cultures. The birds were then mildly ill, survived, and became immune.

Pasteur realized that exposing the bacteria to oxygen had made them less deadly. The idea of using a weakened germ was not new, but the idea of purposely "attenuating"

(weakening) a germ in the laboratory so that it could be used as a safe vaccine was a huge breakthrough.

Other vaccines

Pasteur at once began to look for other diseases to inoculate against. In 1881, he developed a vaccine for anthrax, which he successfully used in sheep, goats, and cows. Then, in 1885, he began to search for a rabies vaccine.

Unlike cholera and anthrax, rabies (unbeknown to Pasteur) is due to a virus, not a bacterium, so it cannot be grown easily in the lab. But the virus mutates quickly, and its virulence can be reduced by passing it through a different species before human use. Pasteur was able to get his attenuated rabies vaccine by drying the spinal cords of rabbits he had infected with the disease.

Following successful trials on dogs, Pasteur was persuaded to test his vaccine on a 9-year-old boy, Joseph Meister, who had been bitten by a rabid dog and was likely to die. Pasteur injected the boy with a daily series of progressively virulent doses of his rabbit-spine concoction. It worked, and the boy recovered. Pasteur insisted that his method would also be called "vaccination," in honor of Jenner, and the name has stuck.

Inspired by Pasteur's success, scientists around the world began to look for other "live, attenuated vaccines," believing that in this way, they could find a vaccine for, and eradicate, every single disease. Live vaccines have since been found for tuberculosis, yellow fever, measles, mumps, and rubella, among other diseases.

Getting it right

The challenge with vaccinations is to find the right vaccine. A vaccine has to trigger the production of the right antibodies, but it clearly should not make the patient ill. Medical scientists have no doubt that the best way of combating most infectious diseases is to find a vaccine. With some diseases, one vaccine seems enough to give long-term immunity. With others, such as influenza, new variations of the virus are appearing all the time, and a new vaccine has to be

developed to combat each one— those vulnerable to winter flu need to get a new vaccination every fall to protect them against that year's version. Other diseases, such as HIV, are very hard to create an effective vaccine for, because HIV attacks a person's immune system.

Vaccination has saved hundreds of millions of lives. Smallpox has been entirely eradicated, and many other infectious diseases are in decline. In the US, for instance, diphtheria declined from 206,939 cases in 1921 to just two cases between 2004 and 2017; whooping cough declined from 265,269 cases in 1934 to 15,609 in 2018; and measles has fallen from 894,134 cases in 1941 to just 372 in 2019.

New diseases are being fought successfully all the time. Since the hemophilus influenzae type b (Hib) vaccine was introduced in the 1990s, for example, the incidence of the disease Hib meningitis, which once killed tens of thousands of children, has declined in Europe by 90 percent and in the US by 99 percent. But globalization has brought new threats, and in 2020, the race to find a vaccine for COVID-19 began. ∎

How vaccination works

When the body is exposed to a pathogen (a disease-causing organism), it reacts by releasing floods of antibodies targeted against that specific germ. It takes a while to produce the right antibodies, and the body may suffer the symptoms of disease before the immune system mounts its counter-attack. Eventually, if the person survives, the germs are beaten and the body recovers.

The next time the body encounters the germ, however, the antibodies are ready to eliminate it before the disease develops. Vaccination primes the immune system by exposing it to weakened, dead, or partial versions of the germ. These "safe" pathogens trigger antibody production but do not cause the disease. With some diseases, a single exposure is enough. With others, immunity needs to be built up gradually with a series of vaccinations or restored with a "booster" jab.

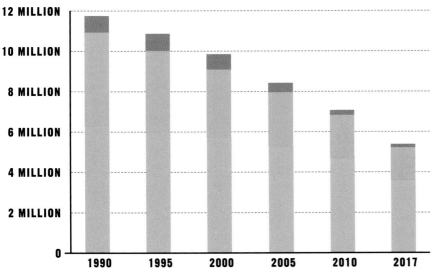

Vaccination has greatly improved the global life expectancy of children under 5. The height of each bar shows the total number of deaths, and the colored sections represent deaths that could have been prevented by vaccines.

Key: Causes of death

■ Causes of death that are preventable by vaccines:
1. Tetanus
2. Whooping cough
3. Measles

■ Causes of death that are partly preventable by vaccines:
1. Meningitis and encephalitis
2. Diarrheal diseases
3. Acute respiratory infections

■ Other causes (not preventable by vaccines)

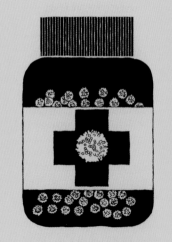

LIKE CURES LIKE
HOMEOPATHY

German physician Samuel Hahnemann first proposed the system of "like cures like" medicine in his 1796 *Essay on a New Principle for Ascertaining the Curative Power of Drugs*. After translating Scottish physician William Cullen's 1781 *Lectures on the Materia Medica* into German, Hahnemann had tested Cullen's observation that taking cinchona bark powder (later isolated as quinine) produced symptoms that were similar to those of malaria, the disease it was known to treat. Hahnemann also experienced malarial symptoms, which led him to the "like cures like" principle. This is the key doctrine of homeopathy, a term Hahnemann coined in 1807.

Hahnemann would prescribe highly diluted solutions of a remedy, as he believed that the lower the dose, the greater its potency. In Britain, Europe, and the US, homeopathy soon became a popular alternative to conventional therapies such as purging and bloodletting; by 1900, there were 15,000 homeopathists in the US.

The system still has many adherents, but conventional medicine warns that there is no reliable evidence to support homeopathy, and it should never be used to treat chronic or serious conditions. As some homeopathic products react with conventional medicines, those considering homeopathy should consult a doctor first. While many users report positive results, these are probably a placebo effect, largely due to the holistic approach of homeopathic practitioners. ∎

> " ... homeopathic products perform no better than placebos.
> **Science and Technology Committee**
> **British House of Commons, 2010**

See also: Ayurvedic medicine 22–25 ▪ Greek medicine 28–29 ▪ Herbal medicine 36–37 ▪ Medieval medical schools and surgery 50–51 ▪ Pharmacy 54–59

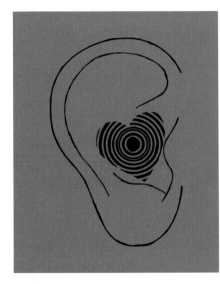

TO HEAR THE BEATING OF THE HEART

THE STETHOSCOPE

IN CONTEXT

BEFORE
17th century BCE Egyptian papyri mention that signs of disease can be heard within the body.

c. 375 BCE Hippocrates suggests shaking patients and pressing an ear against their chest to listen for abnormalities.

1616 William Harvey notes that blood pulsing through the heart "can be heard within the chest."

AFTER
1852 American physician George P. Cammann perfects his design of a flexible binaural (two-earpiece) stethoscope.

1895 In France, obstetrician Adolphe Pinard develops a stethoscope that detects fetal activity in the womb.

1998 3M launches a new Littman stethoscope that electronically amplifies sounds that might go undetected.

I n 1816, French physician René Laënnec invented the stethoscope. He had found the earlier practice of pressing his ear to a patient's chest to listen to the heart and lungs both inefficient and embarrassing—especially when examining women. Laënnec discovered that a piece of paper rolled into a cylinder and pressed against the chest or back made the sounds more clearly audible. His first instrument was a hollow wooden tube $1^{1}/_{3}$ in (3.5 cm) in diameter and $9^{3}/_{4}$ in (25 cm) long, with a small earpiece attached at one end. He called it a stethoscope, from the Greek words *stethos* ("chest") and *skopein* ("to observe").

Widespread use

In 1819, Laënnec published *On mediate auscultation*, which discussed how the sounds of possible heart and lung diseases and defects could be heard through a stethoscope. This work aroused great interest and encouraged widespread use of the instrument over the next 30 years.

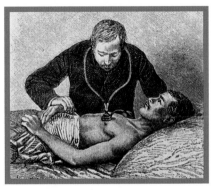

A 19th-century engraving reveals how little the form of stethoscopes has changed. In hospitals, doctors now also use pocket-sized ultrasound scanners.

Improvements made after Laënnec's death in 1826 included a flexible tube, two earpieces, and a dual-head version to press against the back and chest (a hollow bell to detect low-frequency sounds and a diaphragm to pick up high-frequency sounds). American professor David Littman developed a lighter stethoscope with better acoustics in the early 1960s, and in 2015, Palestinian doctor Tarek Loubani remedied a shortage by creating the first 3D-printed model. ∎

See also: Blood circulation 68–73 ▪ Case history 80–81 ▪ Electrocardiography 188–189 ▪ Ultrasound 244 ▪ Pacemakers 257

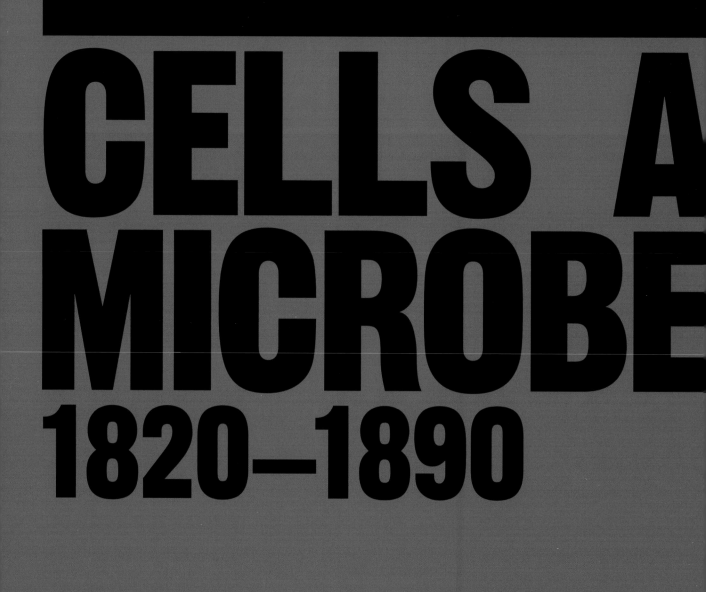

CELLS A
MICROBE
1820–1890

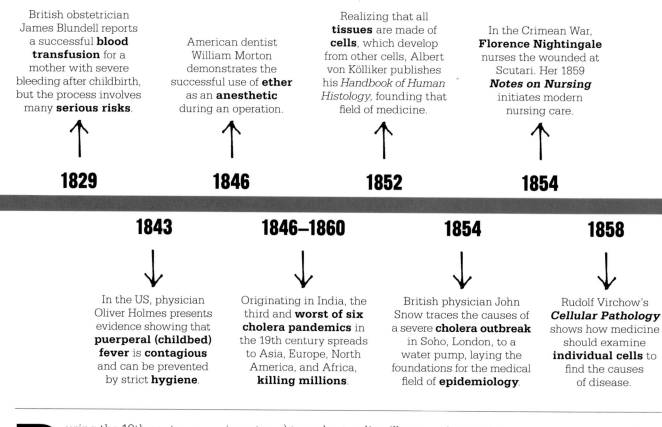

British obstetrician James Blundell reports a successful **blood transfusion** for a mother with severe bleeding after childbirth, but the process involves many **serious risks**.

American dentist William Morton demonstrates the successful use of **ether** as an **anesthetic** during an operation.

Realizing that all **tissues** are made of **cells**, which develop from other cells, Albert von Kölliker publishes his *Handbook of Human Histology*, founding that field of medicine.

In the Crimean War, **Florence Nightingale** nurses the wounded at Scutari. Her 1859 ***Notes on Nursing*** initiates modern nursing care.

1829

1846

1852

1854

1843

1846–1860

1854

1858

In the US, physician Oliver Holmes presents evidence showing that **puerperal (childbed) fever** is **contagious** and can be prevented by strict **hygiene**.

Originating in India, the third and **worst of six cholera pandemics** in the 19th century spreads to Asia, Europe, North America, and Africa, **killing millions**.

British physician John Snow traces the causes of a severe **cholera outbreak** in Soho, London, to a water pump, laying the foundations for the medical field of **epidemiology**.

Rudolf Virchow's ***Cellular Pathology*** shows how medicine should examine **individual cells** to find the causes of disease.

During the 19th century, huge medical progress was made possible by the light microscope. Improvements increased magnifications to many hundreds of times, with far greater clarity. As researchers delved deeper into the body's minuscule secrets, new levels of detail came into focus. In Switzerland, and then Germany, Swiss anatomist Albert von Kölliker studied a vast range of animal materials and moved onto human samples. He observed almost every type of tissue: skin, bones, muscles, nerves, blood, and guts. His first great work, *Handbook of Human Histology*, of 1852, quickly became recommended reading across biology and medicine.

Just six years later, German pathologist Rudolf Virchow applied histology (the study of microscopic anatomy) to understanding illness with his *Cellular Pathology* in 1858. Causes of disease, diagnosis, and progress of treatment could all be achieved by the scrutiny of cells. By now, age-old theories such as the spontaneous generation of life from nonliving matter were fading. In their place came cell theory, with its three key elements: all living organisms are composed of one or more cells; the cell is the basic structural unit of life; and cells arise from preexisting cells.

In France and Germany, further microscopic studies were looking not only at the body's own cells, but at invaders from outside. In the 1850s, French microbiologist Louis Pasteur began to help the local beer and wine industries, whose products suffered from spoiling and souring. Pasteur concluded that tiny organisms—germs—were causing the problems rather than chemical changes or spontaneous generation.

Progress and challenges
Pasteur began to focus on animal diseases, including a blight of silkworms, and cholera and anthrax in farmyard birds and livestock. His microscope-based investigations were inventive and thorough, and he considered that these harmful microorganisms could also cause many human diseases. Gradually, he conceived the notion we now call germ theory.

Around this time, German microbiologist Robert Koch also gained prominence. In 1875, he identified the germ that causes anthrax, *Bacillus anthracis*, followed by those for TB and cholera. Pasteur and Koch also strove to develop

French scientist Louis Pasteur publishes his **germ theory**. He suspects that many diseases are caused by **tiny organisms** that spread in various ways.

French physician Claude Bernard describes his concept of a *milieu intérieur* (constancy of the **internal environment**), which is key to the development of **physiology**.

Joseph Lister reports extremely positive results of using **carbolic acid** as an antiseptic during operations.

Russian researcher Élie Metchnikoff suggests that **white blood cells** are part of the **body's defense mechanism** rather than actually spreading disease.

↑ **1861** ↑ **1865** ↑ **1867** ↑ **1882**

1865 **1865** **1870s** **1884**

↓ ↓ ↓ ↓

Austrian monk Gregor Mendel creates the basis of **genetics** with *Experiments in Plant Hybridization*. Its value is not recognized until 1900.

Elizabeth Garrett-Anderson is the **first woman** to qualify as a doctor in the UK. In 1874, with Elizabeth Blackwell, she inaugurates the **London School of Medicine for Women**.

Rivals Louis Pasteur and Robert Koch announce discoveries identifying the **causes of diseases** including anthrax and cholera, thereby verifying **germ theory**.

French physician Alphonse Laveran first proposes that the **parasite** that causes **malaria** is carried by mosquitoes.

---

vaccines for the diseases they had unraveled. Pasteur successfully developed one for anthrax in 1881.

Away from the microscope, doctors were facing new challenges and had to respond to the continuing effects of industrialization, which brought urbanization and crowded, unsanitary conditions in cities and factories. Disease patterns were changing as a result, with cholera, typhoid, and dysentery all more prominent. Medical organizations were being set up with regulations to govern standards of practice and care. Britain's Royal College of Surgeons became active in 1800, and in 1808, the University of France numbered medicine among its six faculties. Yet these professions were hugely dominated by men. In 1847 in the US, Elizabeth Blackwell seized on a college admissions anomaly to register for a medical degree. She was soon followed by other pioneering women.

Sanitation and surgery

In 1854, British reformer Florence Nightingale and her team of nurses and carers had traveled to Scutari, Turkey, to tend the wounded during the Crimean War. Conditions in the crowded, unsanitary hospital wards were horrific; up to 10 times more men succumbed to disease than to their war wounds. Nightingale's efforts reduced this tally dramatically. On her return to Britain, she continued to lobby for change and in 1859 penned *Notes on Nursing*, generally regarded as the basis of modern nursing practices.

A further field of 19th-century progress was anesthesia. For centuries, surgeons had been restricted by conscious patients screaming in agony and struggling under the knife, and they had to work quickly. The first operations under nitrous oxide, and then ether anesthetic, occurred in the US in the 1840s. The techniques rapidly spread to Europe, with chloroform as the chemical of choice. Surgeons no longer had to rush and could develop more complex procedures.

Despite this, postoperative infections were still a common hazard of surgery. In the 1860s, British surgeon Joseph Lister began to use carbolic acid as an antiseptic against invading micropathogens. His work showed that infections were drastically reduced, yet even this clear evidence was rejected by some in the medical establishment, where dogma continued to hold back progressive practices in medicine. ∎

LET HEALTHY BLOOD LEAP INTO THE SICK MAN

BLOOD TRANSFUSION AND BLOOD GROUPS

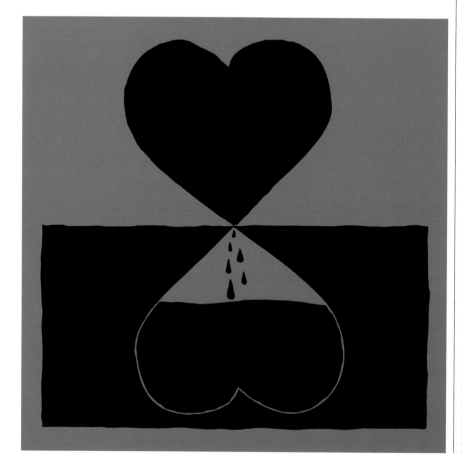

IN CONTEXT

BEFORE
1628 William Harvey publishes *De Motu Cordis et Sanguinis*, in which he describes the circulation of blood.

1665 Richard Lower attempts blood transfusion between two dogs.

1667 Jean-Baptiste Denis transfuses blood from a lamb into a human.

AFTER
1914 Adolph Hustin develops long-term anticoagulants.

1916 US Army medic Oswald Robertson creates "blood depots" during World War I.

1939 Karl Landsteiner and Alexander Weiner discover the Rh blood group system.

There are about 11 pints (5 liters) of blood in an adult human body. Severe blood loss leads to weakness, organ damage, and death. It is a major cause of death from injury and for centuries was a common reason for maternal death in childbirth. The concept of transfusion—replacing lost blood with blood from another person, as British obstetrician James Blundell did in 1829—seemed like an obvious remedy, but the means to do this safely proved elusive until Austrian physician Karl Landsteiner named three blood groups in 1901.

Early experiments

Physicians had written of blood's vital powers, but the first documented blood transfusion was carried out by English physician Richard Lower in 1665. Lower drained the blood of a dog "until its strength

See also: Bloodletting and leeches 52 ▪ Battlefield medicine 53 ▪ Blood circulation 68–73 ▪ The immune system 154–161 ▪ Transplant surgery 246–253 ▪ Monoclonal antibodies 282–283

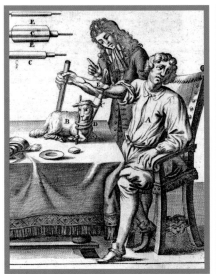

In an early blood transfusion from lamb to man, blood from the carotid artery in the neck of the lamb is transferred into a vein in the man's inner elbow.

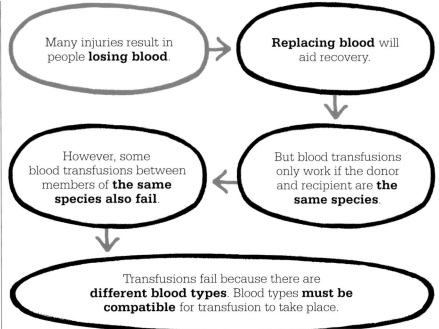

Many injuries result in people **losing blood**.

Replacing blood will aid recovery.

But blood transfusions only work if the donor and recipient are **the same species**.

However, some blood transfusions between members of **the same species also fail**.

Transfusions fail because there are **different blood types**. Blood types **must be compatible** for transfusion to take place.

was nearly gone," then revived it by introducing blood from a second dog. The first dog recovered, but the donor dog died. Following Lower's experiment, physicians in England and France were eager to try the procedure on humans. Given that the outcome for any donor was likely fatal, blood from animals was used instead. The results were inconclusive, and reports of death following transfusion emerged.

French physician Jean-Baptiste Denis faced a murder charge in 1668, when a patient died after he was given lamb's blood. Many doctors condemned the practice, and the Royal Society in London banned it the following year.

Leacock and Blundell

Early in the 19th century, physicians began to reexamine the possibility of human blood transfusion. In 1816,

John Henry Leacock, a plantation owner's son from Barbados, carried out experiments on dogs and cats in Edinburgh, Scotland, and established that the donor and recipient of a blood transfusion had to be the same species. Leacock also created a cross-circulation between two dogs, modifying the rate of blood flow and observing the effects of impeding and then reestablishing the dual circulation. He also recommended human blood transfusion to treat hemorrhage, but whether he carried out any human transfers is unknown.

James Blundell was aware of Leacock's experiments, but he took them a stage further. He discovered that dogs bled to "apparent death" could be revived by transfusions of blood from other dogs. Attempts to use human blood to revive the dogs

were less successful: five of the dogs in his experiment died and only one recovered. Blundell's experiments also differed from Leacock's in that he transfused venous blood rather than arterial »

> ... the blood of one sort of animal cannot, with impunity, be substituted ... in large quantities for that of another sort of animal.
> **James Blundell**
> *Researches physiological and pathological, 1825*

blood and transferred blood with a syringe instead of connecting the donor and recipient using a tube. Blundell calculated the time it took for blood to coagulate in his transfusion method, concluding that blood must not be allowed to remain in the syringe for more than a few seconds.

Human to human

The first documented human-to-human blood transfusion was carried out by Blundell in 1818. Aided by surgeon Henry Cline, Blundell gave a transfusion to a patient suffering from a gastric carcinoma, injecting around 0.7 pints (400 ml) of blood from various donors in small amounts at five-minute intervals. The patient showed an initial improvement but died two days later, although that may have been because he had already been close to death.

Over the next decade, Blundell and his colleagues performed several more transfusions with limited success. Only four out of 10 patients treated survived. The first successful transfusion, reported in *The Lancet* in 1829, was of a woman who recovered from

		DONOR BLOOD TYPE							
		O+	O-	A+	A-	B+	B-	AB+	AB-
RECIPIENT BLOOD TYPE	O+	◆	◆	✕	✕	✕	✕	✕	✕
	O-	✕	◆	✕	✕	✕	✕	✕	✕
	A+	◆	◆	◆	◆	✕	✕	✕	✕
	A-	✕	◆	✕	◆	✕	✕	✕	✕
	B+	◆	◆	✕	✕	◆	◆	✕	✕
	B-	✕	◆	✕	✕	✕	◆	✕	✕
	AB+	◆	◆	◆	◆	◆	◆	◆	◆
	AB-	✕	◆	✕	◆	✕	◆	✕	◆

This chart shows which blood groups are compatible. Type O- is known as the universal donor—it can be given to anyone. However, people with O- can receive blood only from other people with O- blood type. People with type AB+ are universal recipients—they can receive blood from anyone.

Key:
◆ Compatible
✕ Incompatible

severe postpartum hemorrhage after receiving around 0.4 pints (250 ml) of blood drawn from her husband's arm during the course of a three-hour procedure. Realizing the serious risks involved, Blundell advocated transfusion only in the treatment of desperately ill patients. Other physicians who attempted transfusions on patients also reported distressing failure rates.

While a few patients responded positively to the treatment, others died within days.

Blood groups

Physicians did not understand the reason for the different responses to blood transfusions until the beginning of the 20th century. They had observed that when blood from different people was

Karl Landsteiner

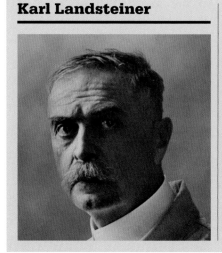

Born in Vienna, Austria, in 1868, Karl Landsteiner was the son of a well-known journalist and newspaper publisher who died when Karl was only 6. Brought up by his mother, Landsteiner studied medicine at the University of Vienna, graduating in 1891. He then spent five years working in laboratories to further his knowledge of biochemistry before going on to practice medicine at Vienna General Hospital.

In 1896, Landsteiner became an assistant to bacteriologist Max von Gruber at Vienna's Institute of Hygiene, where he researched the immune response of blood serum. After discovering blood groups in 1901, he went on to identify the bacterium that caused syphilis, as well as the disease agent that caused polio as a virus. In 1930, he was awarded the Nobel Prize in Physiology or Medicine. Still working at the age of 75, Landsteiner died of heart failure in 1943.

Key work

1928 "On Individual Differences in Human Blood"

mixed in test tubes, the red blood cells sometimes clumped together. It was largely assumed that this was caused by disease and it was not seriously investigated. In 1900, Austrian physician Karl Landsteiner decided to see what happened when healthy blood was combined. He took samples from himself and five of his colleagues and recorded what happened when he mixed them together.

Publishing his results in 1901, Landsteiner classified human blood into three types. He had found that antigens—protein markers on the outside of cells—differed according to the blood type and that blood clumped when the donated red blood cells were of a different type from the recipient's red blood cells. If blood from one blood group was introduced into the body of someone with an incompatible blood group, it would trigger an immunological reaction: the recipient's immune system would

Blood donors in Indonesia give blood during the COVID-19 pandemic. Antibody-rich blood plasma from people who had overcome COVID-19 was given to patients fighting the virus.

attack the alien blood cells, causing them to burst. Accumulated burst cells then created clumps that clogged up the recipient's blood vessels, potentially leading to death.

Landsteiner identified three different blood types: A, B, and C. (The C blood type was later renamed O.) In 1902, one of Landsteiner's students identified a fourth type, AB, and in 1939, Landsteiner and Alexander Weiner discovered the Rh blood group system. Rh+ (Rhesus positive) or Rh- (Rhesus negative) denotes the presence or absence of an inherited protein on the surface of red blood cells, which affects blood compatibility.

New possibilities

Landsteiner's discoveries made safe blood transfusions the norm. The first successful transfusion based on Landsteiner's blood type theory was carried out by Reuben Ottenberg, a physician and hematologist at Mount Sinai Hospital, New York City, in 1907. Knowledge of blood groups paved the way for organ transplants, which are also dependent on the donor and recipient having compatible blood types. ∎

Blood banks

Building on Landsteiner's work, further initiatives soon facilitated the safe storage of blood for transfusion. In 1914, Belgian physician Adolph Hustin found that adding small amounts of sodium citrate to blood stopped it from clotting. Two years later, Peyton Rous and Joseph Turner at the Rockefeller Institute in New York City discovered that blood could be safely stored for 14 days if dextrose (a sugar) was added to the sodium citrate.

In 1916, Oswald Robertson, a medical officer in the US Army, set up the first blood bank. Using the method of Rous and Turner, he created a supply of blood types in order to perform operations on the battlefields of World War I.

The world's first blood donor service—a bank of volunteer donors—was set up in 1921 by British Red Cross worker Percy Oliver. The term "blood bank" was coined by Dr. Bernard Fantus when he set up one in Chicago's Cook County Hospital in 1937.

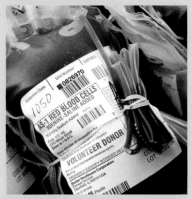

Modern blood banks allow blood to be stored for several weeks after donation. Blood plasma can be stored for up to three years.

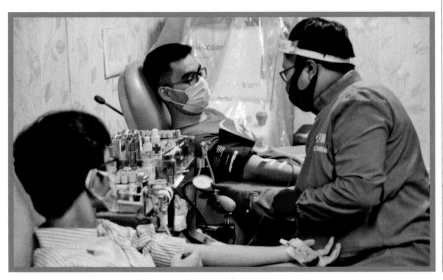

SOOTHING, QUIETING, AND DELIGHTFUL BEYOND MEASURE

ANESTHESIA

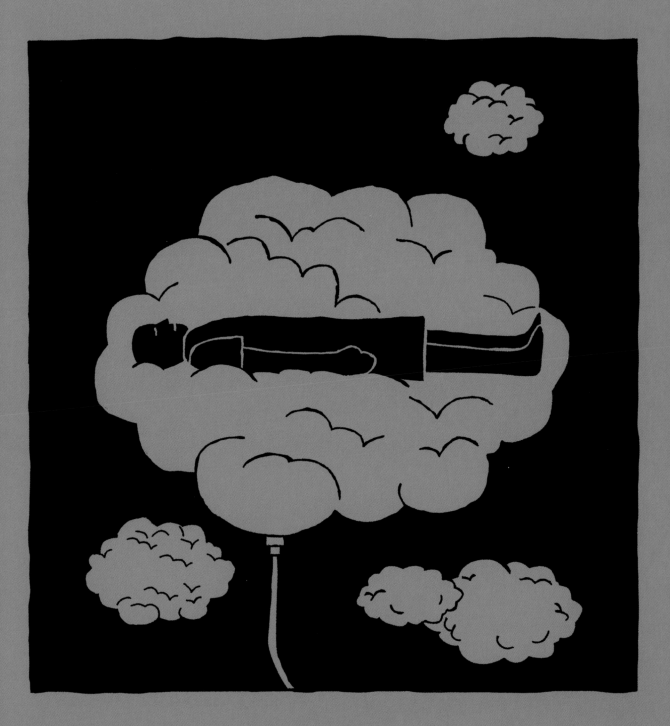

IN CONTEXT

BEFORE

6th century BCE In the *Sushruta Samhita*, the Indian physician Sushruta advocates cannabis and wine to sedate patients during surgery.

2nd century CE Chinese physician Hua Tuo uses an anesthetic containing opium.

c. 1275 In Spain, physician Raymundus Lullius discovers ether, calling it "sweet vitriol."

AFTER

1940s To combat spinal fractures in patients receiving electroconvulsive shock therapy (ECT), American neuropsychiatrist A. E. Bennett uses curare, a muscle relaxant.

1960–1980 Ketamine and etomidate replace earlier barbiturates that could have dangerous cardiac side effects.

1990s Sevoflurane, a safe and effective inhaled anesthetic, becomes widely used.

The use of some form of sedation during surgical operations dates back several millennia. Physicians employed a range of narcotic substances derived from plants, including the mandrake, from whose effects the Greek physician Dioscorides coined the term *anesthesia*, meaning "absence of sensation," in the 1st century CE. However, for most patients undergoing surgery in Europe, there was little effective pain relief until the mid-19th century. British novelist Fanny Burney's harrowing description of her unanesthetized mastectomy in 1811—"suffering so acute that was hardly supportable"—reveals how tortuous such operations were.

In the early 1800s, a new anesthetic agent was emerging in Britain but was not yet in clinical use. In 1798, the young chemist Humphry Davy—later known for his discoveries of chlorine and iodine and his invention of the Davy lamp—had been tasked with investigating the effectiveness of the laughing gas nitrous oxide, discovered by Joseph Priestley 26 years earlier. Davy published a paper describing both nitrous oxide's euphoric effects and its ability to reduce pain—a property he tested on his own erupting wisdom tooth. Davy suggested the possible use of the gas in surgery. His assistant, scientist Michael Faraday, also studied the effects of inhaling ether, whose sedative powers were already known.

Recreational anesthetics

Laughing gas parties and "ether frolics" became the latest trend among Victorian luminaries, often in Davy's own drawing room. Participants who breathed in puffs of the gas reported feelings of intense joy. Lexicographer and physician Peter Mark Roget, the creator of *Roget's Thesaurus*, wrote of a feeling of weightlessness and sinking, while poet Samuel Taylor Coleridge described a sensation like returning from a walk in the snow into a warm room. Yet the leap from party gas to surgical anesthetic was not immediate, probably due to the dosages being difficult to control. Faraday reported in 1818 that one participant anesthetized with ether did not wake up for 24 hours.

In the US around the same time, American medical students and young intellectuals began to engage in the same frolics as those enjoyed by London's society figures. Crawford Long, a physician in Jefferson, Georgia, would inhale ether with friends in the evening and observe the results. The next morning, Long would find new bruises on himself, but he had no memory of the antics that had caused them, nor of the pain they

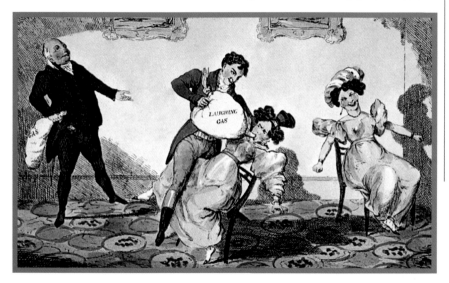

Laughing gas (nitrous oxide) is given to a "scolding wife" in a satirical British engraving from 1830. At that time, the anesthetic's main claim to fame was the euphoria it induced when inhaled.

See also: Plastic surgery 26–27 ▪ Traditional Chinese medicine 30–35 ▪ Herbal medicine 36–37
▪ Antiseptics in surgery 148–151 ▪ Minimally invasive surgery 298 ▪ Nanomedicine 304 ▪ Robotics and telesurgery 305

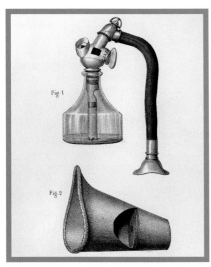

Ether was first used as an anesthetic in a Paris operation in 1846. Early basic masks were soon replaced by more effective models, such as this one, from a 19th-century French medical manual.

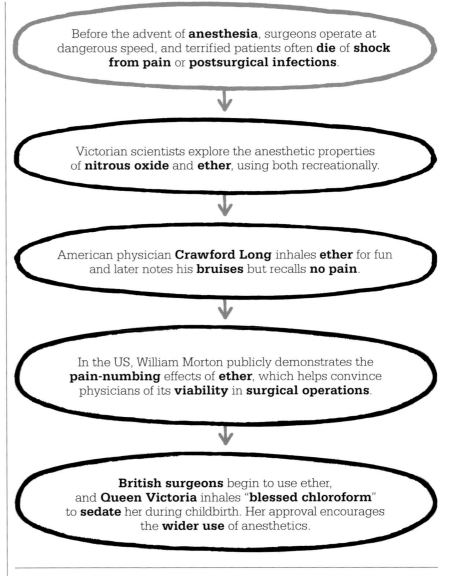

Before the advent of **anesthesia**, surgeons operate at dangerous speed, and terrified patients often **die** of **shock from pain** or **postsurgical infections**.

Victorian scientists explore the anesthetic properties of **nitrous oxide** and **ether**, using both recreationally.

American physician **Crawford Long** inhales **ether** for fun and later notes his **bruises** but recalls **no pain**.

In the US, William Morton publicly demonstrates the **pain-numbing** effects of **ether**, which helps convince physicians of its **viability** in **surgical operations**.

British surgeons begin to use ether, and **Queen Victoria** inhales "**blessed chloroform**" to **sedate** her during childbirth. Her approval encourages the **wider use** of anesthetics.

might have induced. He concluded that ether might prove an excellent agent for eliminating pain during an operation and soon found an opportunity to test his theory.

Early medical use of ether

In 1842, a young man approached Long to ask whether he could remove an unsightly sebaceous cyst from his neck. Long anesthetized his patient with ether and was overjoyed with its success. He began to use it in other operations but did not report his findings until 1849. By this time, others had introduced the effects of the new anesthetics to a wider audience, and Long lost a subsequent legal bid to be declared the discoverer of ether anesthesia.

Horace Wells, a little-known dentist from Hartford, Connecticut, also recognized the potential of nitrous oxide and ether after

watching a demonstration of their effects. To test it on himself, he breathed in nitrous oxide before a fellow dentist extracted his tooth— he experienced no pain. Both he and his business partner William T. G. Morton began to use the gas at his practice. By 1845, Wells felt confident enough to demonstrate the gas at Harvard Medical School.

There, in front of an audience, a medical student agreed to have a tooth extracted. Wells administered the gas, but the student screamed out in pain as soon as the operation began; whether this response was simple theatrics or because Wells used too little nitrous oxide is unknown. The episode sank Wells's career and his reputation. »

Different types of anesthesia

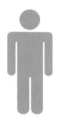

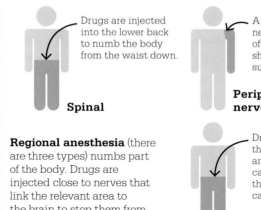

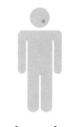

Drugs are injected into the lower back to numb the body from the waist down.

Spinal

A peripheral nerve block is often used in shoulder surgery.

Peripheral nerve block

Drugs to numb the lower body are injected via a catheter (tube) so that repeat doses can be given.

Epidural

A general anesthetic is given via an inhaler, an intravenous injection of anesthetic drugs, or both to sedate the whole body and render the patient unconscious throughout the surgery.

Regional anesthesia (there are three types) numbs part of the body. Drugs are injected close to nerves that link the relevant area to the brain to stop them from transmitting pain signals.

Local anesthesia is often used for a minor skin or dental procedure. The anesthetic is injected at the site to temporarily numb the area.

In October 1846, Wells's colleague Morton gave another demonstration, this time at Massachusetts General Hospital, Boston. He administered ether to a patient so that the attending surgeon John Warren could remove a tumor on his neck. The patient remained unconscious throughout the procedure, which Warren completed without incident. According to legend, Warren turned triumphantly to his audience and declared, "Gentlemen, this is no humbug!" This demonstration of safe, effective pain relief during surgery proved a landmark event.

Battling for recognition

Morton had studied medicine at Harvard after giving up his dentistry work with Horace Wells. It was with Wells that Morton had first seen proof of the pain-relieving qualities of nitrous oxide, and, after learning about the properties of ether from his chemistry professor Charles Jackson, he wondered if it might prove equally effective.

Morton began his ether trials soon after completing his medical training, testing its effects on insects, fish, his dog, and finally

himself. There is no evidence that Jackson was involved in these ether trials, although Morton almost certainly discussed his work with him. As ether anesthesia became more widely used in surgery, the two men's one-time friendship dissolved into a bitter fight over who discovered ether's anesthetic effects. It is said that seeing Morton's tombstone, which read, "Inventor and Revealer of Anesthetic Inhalation," so affected

> " I am inclined to look upon the new application of ether as the most valuable discovery in medical science since that of vaccination.
> **John Snow**
> *On the Inhalation of the Vapour of Ether, 1847* "

Jackson's already fragile mental health that he spent his last seven years in an asylum for the insane.

Further anesthetic agents

News of the American use of anesthesia soon spread. In December 1846, Scottish surgeon Robert Liston became the first doctor in Britain to operate on an anesthetized patient. After amputating the patient's leg, he declared, "This Yankee dodge beats mesmerism [the popular use of hypnotism] hollow!" Liston also found chloroform to be a useful anesthetic. In 1853, royal surgeon John Snow first administered chloroform to Queen Victoria during the birth of Prince Leopold. Her approval (she used it during eight confinements, finding it "delightful beyond measure") silenced earlier objections by some skeptical physicians and instilled public confidence in anesthesia.

As anesthesia became more accepted, surgeons began to use several different gases together—heralding modern medicine's combination of drugs—rather than a potentially more toxic dose of a single drug. They also experimented with local anesthetics, applied to smaller areas of the body, and initially used the South American alkaloid cocaine.

In 1942, Canadian doctor Harold Griffith discovered that curare—a poison South American Indigenous peoples used on the tips of hunting darts—was an effective muscle relaxant. His finding revolutionized anesthesiology because it allowed surgeons safe access to the thorax and abdomen. Before the use of curare, physicians relaxed these areas with high doses of general anesthetic before surgery, which depressed patients' respiration and blood circulation, causing high mortality rates. An injection of curare relaxed muscles sufficiently for a breathing tube to be inserted into the trachea (intubation), so that breathing could be controlled artificially during an operation.

A specialty emerges

By the mid-20th century, the increasing sophistication of surgery required skillful anesthetists, and anesthesiology became a specialized area of medicine. The anesthetist's task is to select the appropriate anesthetic agents, to carefully monitor the patient, and to ensure throughout the surgery that the patient remains oblivious to pain.

Modern drugs have long since replaced ether, but nitrous oxide is still used for dental and other minor operations. Those undergoing long, major operations may receive a general anesthetic, but regional anesthesia can now numb large areas of the body rather than induce total unconsciousness. Key innovations, such as anesthetic machines to induce and maintain a continuous flow of anesthetic and computer-controlled monitors that display information about a patient's breathing and heartbeat, have made anesthesia and the surgery performed much safer for patients. Nanotechnology and ever more rapid automation look set to make future anesthesiology even safer and more effective than it is now. ∎

In general anesthesia, the patient receives an intravenous injection of a drug to cause loss of consciousness, then an inhaled anesthetic to induce or maintain anesthesia.

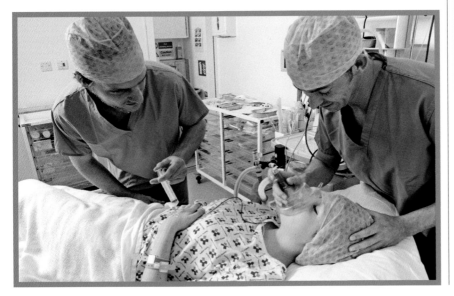

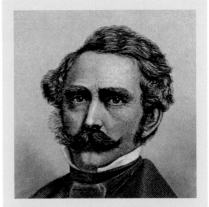

William T. G. Morton

Born in 1819, in Charlton, Massachusetts, William Thomas Green Morton worked as a laborer, salesman, and store owner before training as a dentist. He set up a dental practice with Horace Wells in 1842, but during his engagement to Elizabeth Whitman, he decided to retrain as a doctor. He learned about the effects of ether during the chemistry lectures of Charles Thomas Jackson.

A year after Wells's failed attempt to demonstrate the anesthetic effects of nitrous oxide, Morton staged the first successful demonstration of ether's anesthetic effects, which led to its much wider use in surgery. However, Morton then spent the next 21 years of his life in a costly bid to gain official recognition as the discoverer of ether anesthesia, an honor finally accorded to Horace Wells and the rural Georgia doctor Crawford Long. Morton died in 1868, after suffering a stroke.

Key work

1847 *Remarks on the proper mode of administering sulphuric ether by inhalation*

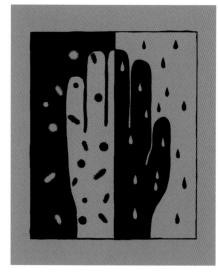

WASH YOUR HANDS

HYGIENE

IN CONTEXT

BEFORE

14th–13th century BCE The prophet Moses sets down laws for the Israelites regarding personal cleanliness for health and religious purification.

c. 400 BCE Hippocrates states the importance of hygiene.

c. 1012 In *The Canon of Medicine*, Ibn Sina associates hygiene and cleanliness with good health throughout life.

AFTER

1858 While studying fermentation, Louis Pasteur links bacteria to decaying organic matter.

1865 Joseph Lister uses carbolic acid (phenol) to cleanse wounds and later reports his successful results in *The Lancet*.

1980s The UK and US issue the first national hand hygiene guidelines for health workers.

Ancient texts that mention frequent bathing and shaving the head to prevent lice indicate that the Egyptians, Greeks, and Romans were well aware that good hygiene mattered, but its crucial health significance was not appreciated for a further 2,000 years. Public health suffered as towns and cities became more populous from the medieval era onward; successive waves of plague killed millions of people. Finally, in the 1840s, two perceptive physicians—Ignaz Semmelweis, a Hungarian working in Austria, and Oliver Wendell Holmes in the US—recognized the link between poor hygiene and contagious diseases.

The quest to save lives

In 1846, Semmelweis began work as an assistant in obstetrics at a teaching hospital in Vienna. At the time, puerperal fever (also known as childbed fever), an infection of the reproductive organs, killed many women within days of childbirth. People attributed it to a "putrid effluvium" in the air, overcrowded neighborhoods, or the poor diet and fatigue that often accompanies poverty. Yet hygiene at the hospital was minimal. Few surgeons scrubbed up before operating or washed their hands between patients.

Semmelweis observed that the mortality rate was two or three times higher in one clinic where physicians and medical students examined women and delivered their babies than in a second where

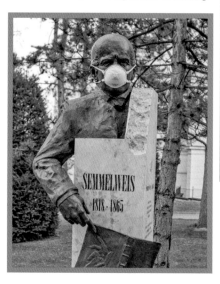

A statue of Semmelweis, erected outside the Medical University in Vienna to commemorate the 200th anniversary of his birth, wears a face mask during the COVID-19 pandemic.

midwives helped women give birth. He noted that, unlike the midwives, the doctors and students carried out autopsies, often handling the corpses of puerperal fever victims, then attending to pregnant women. This, he concluded, was how the disease spread.

When Semmelweis introduced a regime of handwashing in a solution of chlorinated lime for his students and junior doctors in 1847, the mortality rate for the women they attended fell sharply. Despite the evidence, he failed to persuade his senior colleagues that the reduced deaths were due to handwashing. His superior attributed it to a new ventilation system.

A few years earlier, Oliver Wendell Holmes, a brilliant young American physician who studied medicine at Harvard and in Paris, began to research puerperal fever after hearing of a doctor who died a week after performing an autopsy on a fever victim. In his 1843 paper, "The Contagiousness of Puerperal Fever," Holmes sets down the considerable evidence he amassed.

> ❝
> The disease known as puerperal fever is so far contagious as to be frequently carried patient to patient by physicians and nurses.
> **Oliver Wendell Holmes**
> **"The Contagiousness of Puerperal Fever," 1843**
> ❞

It outlines case after case of women contracting and dying of puerperal fever when midwives or doctors had previously attended puerperal fever victims or had conducted autopsies of victims, and includes accounts from a few physicians that strict adherence to hygiene had prevented the disease's spread. In his conclusion, Holmes lays down guidelines for physicians, such as "thorough ablution" and a complete change of clothes after attending autopsies, and waiting "some weeks" after any contact with puerperal fever sufferers before delivering a child.

A lesson finally learned

Both Holmes and Semmelweis were unsung heroes in their time. Their suggestion that physicians with unwashed hands were responsible for so many women's deaths upset their colleagues. Holmes's paper went largely unnoticed until it was republished in 1855 and, for two decades, medical experts in Vienna refused to acknowledge what Semmelweis had clearly shown.

As the work of microbiologists Louis Pasteur in France, Robert Koch in Germany, and Joseph Lister in Britain advanced knowledge and the acceptance of germ theory and antiseptic techniques, the value of handwashing was at last accepted. Its importance in limiting the spread of a highly contagious pandemic disease remains paramount today. ∎

Ignaz Semmelweis

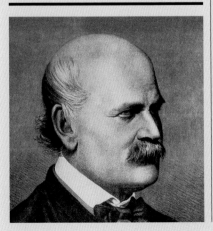

Born in 1818 in Buda (later part of Budapest), Hungary, Ignaz Semmelweis was the fifth of eight children. On his father's advice, he studied law at the University of Vienna in 1837, but he returned to Hungary to study medicine at the University of Pest in 1838.

Semmelweis graduated in 1844, and specialized in obstetrics. As assistant to Professor Johann Klein, he worked in the Vienna General Hospital maternity ward, where in 1846, he made the crucial link between poor hygiene and puerperal fever. However, he lost his post in Vienna in 1848, after taking part in events linked to a failed nationalist uprising in Hungary. Back in Pest, as head of obstetrics at the university, Semmelweis continued to promote his handwashing regime. In later life, he suffered mental health problems and was confined to an asylum in 1865, where he died the same year.

Key works

1849 "The Origin of Puerperal Fever"
1861 *The Etiology, Concept, and Prophylaxis of Childbed Fever*

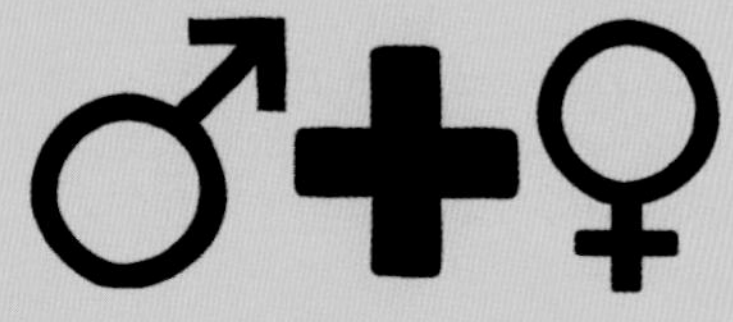

MEDICINE NEEDS MEN AND WOMEN

WOMEN IN MEDICINE

IN CONTEXT

BEFORE

1570 King Henry VIII of England grants a charter establishing the Company of Barber-Surgeons, from which women are barred.

1754 Dorothea Erxleben is the first woman in Germany to earn a medical degree, but she dies just eight years later.

AFTER

1866 The Women's Medical College of Pennsylvania is the first medical school to appoint a female dean.

1876 A British Act of Parliament allows women to train as doctors.

1960 The Pill is introduced. Over the next two decades, the Women's Liberation Movement campaigns for women's rights in all aspects of healthcare and society.

2019 Women make up 50.5 percent of graduates from US medical schools.

In the 1840s, there was no provision for women to attend medical school and qualify as doctors. Elizabeth Blackwell decided to buck this trend by applying to numerous medical schools in the US. After countless rejections, she tried Geneva Medical College in rural New York. The college put the idea to the all-male student body, assuming it would reject it outright. However, as a joke, the students voted "yes," and Blackwell was able to start her studies in 1847. Two years later, she became the first woman to receive a degree from an American medical school. This paved the way for the right of women to become doctors.

Closed to women

Ablaze with scientific discoveries, the 19th century was regarded as a new era of modern medicine, but the profession was still closed to women. Some doctors maintained that higher education might abnormally expand women's brains, while others thought that female doctors would not be able to take the sight of blood. In 1862, the British Medical Journal stated, "It is high time that this unnatural and preposterous attempt ... to establish a race of feminine doctors should be exploded." Women such as Blackwell strongly disagreed.

Challenging the system

Blackwell found a loophole in the British 1858 Medical Registration Act that did not expressly prohibit women with foreign medical degrees from practicing in the UK. She became the first woman to be officially registered by the General Medical Council (GMC) soon after.

Back in the US, Blackwell opened the New York Infirmary for Women and Children in 1857 and, in 1868,

> If the present arrangements of society will not admit of woman's free development, then society must be remodeled ...
> **Elizabeth Blackwell**
> Letter to Emily Collins, 1848

See also: Midwifery 76–77 ▪ Hospitals 82–83 ▪ Nursing and sanitation 128–133
▪ Birth control 214–215 ▪ Hormonal contraception 258

> Women **practice medicine informally** as healers, herbalists, and midwives but are **barred from the professional medical bodies** that emerge during the medieval and Renaissance period.

↓

> Women begin to **exploit loopholes** in legislation to **gain access to medical education** during the 19th century.

↓

> Pioneers such as Elizabeth Blackwell **qualify as doctors** and establish the concept that **women have an equal place with men** in medicine.

a medical college for women next door. This offered a four-year degree with a higher level of clinical training than at existing colleges for men.

British women soon followed Blackwell's lead. Elizabeth Garrett-Anderson became the first female doctor in the UK when she used a loophole in the Charter of the Society of Apothecaries to gain a license to practice medicine in 1865. Four years later, Sophia Jex-Blake and six other women (known as the "Edinburgh Seven") became the first female students at any British university when they were accepted to study medicine at Edinburgh.

In 1874, Garrett-Anderson, Jex-Blake, and Blackwell—now back in England—set up the London School of Medicine for Women, which became the first British institution that allowed women to study and practice medicine. This led to a steady increase in the numbers of women doctors: in 1881, there were only 25 in Britain, but by 1911, this had risen to 495.

Blackwell retired from medicine in 1877, but remained an active campaigner for reform in women's rights, family planning, medical ethics, and preventative medicine. ▪

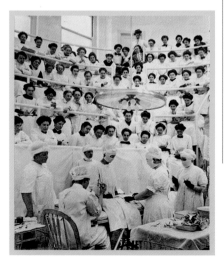

Women attend a class at the Women's Medical College of Pennsylvania in 1911. Founded in 1850, it was one of the earliest institutions authorized to train women as doctors.

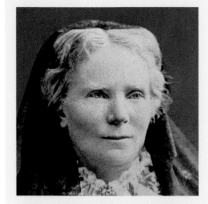

Elizabeth Blackwell

Born in 1821 in Bristol, UK, Elizabeth Blackwell emigrated to the US with her family in 1832. When her father died, leaving the family penniless, Blackwell, aged 17, became a teacher. However, the death of a friend swayed Blackwell in her career choice, and she decided instead to substitute medicine for teaching.

Headstrong in all that she did, Blackwell became the first American woman to graduate from medical school in 1849. She would continue to fight against gender discrimination for the rest of her life on both sides of the Atlantic, working with other pioneering women in medicine, including Sophia Jex-Blake, Elizabeth Garrett-Anderson, Marie Zakrzewska, and her sister Emily Blackwell. In 1907, Blackwell was left disabled after falling down stairs. She died of a stroke three years later.

Key works

1856 *An Appeal in Behalf of the Medical Education of Women*
1895 *Pioneer Work in Opening the Medical Profession to Women*

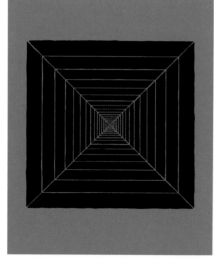

ALL CELLS COME FROM CELLS

HISTOLOGY

istology—the study of the microscopic structure of tissues—has its origins in the 17th century, when Italian, English, and Dutch scientists Marcello Malpighi, Robert Hooke, and Antonie van Leeuwenhoek used primitive microscopes to examine plant and animal tissues. The nascent science stalled for more than a century because of the poor quality of microscope lenses, which produced distorted images, but advanced again with improved lenses in the 1830s.

It was when Swiss anatomist Albert von Kölliker published his *Handbook of Human Histology* in 1852 that histology really came of age. Kölliker was one of the first scientists to realize that all tissues are made up of cells, which do not develop spontaneously, but from other cells. His research placed

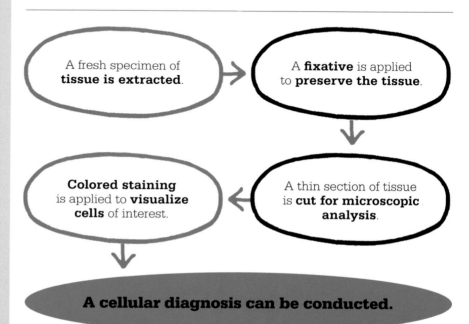

A fresh specimen of **tissue is extracted**. → A **fixative** is applied to **preserve the tissue**.

Colored staining is applied to **visualize cells** of interest. ← A thin section of tissue is **cut for microscopic analysis**.

A cellular diagnosis can be conducted.

microscopic anatomy at the center of medical understanding, and also fed into the new fields of histopathology (the diagnosis of disease at cellular level) and neuroscience.

Perfecting procedures

Kölliker's handbook formalized histological procedures, introducing scientists to the relatively new techniques of fixation, sectioning, and staining samples for analysis.

Tissue samples must be "fixed" to preserve their structure and to inhibit fungal and bacterial growth. Danish pathologist Adolph Hannover used chromic acid solution as a fixative when he made probably the first definitive description of a cancer cell in 1843. Almost 50 years later, German pathologist Ferdinand Blum found that formaldehyde (only discovered in 1859) was an excellent fixative; it is still the most commonly used fixing solution today.

To enable light to pass through samples, they must be very thin. In 1770, Scottish inventor Alexander Cummings built the first microtome to cut slices thin enough to be used

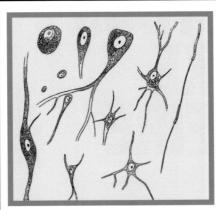

Kölliker's 1852 handbook, with its hand-drawn illustrations of cells observed through a microscope, transformed understanding of tissue structures and the nervous system.

on a microscope slide. Modern ultramicrotomes can now prepare sections as thin as 30 nanometers.

Staining highlights important tissue features and differentiates between cell structures, as the stain chemically binds to some substances but not others. Advances in chemical processes and dye synthesis in the mid-19th century improved histological staining methods. In

1858, German anatomist Joseph von Gerlach achieved the differential staining of a cell's nucleus and cytoplasm, and in the 1880s, Kölliker made use of Italian biologist Camillo Golgi's new silver staining method to study the structure of nerve cells. Combining the dye hematoxylin with the acid compound eosin in the 1890s also produced an effective tissue stain, which is still in use today.

Tied to technology

By the end of the 19th century, the availability of reliable microscopes, improvements in the processing of samples, and the work of scientists such as Kölliker had initiated a modern age of medical histology. Further technological innovations, such as the electron microscope, allowing analysis of tiny cellular structures; microscopes that allow 3D imaging of cells; and optical coherence tomography (OCT), which uses infrared light to generate cross-sectional images with microscopic resolution, continue to advance the field. ▪

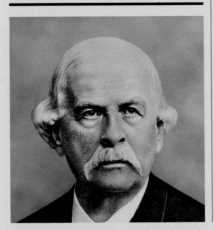

Albert von Kölliker

Born in Zurich, Switzerland, in 1817, Rudolph Albert von Kölliker studied medicine at the University of Zurich, where he developed an interest in embryology. Appointed professor of anatomy at Zurich in 1844, he transferred to the University of Würzburg, Germany, shortly afterward. There, he taught and researched for the rest of his career, making advances in the microscopic study of tissues.

Among his many discoveries, Kölliker suggested that cell nuclei may carry the key to heredity, was one of the first to notice bodies within striated muscle

cells that would later be identified as mitochondria, and demonstrated that nerve fibers are elongated parts of nerve cells. Continuing to conduct research into his late 80s, Kölliker died in 1905.

Key works

1852 *Handbook of Human Histology*
1861 *Embryology of Man and Higher Animals*

THEY MISTOOK THE SMOKE FOR THE FIRE

EPIDEMIOLOGY

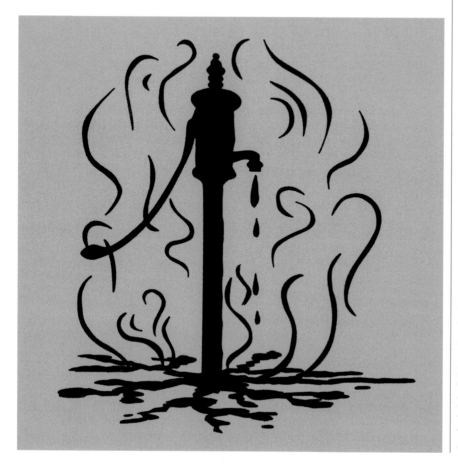

Cholera is a gastrointestinal infection that is still a major global health problem today in areas with inadequate sanitation. The symptoms include diarrhea, nausea, and vomiting, which can result in severe dehydration and death. John Snow's systematic study of its spread in 19th-century London changed understanding about the causes of disease, how diseases are transmitted, and how best to study this process, establishing the field of epidemiology.

Something in the air?
The idea that disease was caused by a miasma, or "something bad in the air," had persisted for centuries. The alleged corruption of the air was attributed to causes such as

See also: Roman medicine 38–43 ▪ Medieval medical schools and surgery 50–51 ▪ Case history 80–81 ▪ Anesthesia 112–117 ▪ Hygiene 118–119 ▪ Nursing and sanitation 128–133 ▪ Germ theory 138–145 ▪ Virology 177 ▪ Pandemics 306–313

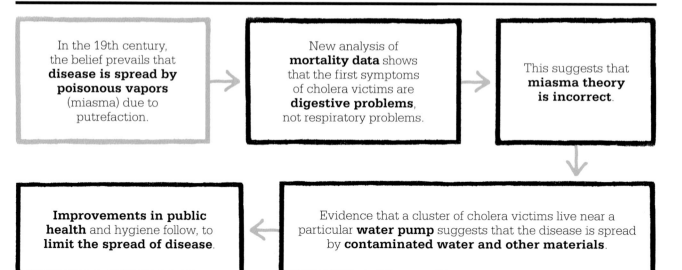

In the 19th century, the belief prevails that **disease is spread by poisonous vapors** (miasma) due to putrefaction.

New analysis of **mortality data** shows that the first symptoms of cholera victims are **digestive problems**, not respiratory problems.

This suggests that **miasma theory is incorrect**.

Evidence that a cluster of cholera victims live near a particular **water pump** suggests that the disease is spread by **contaminated water and other materials**.

Improvements in public health and hygiene follow, to **limit the spread of disease**.

decay of waste organic matter, "exhalations" from swamps and marshes, or ill winds bringing bad air from other places. People noted the coincidence of the outbreak of disease with the summer months, when smells of decomposing waste were pervasive. In an attempt to combat the spread of infection, ineffective interventions were pursued, such as lighting bonfires, in the hope that the smoke would halt both plague and cholera.

By the mid-19th century, bad smells and the spread of disease were a serious public health issue as fast-expanding cities, unable to properly dispose of large quantities of human and industrial waste, used streets as open drains and waterways as open sewers.

In Britain, debate still raged as to the origin of diseases such as cholera. The sanitation reformer Thomas Southwood Smith; public health reformer Edwin Chadwick; and Florence Nightingale, the founder of modern nursing, were all staunch proponents of the miasma

theory. Southwood Smith in his role as physician at the London Fever Hospital was convinced that there was a link between the slum conditions many endured in cities and the contagious diseases they suffered from. These views were echoed by Chadwick, who was a close acquaintance.

Chadwick believed that there was no mystery to the origins of disease: it came from environmental

> 66
>
> The annual loss of life from filth and bad ventilation are greater than the loss from death or wounds in any wars …
> **Edwin Chadwick**
>
> 99

causes such as poor sanitation, and these factors could be rectified. He saw improving living conditions as making sound economic sense—men who were ill could not work after all.

In 1838, Chadwick, assisted by Southwood Smith among others, began work on reports for the Poor Law Commission. Southwood Smith advocated fumigation and improved ventilation in buildings; others pointed out the importance of removing "nuisance occupations" (such as slaughterhouses) from residential areas and of improving drainage, sewers, and cesspools to prevent the spread of disease.

Chadwick's *Report on the Sanitary Condition of the Labouring Population of Great Britain* was published in 1842 to enthusiastic endorsement from newspapers such as *The Times*. Detailing the cramped and insanitary living conditions found across the country, it led to an urgent demand for change.

In 1848, the government set up a General Board of Health, its members including Chadwick » and Southwood Smith, to tackle the problem. When a new cholera outbreak struck London in the board's first year of operation, they instigated emergency measures to remove waste and clean the streets.

Tracking contagion

In 1853, Thomas Wakley, editor of *The Lancet*, wrote on the subject of cholera: "Is it a fungus, an insect, a miasma, an electrical disturbance, a deficiency of ozone …? We know nothing; we are at sea in a whirlpool of conjecture." In August 1854, a severe outbreak of cholera hit the Soho area of London. Thousands of people succumbed to the illness and at least 600 died. John Snow, a doctor working in Soho at the time of the outbreak, began to formulate his own ideas about its cause.

Snow had previous experience of cholera. During an outbreak of the disease that spread across the

northeast of England in 1831, he had attended to sufferers who worked in the Killingworth Colliery near Newcastle upon Tyne. He noted that many of the miners succumbed to cholera while working beneath the ground and wondered how this squared with transmission by miasma. He suspected that transmission was by a different route. The observations he made at this time laid the foundations for his later work.

In September 1848, Snow attempted to track the progress of an outbreak in London to determine how the disease was spread. He discovered that the first victim, a merchant seaman, had arrived from Hamburg by ship on September 22, had quickly developed cholera symptoms and had died. Snow learned that, just a few days after the seaman's death, his room was rented to a second man who also

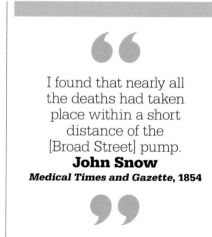

> I found that nearly all the deaths had taken place within a short distance of the [Broad Street] pump.
> **John Snow**
> *Medical Times and Gazette*, 1854

contracted cholera and died. Snow viewed this second death as strong evidence of contagion.

As more cases developed, Snow found that all victims reported that their first symptoms were digestive problems. He believed this showed that the disease must be transferred via polluted food or water. If miasma was the vector, then, he reasoned, the first symptoms should surely have affected the respiratory system, not the digestive. He suspected that the extreme diarrhea that was a feature of the disease might be the source of infection. Just a few drops contaminating the water supply had the potential to spread the disease over a whole community.

In August 1849, Snow published a pamphlet entitled *On the Mode of Communication of Cholera*, setting out his arguments and evidence to support his theory. He cited the case of a London street in which

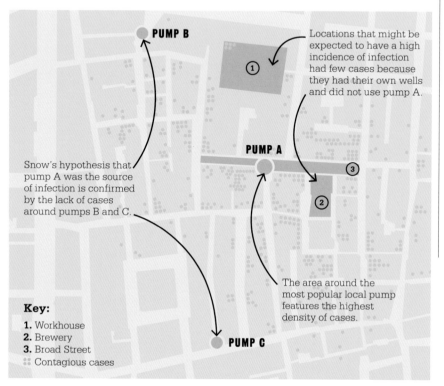

Locations that might be expected to have a high incidence of infection had few cases because they had their own wells and did not use pump A.

Snow's hypothesis that pump A was the source of infection is confirmed by the lack of cases around pumps B and C.

The area around the most popular local pump features the highest density of cases.

Key:

1. Workhouse
2. Brewery
3. Broad Street
::: Contagious cases

John Snow compiled a spot map to log cholera cases, showing the distribution of infection. This new method of statistical disease mapping allowed Snow to compare different groups of people and has become a key component of modern epidemiology.

John Snow

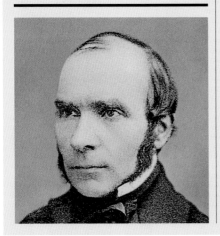

The eldest of nine children, John Snow was born in York, UK, in 1813. His father was a coal-yard laborer, and the family home was in one of York's poorer areas. Aged 14, Snow was apprenticed to a surgeon and in 1836 moved to London to begin his formal medical education, graduating from the University of London in 1844.

In 1849, Snow published his ideas on cholera's transmission, contending that the prevailing miasma theory was wrong. He backed up these claims with his study of the 1854 Soho outbreak. As well as epidemiology, Snow was a pioneer in the field of anesthetics. In 1853, he attended the birth of Prince Leopold, giving his mother, Queen Victoria, chloroform to ease her birth pains.

Snow was a vegetarian and teetotaler who campaigned for temperance societies, but his chronic health problems may have contributed to his early death, aged just 45, in 1858.

Key work

1849 *On the Mode of Communication of Cholera*

many residents on one side became cholera victims, while on the other side only one person succumbed. Snow reported that dirty water, emptied into a channel by the inhabitants of the first houses, got into the well from which they drew their water. He believed that to prevent cholera epidemics, wells and freshwater pipes would have to be isolated from pipes carrying waste, but his ideas gained little traction with his fellow medics.

The Broad Street pump

As the 1854 Soho outbreak took hold, Snow believed that the source of the infection was to be found in the water supply. By talking to local residents and using information from local hospital and public records, he marked each residence where cholera had occurred on a map of the area and found that they centered on one particular water pump in Broad Street. Today, this type of map, showing the geographic distribution of cases, is called a spot map. Snow theorized that the pump was the source of the epidemic. In a letter to the *Medical Times and Gazette,* he wrote: " … there has been no particular outbreak or prevalence of cholera in this part of London except among the persons who were in the habit of drinking the water of the above-mentioned pump well."

Snow took his findings to the local council and convinced them to remove the handle from the pump, making it unusable. Shortly after, the outbreak ended. It was later found that the source of the outbreak was the discarded soiled diapers from a baby who had contracted cholera elsewhere, which had been dumped in a cesspit near the pump.

Hand pumps like the one on Broad Street were not the only source of water. Snow began to

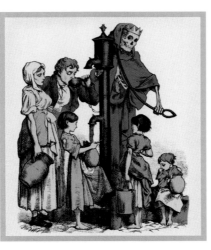

investigate incidences of cholera in South London and linked them to the Southwark and Vauxhall water companies, which were supplying mechanically pumped water from sewage-polluted sections of the Thames and delivering it to homes.

Snow's detailed statistical analysis proved to be a compelling way of demonstrating the correlation between the quality of the water source and cholera cases. Shortly after the end of the outbreak, Snow presented his views to the Medical Society of London, only to have them rejected by leading doctors.

It would be several more years before the germ theory of disease would begin to find acceptance, when it was proved by French chemist Louis Pasteur. Sadly, Snow did not live to see his theories vindicated, as he died in 1858 following a stroke. It was not until 1884 that Robert Koch identified the comma-shaped bacillus, *Vibrio cholerae*, which causes cholera. ∎

An 1866 satire on London's polluted water supply indicates a shift from the belief that diseases are spread by airborne "miasma" to a realization that they are caused by specific organisms.

A HOSPITAL SHOULD DO THE SICK NO HARM

NURSING AND SANITATION

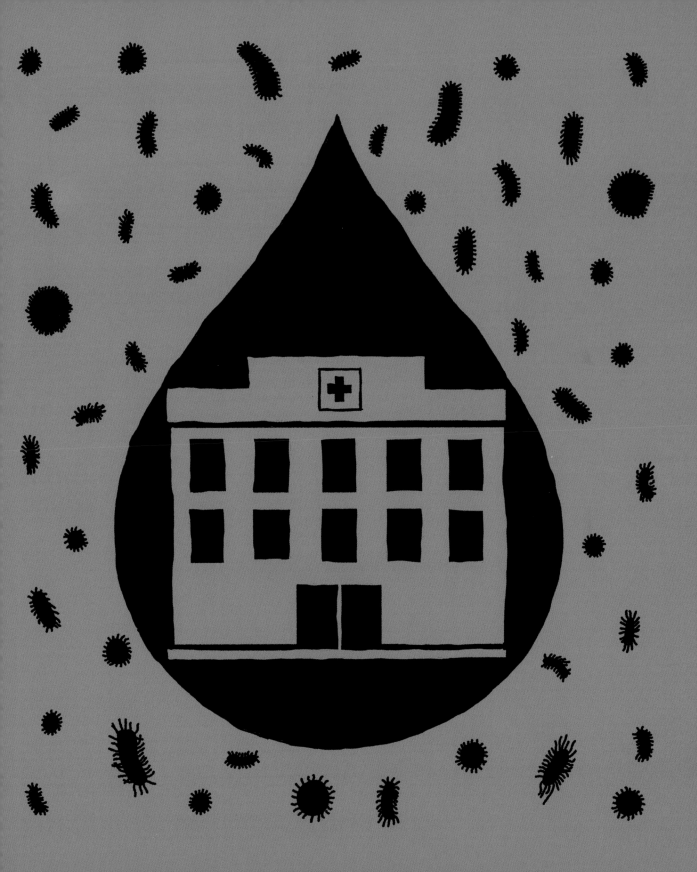

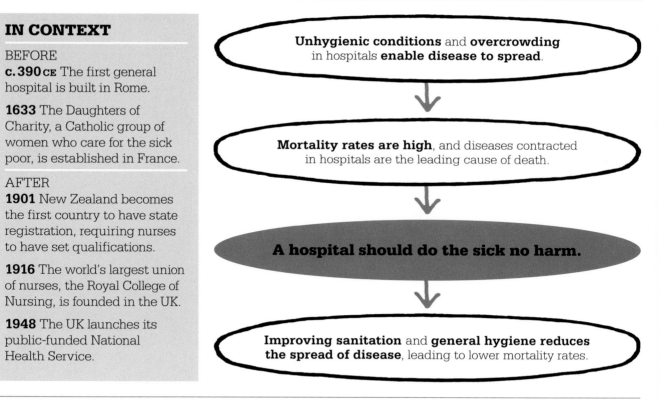

Unhygienic conditions and **overcrowding** in hospitals **enable disease to spread**.

Mortality rates are high, and diseases contracted in hospitals are the leading cause of death.

A hospital should do the sick no harm.

Improving sanitation and **general hygiene reduces the spread of disease**, leading to lower mortality rates.

E xactly when nursing care first began is impossible to say. Caring for the sick and injured is a natural part of human existence, but for a long time, it was tied up with religious beliefs, with nursing often being carried out in Europe by members of holy orders, such as nuns and monks. In the Islamic world, Rufaida Al-Aslamia (c. 620 CE) is thought to be the first nurse who treated casualties and trained other women in hygiene. Yet the history of modern nursing really begins with Florence Nightingale— a tireless social reformer who not only took a scientific approach to nursing, but also saw the need for medicine to be based on statistics.

Nursing in the mid-19th century was not considered to be a suitable profession for an educated woman, and Nightingale's wealthy family were opposed to her gaining any hospital experience. It was while on a tour of Europe and Egypt with family friends that Nightingale had the opportunity to study different hospital systems. In early 1850, she began training at the Institute of St. Vincent de Paul in Alexandria, Egypt. This, and further training in Germany and France, taught her observation and organization, as well as nursing care. On returning to London in 1853, Nightingale took up the position of superintendent at the Institution for Sick Gentlewomen in Distressed Circumstances. Here, she honed her administrative and nursing skills, and soon improved conditions at the institution.

Lady with the lamp

In March 1854, the Crimean War began when Britain, France, and Turkey declared war on Russia. British military medical facilities faced harsh criticism in the press, which described them as ineffective and incompetent. Nightingale, who had been on the verge of taking up a post as superintendent of nurses at King's College Hospital, London, was invited to take on the role of nursing administrator, overseeing the deployment of nurses to British military hospitals.

Nightingale arrived in Scutari, near Constantinople (now Istanbul), in November 1854, accompanied by 38 nurses and 15 nuns. She found soldiers crowded together on bare floors, with little ventilation or food, operations carried out in unhygienic conditions, inadequate supplies of medical equipment, and diseases such as cholera and typhus running rampant in the hospitals.

At first, the male army doctors resented the intrusion as an attack on their professionalism. But the nurses soon proved their value when, a few days after their arrival, an influx of injured soldiers from

> All were swarming
> with vermin, huge lice
> crawling all about their
> persons and clothes. …
> Several were completely
> prostrated by fever
> and dysentery.
> **Henry Bellew**
> **British assistant surgeon describing**
> **Scutari hospital, January 1855**

major battles threatened to overwhelm the hospital. Using funds supplied by *The Times* newspaper, Nightingale bought equipment for the hospital and pressed soldiers' wives into service cleaning and laundering. She addressed not only the soldiers' physical needs, but also their psychological ones, helping them write letters and finding ways to keep their minds off their situation.

Disease played a major role in the Crimea; in the winter of 1854–1855, 23,000 troops were unfit for duty due to sickness. A Sanitary Commission sent out by the UK government to investigate conditions in 1855 found that the hospital at Scutari had been built over a broken sewer, and the patients were drinking contaminated water.

This scene from the military hospital at Scutari during the Crimean War shows Florence Nightingale inspecting the wards at night, holding her iconic lamp.

With Nightingale's cooperation, the sewers were fixed and flushed out, toilets and washing facilities upgraded, and overcrowding in the hospitals reduced. Only then did the appalling death rate begin to drop. Mortality fell from 41 percent when Nightingale first arrived to just 2 percent by the end of the war. Her experiences in the Crimea led Nightingale to campaign for better sanitation in hospitals generally when she returned to Britain.

Reports of the achievements of Nightingale and her nurses in combating the squalid conditions in the Crimea made Nightingale a national celebrity. She became known as "the lady with the lamp," a description that originated in an article published in *The Times*: "When all the medical officers have retired for the night, and silence and darkness have settled down upon these miles of prostrate sick, she may be observed alone, with a little lamp in her hand, making her solitary rounds."

Despite contracting "Crimean fever," a debilitating condition that would affect her for the rest of her life, Nightingale returned from the Crimean War in 1856, determined that the catastrophic loss of life she had witnessed be prevented in future. Backed by Queen Victoria, she persuaded the government to establish a royal commission into the state of health in the army.

Numbers in pictures

A talented student of mathematics from an early age, Nightingale collected data and organized a record-keeping system. Together with her friend William Farr, the UK's leading statistician, and John Sutherland of the Sanitary Commission, she embarked on an analysis of army mortality rates in the Crimean hospitals. They established that the leading cause of death among the soldiers was not combat, but disease—often diseases that could be prevented by good hygiene. Injured soldiers were seven times more likely to die of infections caught in the hospitals than from injuries sustained on the battlefield.

Nightingale realized that the data was best presented visually, "to affect thro' the eyes what we »

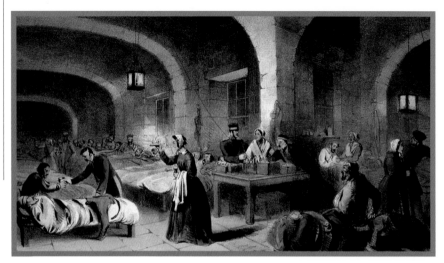

fail to convey to … the public through their word-proof ears." What she came up with was the coxcomb, or polar area, graph—a variation on the pie chart. The pie was split into 12 slices, one for each month, larger or smaller according to the number of deaths, and color-coded to indicate the causes of death. Nightingale's graphs of patient mortality would influence the development of epidemiology—the branch of medicine that deals with the appearance, distribution, and control of epidemic diseases.

Today, the use of graphical data is the norm, but Nightingale was one of the first people to use data visualization to influence public policy. The royal commission report produced from her findings suggested the creation of a statistical department to track rates of disease and mortality, identifying problems so they could be dealt with promptly.

In 1858, in recognition of her work, Nightingale became the first female member of the UK's Royal Statistical Society. During the 1860 International Statistical Congress, she advocated the collection of hospital statistics so that outcomes could be compared by hospital, region, and country—the first model for the systematic collection of hospital data. She also pressed, unsuccessfully, for questions on health to be added to the 1861 UK population census, believing that this would provide an invaluable overview and a source of data to guide public policy on health.

Training nurses

The Nightingale Training School and Home for Nurses, based at London's St. Thomas's Hospital, welcomed its first 10 students in 1860. Financed by the Nightingale Fund, a public contributions fund

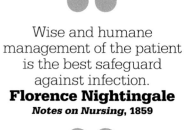

> Wise and humane management of the patient is the best safeguard against infection.
> **Florence Nightingale**
> *Notes on Nursing*, 1859

set up during Nightingale's time in the Crimea, the school aimed to provide nurses with practical training in hospitals specially organized for that purpose. It was largely due to the foundation of the school that Nightingale was able to transform nursing into a respectable and responsible career, and the school provided a model that would later be adopted worldwide. The Nightingale Fund also financed the setting up of a school for midwives at King's College Hospital in 1862.

When Nightingale published *Notes on Hospitals* and *Notes on Nursing* in 1859, the UK had no health service, and private healthcare was beyond the means of most. She believed that everyday knowledge of sanitation was vital in preventing the spread of disease, and *Notes on Nursing* was intended to educate the public as much in improving health standards as in caring for the sick.

Nightingale's focus on sanitation and healthcare also extended to reforming the nursing services offered to the poorest members of society in workhouse infirmaries. These institutions had scant medical care of any kind, relying on untrained nurses who were

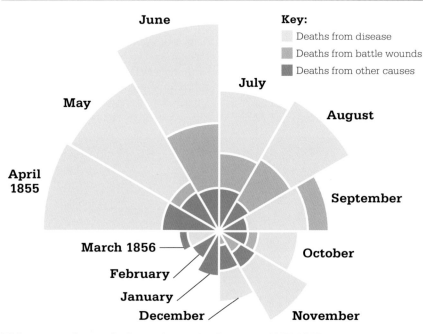

Key:
- Deaths from disease
- Deaths from battle wounds
- Deaths from other causes

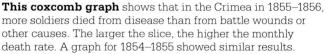

This coxcomb graph shows that in the Crimea in 1855–1856, more soldiers died from disease than from battle wounds or other causes. The larger the slice, the higher the monthly death rate. A graph for 1854–1855 showed similar results.

Florence Nightingale with students from the Nightingale Training School at St. Thomas's, photographed in 1866 at the home of her brother-in-law and supporter, Sir Harry Verney.

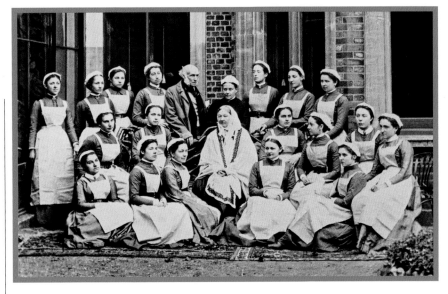

themselves workhouse inmates. Thanks to Nightingale's persistence and funding from philanthropist William Rathbone, the first attempts to staff a workhouse infirmary with trained nurses took place in 1865 in Liverpool. Twelve nurses trained at the Nightingale school, assisted by 18 probationers, were placed in the workhouse infirmary. Gradually, the nursing system was taken up by other infirmaries.

Campaign for healthcare

Nightingale believed that the sick were best cared for at home, so she also advised Rathbone to start a training school and home for nurses at Liverpool's Royal Infirmary. Opened in 1862, the school formed the basis of a district nursing system, where nurses went out to visit the ill in their homes.

Nightingale's own poor health prevented her from practicing as a nurse, but she remained a tireless campaigner, writing thousands of letters and publishing around 200 books, reports, and pamphlets. She advised on healthcare in India, where her reforms led to a sharp decline in mortality among British soldiers, as well as improved sanitation in rural communities. She was a consultant to the US government during the Civil War, inspiring the formation of the US Sanitary Commission, and acted as a mentor to Linda Richards, who was America's first professional nurse. Florence Nightingale's lasting legacy is the role she played in setting nursing on the road to becoming a modern, professional career in the field of medicine. She was also key in driving improvements in public hygiene and sanitation, extending life expectancy for thousands. Medical science has made huge strides since her lifetime, but her practical, evidence-based approach to healthcare is still relevant in today's health services. ∎

Florence Nightingale

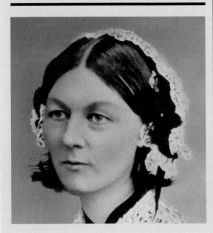

Named after the Italian city of her birth, Florence Nightingale was born in 1820, while her parents were touring Europe. Her father took particular interest in her education, teaching her history, philosophy, and mathematics. From an early age, she loved to collect and organize data—she used lists and tables to document her impressive shell collection.

Despite some family opposition, Nightingale trained as a nurse, seeing it as her calling to combat suffering. She led a team of nurses in the Crimea during the war, returning home a celebrity in 1856. Although she was largely housebound from 1858 due to the illness she had contracted in the Crimea, Nightingale used her fame to work on reforming health and social care in Britain. She was the first woman to be awarded Britain's Order of Merit, and her ideas of nursing practice still underpin the profession today. She died in 1910, aged 90.

Key works

1859 *Notes on Hospitals*
1859 *Notes on Nursing*

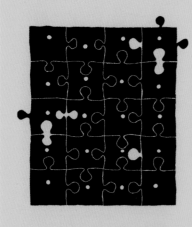

DISTURBANCES AT THE CELLULAR LEVEL
CELLULAR PATHOLOGY

IN CONTEXT

BEFORE
1665 In *Micrographia*, English physicist Robert Hooke coins the term "cells" to describe the microscopic boxlike units in cork wood.

1670s Dutch scientist Antonie van Leeuwenhoek observes single-celled "animalcules."

1838–1839 In Germany, scientists Matthias Schleiden and Theodor Schwann propose that cells are the basic building blocks of all living things.

AFTER
1857 Albert von Kölliker describes mitochondria, which release energy to the cell.

1909 In Russia, scientist Alexander Maximow uses the term "stem cell" and proposes that all types of blood cell come from a single ancestor cell.

1998 American researchers James Thomson and John Gearhart isolate and culture human embryonic stem cells.

The study of diseases in terms of cell abnormalities, known as cellular pathology, is central to modern medical diagnosis and treatment. The field owes much to 19th-century German pathologist Rudolf Virchow, who insisted that science should look beyond organs and tissues and examine individual cells to find the causes of disease.

In 1855, Virchow popularized the key tenet of cell theory that all cells are derived from other cells (*omnia cellula e cellula*) as a result of division—an idea first posited by Polish–German physiologist Robert Remak three years earlier. Virchow went on to discover that disease occurs when normal cells produce abnormal cells, leading him to the conclusion that all diseases arise at the cellular level.

Virchow was the first to explain that cancer develops from cell abnormalities, and he described and named leukemia, a potentially fatal disease in which the blood produces too many leukocytes (white blood cells). He also coined the terms "thrombus" (a clot of coagulated blood) and "embolism" (when a blood clot blocks an artery) and showed that a blood clot in the leg could travel to the lung, causing a pulmonary embolism. His 1858 work *Cellular Pathology* became a bible for pathologists for many years.

Rapid scientific advances
Virchow's groundbreaking work on cells paved the way for further progress in understanding disease in the late 19th and 20th centuries. Histopathology—the microscopic examination of tissue to study disease—became an increasingly important area of research and diagnosis, advanced by the use of more effective dyes to stain tissue.

> We must endeavor to ... take [the cell] apart and find out what each portion contributes to cellular function and how these parts go wrong in disease.
> **Rudolf Virchow, 1898**

See also: Histology 122–123 ▪ Cancer therapy 168–175 ▪ Targeted drug delivery 198–199 ▪ Cancer screening 226–227 ▪ Stem cell research 302–303

From his study of cells, Virchow's distinguished pupil Friedrich von Recklinghausen explored a variety of bone and blood disorders, while Edwin Klebs, another of Virchow's students, uncovered links between bacteria and infectious disease and discovered the diphtheria bacillus. In 1901, in another major advance, Austrian immunologist Karl Landsteiner identified the A, B, and O blood groups, documenting the cellular differences between types.

The cell research of Greek American physician George Papanicolaou, who identified cervical cancer cells in vaginal smears in the 1920s, led to mass cervical "Pap smear" tests from the 1950s onward. Screening tests for other cancers followed. Since the 1950s, increasingly advanced diagnostic equipment and new techniques have helped scientists explore DNA, analyze cell nuclei, discover embryonic stem cells, and shed light on gene-based diseases.

Ever-tinier cell components

Today's specialists use powerful electron microscopes to assess changes in the size, shape, and appearance of a cell's nucleus that may indicate cancer, precancer, or other diseases. In tissue samples, they study the interaction of cells and identify any abnormalities.

Diagnosis is not the only goal, however. By studying ever-tinier cell molecules, scientists can better understand disease processes, while cell therapy—the insertion of viable cells to combat mechanisms that cause disease—may soon offer real hope to those suffering from thus far incurable disorders. ∎

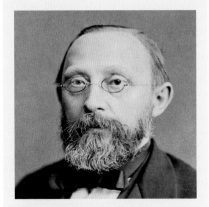

Rudolf Virchow

Born in Pomerania (now part of Poland) in 1821, Virchow graduated in medicine from the University of Berlin and learned much about pathology while working in the city's Charité Hospital. In 1848, he took part in Germany's failed revolutionary uprising and was banished from Berlin. He was soon offered a position at the University of Würzburg in Bavaria, where he shared ideas with Swiss histologist Albert von Kölliker.

Returning to Berlin in 1855, Virchow continued his innovative work on cellular pathology; campaigned vigorously for public health; established the city's water supply and sewerage system; and, from 1880 to 1893, was a member of the German Reichstag (parliament). After jumping from a streetcar and breaking his femur, Virchow died of an infection in 1902.

Key works

1854 *Handbook on Special Pathology and Therapeutics*
1858 *Cellular Pathology as Based upon Physiological and Pathological Histology*
1863–1867 *Pathological Tumors*

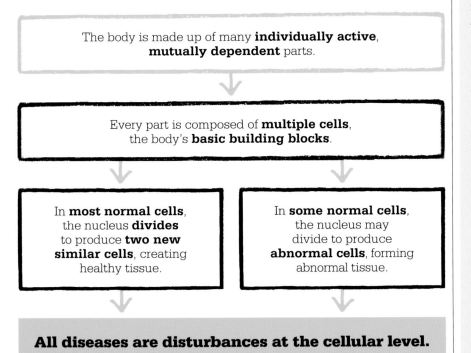

The body is made up of many **individually active, mutually dependent** parts.

⬇

Every part is composed of **multiple cells**, the body's **basic building blocks**.

⬇ ⬇

In **most normal cells**, the nucleus **divides** to produce **two new similar cells**, creating healthy tissue.

In **some normal cells**, the nucleus may divide to produce **abnormal cells**, forming abnormal tissue.

⬇ ⬇

All diseases are disturbances at the cellular level.

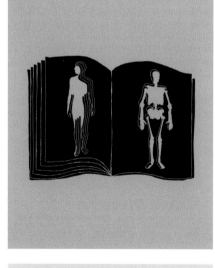

MAKE YOURSELVES MASTERS OF ANATOMY
GRAY'S ANATOMY

IN CONTEXT

BEFORE
1543 Andreas Vesalius publishes *De Humani Corporis Fabrica*, which marks the birth of modern anatomy.

1780s A rapid rise in the number of European medical schools increases demand for detailed anatomical knowledge through dissection. "Body-snatching" from cemeteries becomes common.

1828 Irish anatomist Jones Quain publishes his three-volume *Elements of Anatomy*, which becomes the standard textbook on anatomy.

1832 Parliament's Anatomy Act gives surgeons, medical students, and anatomists the legal right to dissect donated bodies in the UK.

AFTER
2015 The 41st edition of *Gray's Anatomy* is published; it is the first edition to include additional online content.

British surgeon Henry Gray became a lecturer in anatomy at St. George's Hospital Medical School, London, in 1853. Wanting to create an accurate, authoritative, low-cost textbook for his students, Gray enlisted the help of a colleague, Henry Vandyke Carter, to draw the illustrations. Published in 1858, the 750-page tome described the human body in vast anatomical detail, using 363 images. Originally titled *Anatomy: Descriptive and Surgical*, then *Anatomy of the Human Body*, the book is still in print today and, since 1938, is known as *Gray's Anatomy*.

A pioneering textbook
Working side by side over 18 months, Gray and Carter conducted detailed dissections on unclaimed cadavers from hospitals and workhouses. Gray used his scalpel to strip back the human body's many layers,

Gray's book was unique in including anatomical labels within its illustrations and in using life-sized representations to aid understanding.

while Carter meticulously recorded every tendon, muscle, bone, and tissue with his pencils. The illustrations, which emphasized the functionality and form of each body part, were key to the book's success.

Cleverly published to coincide with the start of the academic year, and priced below its competitors, Gray's book was an instant success. Its detail, accuracy, and clarity led to enduring popularity, and it has remained the most comprehensive guide to anatomical knowledge for physicians. ■

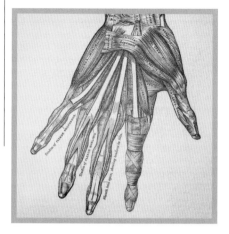

See also: Roman medicine 38–43 ▪ Anatomy 60–63 ▪ Blood circulation 68–73 ▪ Physiology 152–153

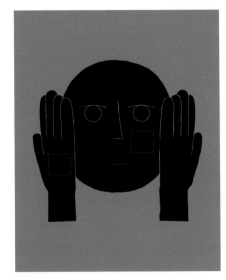

ONE MUST REPLACE THE SCARRING TISSUE
SKIN GRAFTS

IN CONTEXT

BEFORE
1663 English physician Walter Charleton attempts the first recorded skin graft on a dog.

1785 Italian physiologist Giuseppe Baronio begins researching skin grafts using a variety of animals and proves that they are feasible.

1817 British surgeon Astley Cooper performs the first documented successful skin graft on a human.

1869 Jacques-Louis Reverdin pioneers the pinch graft using tiny particles of skin.

AFTER
1929 American surgeons Vilray Blair and James Brown improve split-thickness graft techniques to enable grafts of varying dermal thickness.

1939 American surgeon Earl Padgett and engineer George Hood pioneer a mechanical "dermatome" for accurately harvesting large skin grafts.

I n 1874, German surgeon Karl Thiersch published the results of his experiments with skin grafts. His groundbreaking results showed that the best outcome was achieved by removing granulation tissue—the new tissue that forms on the surface of a wound—before applying a razor-thin, uniform graft, using skin taken from the patient's own body (an autograft). Autografts using the full thickness of skin had been attempted previously but often failed because underlying fat and tissue layers prevented new blood vessels forming between the wound site and the graft.

Split-thickness success

Five years earlier, in 1869, Swiss surgeon Jacques-Louis Reverdin had shown that tiny skin fragments, later named "pinch grafts," could be applied successfully to burns, ulcers, and open wounds. Thiersch was able to build on this principle, using new surgical instruments that allowed him to harvest larger and thinner grafts than previously possible. These grafts had quicker attachment and survival rates and produced less scar tissue at the site of the graft and minimal damage at the donor site, making it possible to harvest as much skin as needed for a repair. Called a "split-thickness" graft because it uses only part of the thickness of the skin, Thiersch's technique transformed outcomes in reconstructive surgery and became the standard procedure for repairing large expanses of skin. ∎

> [Thiersch] possessed not only the necessary firmness of eye and hand, but also a sovereign calmness …
> **Obituary**
> *Popular Science Monthly*, **1898**

See also: Plastic surgery 26–27 ▪ Transplant surgery 246–253 ▪ Nanomedicine 304 ▪ Face transplants 315

LIFE IS AT THE MERCY OF THESE MINUTE BODIES

GERM THEORY

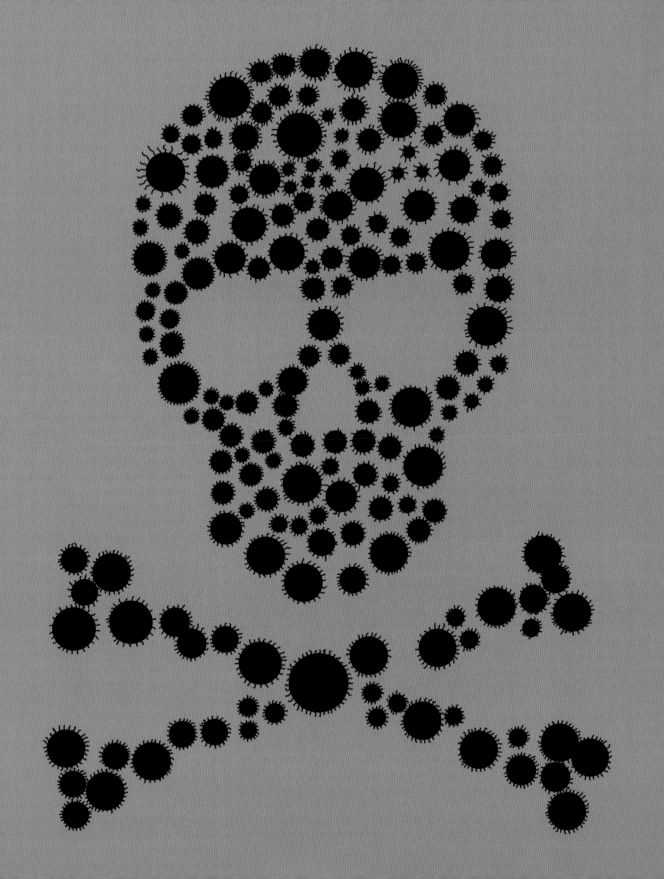

IN CONTEXT

BEFORE

1656 Athanasius Kirchner identifies microscopic worms in the blood of plague victims.

1670s Under his microscope, Antonie van Leeuwenhoek sees bacteria or "animalcules."

AFTER

1910 Paul Ehrlich develops Salvarsan, the first drug to be targeted at a germ, the syphilis bacterium.

1928 Alexander Fleming discovers penicillin, the first effective antibiotic.

1933 H1N1, a virus of avian origin, is named as the cause of the 1918–1919 flu pandemic.

2016 Facebook founder Mark Zuckerberg and Priscilla Chan launch the Chan Zuckerberg Initiative—to cure, prevent, or manage all human disease by the end of the century.

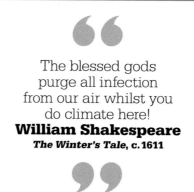

> The blessed gods
> purge all infection
> from our air whilst you
> do climate here!
> **William Shakespeare**
> *The Winter's Tale, c. 1611*

Germ theory asserts that a host of diseases, from smallpox to tuberculosis, are caused by germs—minuscule organisms, such as bacteria, that are mostly too small to be seen with the naked eye. Each disease is linked to a particular kind of germ. People get sick when the germ, or "pathogen," enters the body and multiplies, triggering the symptoms of the disease.

French chemist Louis Pasteur published his theory that microbes might be to blame in 1861, but in the 1870s, experiments conducted by Pasteur and German physician

Robert Koch proved the germ theory beyond doubt. Since then, hundreds of infectious diseases have been linked to particular germs. The first priority for medical scientists today when a new transmissible disease emerges is to identify the germ responsible.

Early theories

Ancient physicians were aware that many diseases are contagious and speculated over their causes. More than 2,500 years ago in India, followers of the Jainist religion believed that minute beings called *nigoda*, which were thought to pervade the Universe, caused diseases such as leprosy. During the 1st century BCE, Roman scholar Marcus Terentius Varro advised his readers to take precautions in the neighborhood of swamps "because there are bred certain minute creatures which cannot be seen by the eyes, which float in the air and enter the body through the mouth and nose and there cause serious

Doctors in the medieval era wore a beaked mask filled with herbs to protect themselves from miasmas— the foul odors thought to cause disease until well into the 19th century.

diseases." Later, the Roman physician Galen described plague as being spread by "seeds of plague" that are carried on the air and lodge in the body.

In the medieval era, two Islamic physicians who witnessed outbreaks of the Black Death in 14th-century Andalusia drew similar conclusions about disease. In his *Kitab al-Tahsil* (*Book of the Pest*), Ibn Khātima suggested that plague was spread by "minute bodies." In another treatise on the plague, Ibn al-Khatib explained how such entities spread the disease through contact between people, remarking that individuals "who kept themselves in isolation" remained in good health.

For a long time, the air itself was believed to spread disease— especially damp, misty air near ditches and swamps. This odorous mist was called a miasma (ancient Greek for "pollution"). The Roman architect Vitruvius, writing in the 1st century BCE, thought it unwise to build a city anywhere near swamps, saying that morning breezes would blow miasmas from the marshes,

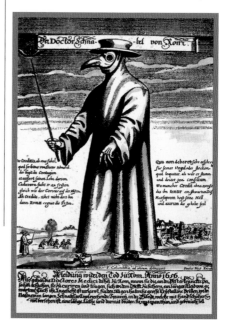

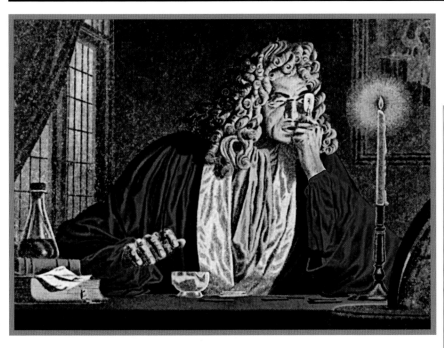

Antonie van Leeuwenhoek uses his newly invented microscope to view the microorganisms he called "animalcules." The single lens was a tiny glass bead held between two metal plates.

along with the poisonous breath of swamp creatures, into the city and make people ill. In ancient China, under imperial rule from the 3rd century BCE onward, prisoners and insubordinate officials were exiled to the damp and humid mountains of southern China in the hope that they would fall ill and die from the noxious air.

Little worms

The microscope, invented by Dutch spectacle-maker Zacharias Janssen around 1590, revealed a new world of tiny organisms too small to see with the naked eye. In 1656, German priest and scholar Athanasius Kirchner examined the blood of plague victims in Rome through a microscope and saw "little worms" that he believed caused the disease. He may have seen blood cells rather than the *Yersinia pestis* bacterium that causes plague, but he was right to say that microscopic organisms

cause plague. He outlined his germ theory in 1658 and recommended protocols to stop its spread: isolation, quarantine, and the burning of clothes worn by victims.

In the 1660s, Dutch scientist Antonie van Leeuwenhoek made a microscope that could magnify objects 200 times. He discovered that clear water is not clear at all, but teeming with tiny creatures, and that these minuscule organisms are almost everywhere. In 1683, Leeuwenhoek viewed bacteria wriggling in plaque from the teeth of his wife and daughter. He drew the shapes of the bacteria he saw: round (coccus), spiral (spirillum), and rod (bacillus). This was the first depiction of bacteria.

Increasing evidence

In spite of Leeuwenhoek's discovery of bacteria, the miasma theory still continued to hold sway until the early 1800s, when Italian

entomologist Agostino Bassi began to investigate muscardine disease, which was devastating the Italian and French silkworm industries. In 1835, after 28 years of intense study, Bassi published a paper showing the disease was caused by a microscopic, parasitic fungus and that it was contagious. He demonstrated that the organism *Beauveria bassiana* spread among the silkworms through contact and infected food. He also suggested that microbes were the cause of many other diseases in plants, animals, and humans.

Over the next few decades, the germ theory gathered support. In 1847, Hungarian obstetrician Ignaz Semmelweis insisted on strict hygiene in labor wards, where puerperal (childbed) fever »

> I now saw very distinctly that these were little eels or worms … the whole water seemed to be alive with the multitudinous animalcules.
> **Antonie van Leeuwenhoek**
> **Letter to German natural philosopher Henry Oldenburg, 1676**

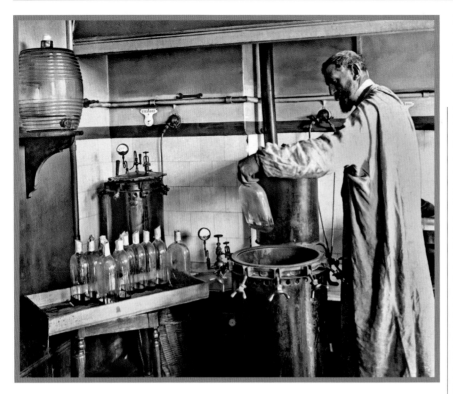

Louis Pasteur works in his laboratory, c. 1880. Originally a chemist before turning to biology, Pasteur was a meticulous experimenter who guarded against error.

afflicted many new mothers (although at the time his advice was largely ignored). He argued that it was "cadaverous particles" spreading the disease, transmitted from the autopsy room to the obstetric wards on the hands of physicians. Instituting handwashing with a chloride of lime solution dramatically reduced mortality rates.

In 1854, a cholera epidemic hit London's Soho district. British physician John Snow was not convinced that the miasma theory explained the outbreak, because some victims were clustered in a very small area while others were scattered far away.

After conducting detailed research, Snow demonstrated that all the victims, including those living further afield, had drunk water from a particular water pump in Soho that had been contaminated by human excrement. The city authorities were unconvinced by Snow's explanation but began to make improvements to London's water supply nonetheless.

Cholera also hit Florence, in Italy, that year. Anatomist Filippo Pacini examined mucus lining the guts of some of its victims and discovered a bacterium common to all of them—*Vibrio cholerae*. This was the first clear link between a particular pathogen and a major disease. Despite republishing his findings several times, Pacini was ignored by the medical establishment, which continued to favor the miasma theory.

Pasteur's experiments

Semmelweis and Snow had shown that clean hands and good drains can reduce the spread of disease, and it became increasingly clear that bad air was not to blame. Within a few years, Louis Pasteur began a series of experiments that proved germ theory conclusively.

Pasteur's interest in microbes had begun in the 1850s, when he was studying the fermentation of wine and beer. People had assumed that fermentation was a chemical reaction, but Pasteur showed that tiny round microbes called yeast are responsible. However, it has to be the right type of yeast: another kind that makes unwanted lactic acid ruins the wine. Pasteur found that by heating the wine gently to about 140°F (60°C), he could kill the harmful yeast while leaving the good yeast undamaged. "Pasteurization" is now widely used not only in the wine industry, but to destroy potential pathogens in milk, fresh fruit juice, and other foods.

Pasteur wondered how such microbes appear in substances in the first place. Most people still believed in the idea of spontaneous generation—that maggots and mold simply appear out of nowhere when food decays. In 1859, Pasteur showed that these microbes came from the air. He boiled meat broth in a flask with a bent "swan" neck so that no air could get in, and the

> In the field of observation, chance favors only the prepared mind.
> **Louis Pasteur, 1854**

broth stayed clear. When he broke the tip of the neck so that air could enter the flask, the broth quickly went cloudy; the microbes were multiplying. Crucially, Pasteur had demonstrated that the broth could be contaminated and ruined by microbes in the air, suggesting that disease might very well be spread in a similar way.

Disease prevention

A few years later, in 1876, Pasteur was asked to find a solution to pébrine disease, which was killing silkworms and devastating the silk industry of southern France. Helped by reading Bassi's work from 30 years earlier, he quickly discovered that a tiny parasite was to blame. Pasteur recommended a drastic solution—destroying all the infested worms, and the mulberry trees on which they fed, and starting again. The silk makers took his advice and the industry survived.

By now, Pasteur was convinced that germs were to blame for many infections and began to study how diseases spread among humans and animals. In Scotland, surgeon

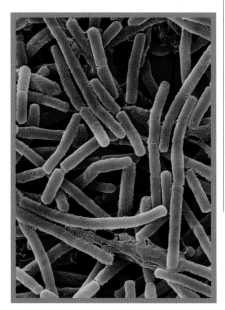

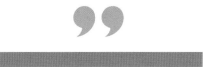

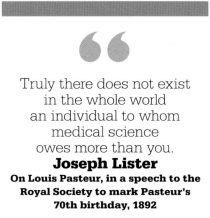

Truly there does not exist in the whole world an individual to whom medical science owes more than you.
Joseph Lister
On Louis Pasteur, in a speech to the Royal Society to mark Pasteur's 70th birthday, 1892

Joseph Lister, who had read about Pasteur's earlier work on microbes, realized that surgical operations are much safer if wounds are cleaned and dressings sterilized to destroy microbes. With this "antiseptic" procedure, death rates among Lister's patients fell by two-thirds between 1865 and 1869.

Germ theory proved

In 1876, Robert Koch announced that he had identified the germs that cause the barnyard animal disease anthrax. He extracted the bacteria *Bacillus anthracis* from the blood of a sheep that had died from anthrax, then left them to multiply in a culture dish of food—initially the liquid from an ox's eye, but later a broth of agar and gelatin. Koch then injected the bacteria into a mouse. The mouse died of anthrax, too, proving that the bacteria had caused the disease. Pasteur immediately »

Bacillus anthracis is a rod-shaped bacterium that causes anthrax, a serious disease that produces skin lesions, breathing difficulties, vomiting, and shock.

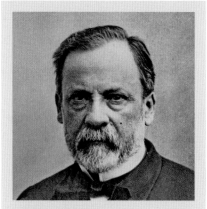

Louis Pasteur

Pasteur was born in Dôle, the French Pyrenees, in 1822. As a boy, he preferred art to science, but at the age of 21, he went to the *École normale supérieure* in Paris to train as a science teacher. A year after graduating, he delivered a brilliant paper on molecular asymmetry to the Academy of Sciences, for which he won the Légion d'honneur.

In 1854, aged 32, Pasteur was made head of science and professor of chemistry at the University of Lille, where several local distilleries asked him for assistance with the process of fermentation. This formed the basis of his interest in microbes and germ theory. By 1888, Pasteur was world famous, and money was raised to create the Pasteur Institute in Paris for the further study of microorganisms, diseases, and vaccines. When he died in 1895, Pasteur was given a state funeral and was buried in Notre-Dame Cathedral.

Key works

1866 *Studies on Wine*
1868 *Studies on Vinegar*
1878 *Microbes organized, their role in fermentation, putrefaction and contagion*

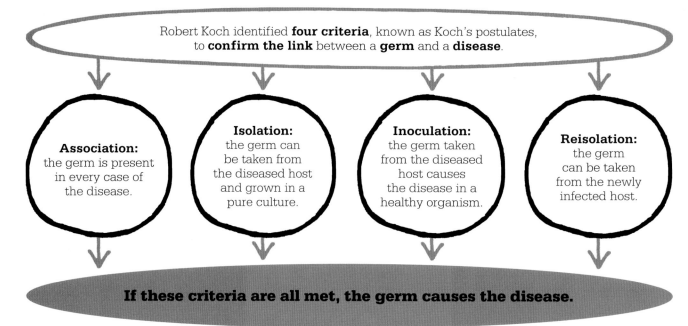

Robert Koch identified **four criteria**, known as Koch's postulates, to **confirm the link** between a **germ** and a **disease**.

Association: the germ is present in every case of the disease.

Isolation: the germ can be taken from the diseased host and grown in a pure culture.

Inoculation: the germ taken from the diseased host causes the disease in a healthy organism.

Reisolation: the germ can be taken from the newly infected host.

If these criteria are all met, the germ causes the disease.

ran his own tests. He confirmed Koch's findings and also showed that the germs could survive in soil for long periods, proving that healthy animals could pick up the disease from a field that had previously been occupied by infected livestock.

Pasteur went on to develop a vaccine against the disease after realizing that heating the bacteria produced a weakened form of the pathogen that was potent enough to provoke a defense in the body of the sheep but not strong enough to cause disease.

Koch's postulates

The bacterium that causes anthrax, *Bacillus anthracis*, is a tiny rod-shaped organism that is visible only under a microscope. Pasteur and Koch had shown that despite its tiny size, *Bacillus anthracis* can kill animals and also people. It multiplies in the body, releasing a toxin or interfering with the body's functions. Such an invasion is called an infection. Not every infection by

a pathogen will cause a disease, and not everyone's body responds in the same way, but the link is clear.

Pasteur had proved that air can transmit microbes, and he and Koch had shown that these microbes may cause disease. Koch then went on to show that there is an army of

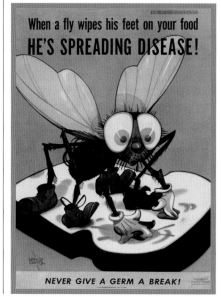

When a fly wipes his feet on your food
HE'S SPREADING DISEASE!

NEVER GIVE A GERM A BREAK!

pathogenic microbes that are to blame for all infectious diseases. In the 1880s, Koch provided medical scientists with a series of four steps for confirming the link when they came to investigate a disease for the first time. Koch's postulates still underpin the more extensive criteria used today to establish the causes of contagious diseases.

By 1882, Koch had identified the germ responsible for tuberculosis (TB)—*Mycobacterium tuberculosis*, or Koch's bacillus—which is transmitted through tiny droplets released into the air, mainly through coughing or sneezing. Next, he turned his attention to finding the germ responsible for cholera, visiting Egypt and India to acquire samples. By 1884, he had identified the cause to be the comma-shaped bacterium

A US government poster from 1944 warns against the spread of germs. Flies were linked to outbreaks of dysentery and other infectious diseases during World War II.

Vibrio cholerae, confirming Pacini's discovery 30 years earlier. Koch took his findings one stage further by linking *Vibrio cholerae* with contaminated water and then suggesting several measures that would prevent its spread.

Find and destroy

By the late 19th century, many scientists were actively searching for the microbes that cause disease. It is now known that 99 percent of microbes are completely harmless and many, such as those found in gut flora, are beneficial. However, around 1,500 have been identified as pathogens, with more discovered each year. The main pathogens are bacteria, viruses, fungi, and protozoa (single-celled organisms that are responsible for many diseases, including amoebic dysentery).

Knowing that diseases are caused by germs transformed the fight against them. It clarified the measures needed to prevent their spread, such as hygiene, sanitation, and quarantining, and it quickly led to an understanding of how vaccines confer immunity. It also promoted the development of drugs, such as antibiotics and antivirals, to target

Some ways that germs enter the body

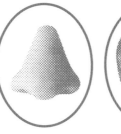 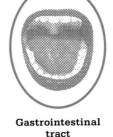 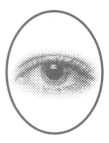

Airways
Airborne pathogens in evaporated droplets or dust particles can be breathed in. They include the influenza virus.

Gastrointestinal tract
Consumption of contaminated food or water causes many diseases, including salmonella and cholera.

Cuts in the skin
Pathogens can enter the body through wounds or bites. They include *Clostridium tetani*, which causes tetanus.

Eyes
Rubbing eyes with hands that have touched infected surfaces can transfer pathogens such as cold viruses into the body.

specific microbes—stopping the disease rather than just addressing its symptoms.

From the mid-20th century, new diagnostic tools and advances in biochemistry and genetics further transformed health in the developed world. In 1900, for example, the infectious diseases pneumonia, TB, influenza, and enteritis with diarrhea were the three leading causes of death in the US, taking the lives of 40 percent of children aged under 5. A century later, these diseases killed far fewer people, with diseases that are not infectious, notably heart disease, overtaking them. Yet infectious diseases still killed 10 million people in 2017 alone—many of them in developing countries, where poor nutrition and sanitation and limited access to health care allow avoidable and treatable diseases to thrive. Here, poverty-related diseases, such as diarrhea, TB, and malaria, are more lethal than incurable diseases. ∎

Robert Koch

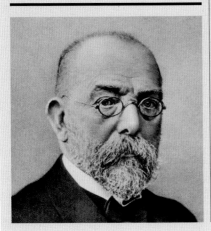

Born in Clausthal, in Germany's Harz Mountains, in 1843, Robert Koch studied medicine at the University of Göttingen. He served as an army surgeon in the Franco-Prussian War (1870–1871) before becoming district medical officer for Wollstein (now Wolsztyn in Poland) between 1872 and 1880.

Applying Louis Pasteur's ideas on germ theory, Koch began his research on anthrax bacteria in a custom laboratory in his home. This marked the start of a period of intense rivalry between the two men as they vied to identify new microbes and develop vaccines.

Koch conclusively proved that Pasteur's germ theory explained the cause and spread of disease. He became professor of hygiene at the University of Berlin in 1885, and surgeon general in 1890. For his research on TB (which used to kill one in seven people in the West), he received the Nobel Prize in Physiology or Medicine in 1905. Koch died in Baden-Baden in 1910.

Key work

1878 *Investigations of the Etiology of Wound Infections*

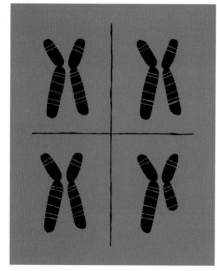

A GENETIC MISPRINT

INHERITANCE AND HEREDITARY CONDITIONS

Austrian monk Gregor Mendel laid the basis for our understanding of inheritance by meticulously studying pea plants in his monastery garden. He selectively bred thousands of plants between 1856 and 1863, studying specific features or traits such as plant height, flower color, and pod shape. Mendel showed that these traits were not the result of blending or merging, but "factors" (later called genes) inherited from parent plants. He also noted that each factor had different versions, now known as alleles.

Most organisms, from pea plants to humans, have two sets of genes, one from each parent, and two alleles for each trait. Mendel devised three laws that govern how these alleles are passed on. His law of segregation states that alleles for a trait are allocated randomly to offspring rather than in any regular pattern. His law of independent assortment says that traits are inherited separately—the allele for flower color, for example, passes on independently of that for pod shape.

Mendel's law of dominance asserts that one allele, termed dominant, can override or overpower another, known as recessive. When peas with purple flowers were bred with white-flowered peas, the next generation had purple flowers. Mendel deduced that the purple allele for flower color dominated the recessive white allele. For a pea plant to have white flowers, it must have two recessive alleles, one inherited from each parent plant.

Ideas rediscovered

Mendel published his research in 1865, but it remained obscure until 1900, when it was rediscovered by three botanists: Hugo de Vries in Holland, Carl Correns in Germany,

> 66
> … [recessive traits] recede or disappear entirely in the hybrids, but reappear unchanged in their progeny …
> **Gregor Mendel**
> *Experiments in Plant Hybridization, 1865*
> 99

See also: Color vision deficiency 91 ▪ Cellular pathology 134–135
▪ Genetics and medicine 288–293 ▪ Gene therapy 300

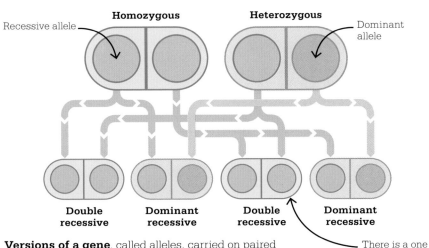

Homozygous   Heterozygous

Recessive allele

Dominant allele

Double recessive   **Dominant recessive**   **Double recessive**   **Dominant recessive**

There is a one in two chance that a child will inherit the recessive trait.

Versions of a gene, called alleles, carried on paired chromosomes, determine inherited traits. One allele is inherited from each parent, and some alleles dominate or overpower other (recessive) genes. Individuals with identical alleles are termed homozygous; those with varying alleles are heterozygous.

and Erich Tschermak in Austria. Their discussion of Mendel's work had an immediate impact and fueled the studies of British biologist William Bateson. Bateson went on to republish Mendel's original papers and to popularize his ideas, establishing the field of genetics.

Hereditary conditions
Mendel's original ideas guided medical understanding of genetic conditions, explaining why some run in families, are sex-specific, or skip a generation. Huntington's disease is due to a dominant mutated allele that overpowers the normal one. Cystic fibrosis is recessive, so it needs two recessive alleles to occur, one from each parent.

Some conditions are sex-related, such as the blood-clotting disorder hemophilia, which more commonly affects men. A recessive allele on the X sex chromosome causes it. Men have two sex chromosomes, XY—the X is from the mother and the Y from the father. If the X chromosome carries the allele for the condition, it cannot be counteracted by a dominant allele because the Y chromosome does not have this gene. Women have two X chromosomes, XX, so they must receive two recessive alleles to be affected, which is exceptionally rare. Affected women are "carriers," who can transmit the condition to their offspring, but they usually have no symptoms themselves.

Genetics is now known to be more complex than Mendel could have imagined. There are currently more than 5,000 known inherited conditions, and many traits depend not on a single "factor" or gene, but on several, even hundreds, working together. There are some alleles that are neither dominant nor recessive, but codominant (expressed to an equal degree). Yet Mendel's pea plants laid the foundations for a new understanding of genetics and inherited medical conditions. ▪

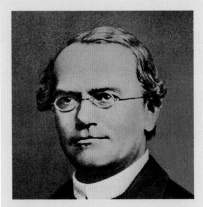

Gregor Mendel

Christened Johann, Mendel was born in Silesia, then part of the Austrian Empire, in 1822. Excelling in math and physics at university, he joined St. Thomas's Monastery in Brünn (now Brno, in the Czech Republic) as an Augustinian monk in 1843. Here, he took the name Gregor.

In 1851, the monastery sent Mendel to the University of Vienna to continue his studies. He worked under Austrian physicist Christian Doppler, and also learned much about the physiology of plants using microscopy. After returning to Brünn, Mendel embarked on his inheritance project using pea plants and presented the results in 1865. Two years later, he became the monastery's abbot but still continued to devote time to research, studying bees and the weather. In his later years, Mendel suffered from a painful kidney disorder. After his death in 1884, the rediscovery of his ideas in 1900 led to his posthumous recognition as the father of genetics.

Key work

1865 *Experiments in Plant Hybridization*

IT IS FROM PARTICLES THAT ALL THE MISCHIEF ARISES

ANTISEPTICS IN SURGERY

IN CONTEXT

BEFORE
c. 1012 Persian polymath Ibn Sina establishes early ideas about germ theory.

1850s Louis Pasteur suggests that microorganisms could cause food and drink to spoil.

1861 Pasteur publishes his germ theory of disease.

AFTER
1880s Robert Koch shows that steam sterilization is as effective at killing germs as antiseptics.

1890s Gustav Neuber establishes sterilization and aseptic methods in his operating theater.

1940s The mass use of antibiotics helps surgeons tackle infection by killing microorganisms from inside the body.

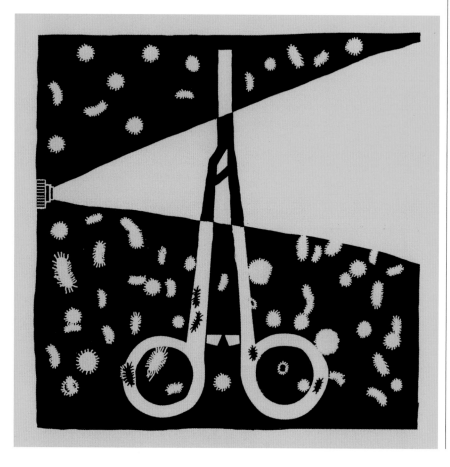

Operating rooms in the mid-19th century were dirty, dangerous places where surgeons seldom washed their hands or took precautions to prevent patients' wounds becoming infected. Unsterilized surgical instruments, made of ivory or wood, were difficult to keep clean, and operating tables were not usually wiped down between procedures. Surgeons sported blood-encrusted operating aprons and took pride in the "good old surgical stink" that surrounded them.

The discovery of anesthesia in 1846 meant that patients no longer had to be awake during operations, nor did they have to be subjected to procedures in which—to reduce

See also: Anesthesia 112–117 ▪ Hygiene 118–119 ▪ Nursing and sanitation 128–133 ▪ Germ theory 138–145
▪ Malaria 162–163 ▪ Antibiotics 216–223

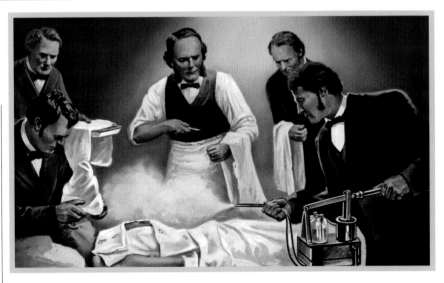

Joseph Lister (center) directs an assistant who is using carbolic spray to clean the surgeons' hands, their instruments, and the air around them during an operation.

the chances of a patient dying from shock or blood loss—speed was prized over skill. Surgery was now pain-free, allowing more time for complicated procedures. But it also led to a dramatic rise in the number of deaths from infection caused by unsterilized surgical conditions.

Doctors of the time were unaware that the microorganisms now known as germs should be prevented from entering an open wound during surgery. Most were baffled by the high numbers of postoperative patients succumbing to infection—especially those who had had a limb amputated.

Invisible killer

This was the environment that young British physician Joseph Lister encountered in 1861, when he became surgeon to the Glasgow Royal Infirmary in Scotland. Lister was placed in charge of the Male Accident Ward, one of several wards in the new surgical block. It had been constructed in the hope of reducing the high death rate from "hospital disease" (today called operative sepsis: the infection of blood by germs). But the newness of the building did nothing to stem the tide of deaths. Lister determined to discover the underlying cause of the infections.

Up until that point, many in the medical profession believed that disease was spread by bad air (miasma), while others thought it was transferred by something in the body (contagionism). Lister proposed that sepsis was spread by an airborne dustlike substance, although he did not consider that this dust would be living. It was not until he read the work of French bacteriologist Louis Pasteur in »

Joseph Lister

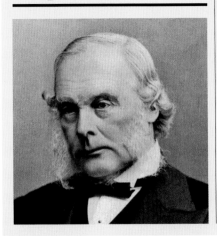

Born in 1827, in Essex, UK, Joseph Lister was brought up a Quaker. His father taught him how to use a microscope, which Lister used for his later trials on infected human tissue. After graduating from London's University College in 1852, he became an assistant to Edinburgh surgeon James Syme. In 1856, Lister married Syme's daughter Agnes, who also became his lifelong laboratory partner.

Lister worked as a surgeon in Edinburgh and Glasgow before moving to London in 1877. He was professor of clinical surgery at King's College Hospital for 16 years, until he retired in 1893. Despite winning numerous honors, including the Order of Merit, and being the first surgeon to be made a peer in the House of Lords, Lister led a somewhat reclusive existence. He died in 1912, and was buried in London after a funeral at Westminster Abbey.

Key work

1867 "On the Antiseptic Principle in the Practice of Surgery"

In the early 19th century, **operations** in Britain are carried out in **filthy conditions** using **unsterilized instruments**. **Nearly half of all patients die** following surgery.

⬇

Joseph Lister postulates that if **"floating particles,"** or **microorganisms**, can cause food and drink to spoil, they might also be **infecting patients' wounds**.

⬇

Lister uses **antiseptic spray** and antiseptic-soaked bandages **during surgery** to **kill these microorganisms** and prevent them from getting into open wounds.

⬇

Surgical mortality rates improve dramatically.

1865 that he began to make the connection between germs and surgical infection.

Pasteur had discovered the role of microorganisms in disease after studying the fermentation of beer and milk. He proved that food and drink were not spoiled by oxygen in the air, but by microbes that appeared and thrived over time within oxygen-rich environments.

Blocking bacteria

Lister seized on Pasteur's germ theory and decided to apply it to surgical infections. Pasteur had suggested that microorganisms could be eliminated through heat, filtration, or exposure to chemicals. As the first two methods were unworkable for wounds, Lister began experimenting with chemicals on infected human tissue under a microscope. His ultimate aim was to prevent germs from entering an open wound by creating a chemical barrier between the wound and its surroundings. He would later call this chemical an "antiseptic."

Carbolic acid, which was being used to clean Scotland's worst-smelling sewers, proved to be an effective antiseptic. Lister found that adding diluted carbolic acid to infected wounds was a good way to prevent the development of gangrene. He then reasoned that spraying a carbolic solution onto surgical instruments, a surgeon's hands, and postoperative bandages would also effectively block the transmission of germs from these objects into a patient's wounds.

In 1865, Lister was able to test his theories on an 11-year-old boy who had presented at the infirmary with an open fracture, after a cart ran over his leg. Open fractures, where the bone had broken the skin, were often death sentences at that time, as the necessary surgery invariably led to infection. In most cases, surgeons would try to offset this risk by amputating the limb altogether, which also came with great mortal risk. Lister, however, set the boy's leg and applied a bandage soaked in carbolic acid to the wound. A few days later, there was no sign of infection, and the bone showed itself to be healing. The boy was discharged five weeks later, having made a full recovery.

Lister continued his clinical work with carbolic acid and, in 1867, published his findings in the article, "On the Antiseptic Principle in the Practice of Surgery," in the *British Medical Journal*. His results made for startling reading. Between 1865 and 1869, surgical mortality caused by infected wounds fell by two-thirds in Lister's Male Accident Ward.

Overcoming skepticism

Despite Lister's demonstrable successes, there was immediate opposition to his theories. For many surgeons, Lister's techniques simply slowed surgery down, which improved the likelihood of death through blood loss. Surgeons also

> ... since the antiseptic treatment has been brought into full operation ... my wards ... have completely changed their character ...
> **Joseph Lister**
> **Speech at the Dublin meeting of the British Medical Association, 1867**

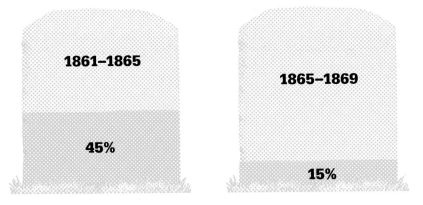

1861–1865

45%

1865–1869

15%

When Joseph Lister took charge of the new Male Accident Ward at the Glasgow Royal Infirmary in Scotland, almost half of all patients were dying from postoperative infection. After Lister introduced his antisepsis method, the mortality rate on the ward dropped to 15 percent.

remained unconvinced that Lister's antisepsis system—antiseptic sprays and washes as barriers to infection—constituted any kind of advance. The spray hurt surgeons' eyes and could damage healthy tissue, as well as infected tissue.

In 1869, Lister succeeded his friend James Syme as professor of Edinburgh University's clinical surgery, where he continued his work on germ theory. His ideas brought acclaim on a lecture tour of German surgical centers in 1875, but were met with strong criticism in the US the following year.

Undeterred, Lister continued to publish his findings in articles for the *British Medical Journal* and *The Lancet*. But he was not a naturally gifted writer, and his refusal to print statistics did not endear him to his readers or peers. For many in the medical profession, Edinburgh was considered a second-rate center of surgical expertise when compared to London. Lister would have to prove himself in the capital.

Lister's chance came in 1877, when he became professor of clinical surgery at London's King's College Hospital. Here, he captured the attention of colleagues by wiring a patient's fractured kneecap. First, he turned the single fracture into a compound one, greatly increasing the risk of infection and death. By using his antisepsis techniques, however, Lister was able to treat the wound, and the patient recovered. Few could now dispute that these antiseptic methods provided anything but lifesaving value to surgical procedures.

Royal approval

In 1871, Lister further enhanced his reputation by lancing a large abscess in Queen Victoria's armpit. During the procedure, carbolic acid was accidentally sprayed into the queen's eyes. Lister had introduced the use of a carbolic steam spray after theorizing that the air around an operating table might also contain germs. Luckily, the queen suffered no lasting effect, and Lister later abandoned this practice.

Lister's operation on Queen Victoria might have had a very different outcome without the use of antiseptic to prevent infection. His success won him the role of personal surgeon to the queen in 1878.

By the time Lister retired from surgery in 1893, his contributions to safe surgical practice were universally accepted. Among the scientists researching ever safer ways of controlling infection was German bacteriologist Robert Koch. Asepsis, Koch's system of keeping a surgical environment free of germs through heat, antiseptics, and soap and water, was a natural evolutionary advance on the antisepsis methods pioneered by Lister.

Koch demonstrated that dry heat and steam sterilization were just as effective as antiseptics at killing germs. Expanding this theory further, German physician Gustav Neuber introduced sterile gowns, rubber gloves, and face masks to surgery. Easy-to-disinfect floors and walls in operating rooms were to follow.

These practices remain the key tenets of safe surgical procedure today, with the sterilization of instruments and the operating environment in general being of paramount importance. The theory behind them stems directly from Lister's findings in the 1860s—that germs must not gain entry to any wound during an operation. ■

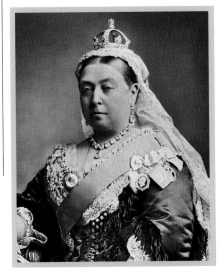

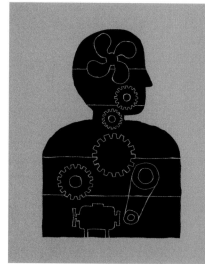

THE FIELD OF VITAL PHENOMENA

PHYSIOLOGY

hysiology is the study of the functions of an organism, as opposed to the study of its structure (anatomy). An approach to medicine first advocated in the mid-19th century by a number of German physicians and French physician Claude Bernard, it takes account of the biological systems of organisms at cellular, tissue, and whole-body levels.

A scientific approach

Physiology arguably began in 1628, when William Harvey published his findings on the circulation of the blood, deduced from meticulous experiments, yet the scientific approach to medicine was slow to evolve. It was dramatically bolstered by cell theory, the principle that all organisms are composed of units called cells, formulated by German botanist Matthias Schleiden and physician Theodor Schwann in 1838–1839. This paved the way for Johannes Müller, Justus von Liebig, and Carl Ludwig to put physiology on a sound experimental footing.

Justus von Liebig's laboratory at the University of Giessen, Germany, was one of the first purpose-built laboratories designed for teaching and research.

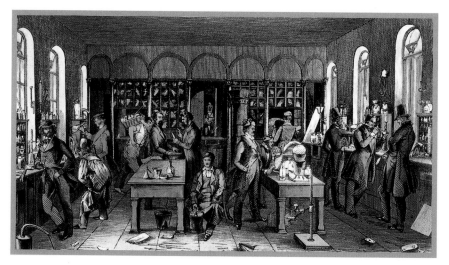

See also: Anatomy 60–63 ▪ Blood circulation 68–73 ▪ Histology 122–123
▪ Cellular pathology 134–135 ▪ Diabetes and its treatment 210–213

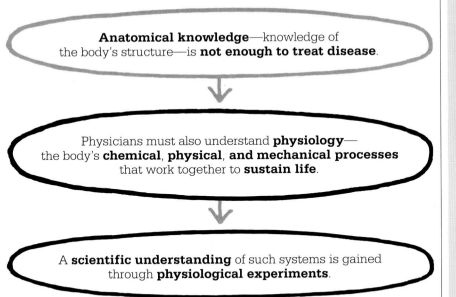

Anatomical knowledge—knowledge of the body's structure—is **not enough to treat disease**.

↓

Physicians must also understand **physiology**—the body's **chemical, physical, and mechanical processes** that work together to **sustain life**.

↓

A **scientific understanding** of such systems is gained through **physiological experiments**.

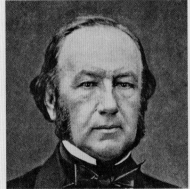

Claude Bernard

The son of a winegrower, Bernard was born in 1813 in Saint-Julien, a village in the Rhône department of eastern France. On leaving school, he became a pharmacist's apprentice and later enrolled at the Faculty of Medicine in Paris, graduating in 1843. Two years later, he entered a marriage of convenience with Marie Martin. Her dowry helped finance his scientific experiments, though she left him after he vivisected the family dog.

In 1847, Bernard was appointed deputy to François Magendie at the Collège de France, in Paris, succeeding him as full professor in 1855. In 1868, Bernard became professor of general physiology at the Museum of Natural History of the Jardin des Plantes and was admitted as a member of the Académie Française the same year. He died in Paris in 1878.

Key works

1865 *An Introduction to the Study of Experimental Medicine*
1878 *Lectures on the phenomena of Life Common to Animals and Plants*

Müller was particularly interested in the effect of stimuli on the sense organs and provided insights into the nerve pathways of reflex actions. Liebig and Ludwig made precise measurements of functions such as respiration and blood pressure and carried out chemical analyses of body fluids.

Experimental medicine

Claude Bernard was one of the founders of experimental medicine. He viewed test-tube experiments as being too limited and thought vivisection (or animated anatomy, as it was then called) was the only way to understand the complexities of organisms.

Bernard studied the effects of poisons such as carbon monoxide and curare on the body. He showed how carbon monoxide combined with hemoglobin in the blood causes oxygen starvation, and that curare attacks the motor nerves, causing paralysis and death, but has no effect on the sensory nerves. He also performed groundbreaking work on the role of the pancreas in digestion and the function of the liver as a store for glycogen, a starchy substance that can be broken down into glucose (sugar) if the body requires energy.

One of Bernard's most important insights was his concept of a *milieu intérieur* (internal environment), which describes the self-regulating mechanisms that keep the internal environment of an organism in equilibrium when the external environment is constantly changing. Developed in 1865, it describes the relationship between cells and their environment as being fundamental to the understanding of physiology. It is the underlying principle of what would be called homeostasis by American physiologist Walter B. Cannon in the 1920s. A small part of the lower front brain called the hypothalamus plays a key role in maintaining homeostasis. ▪

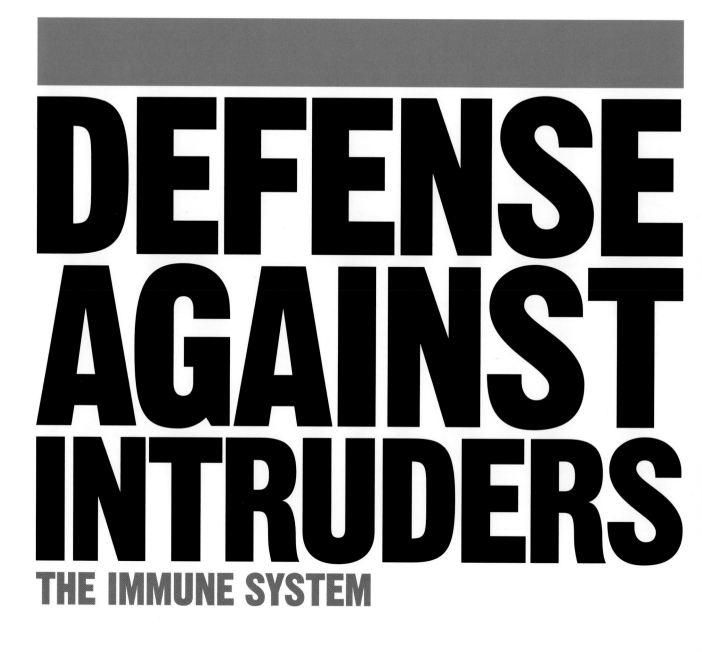

DEFENSE AGAINST INTRUDERS

THE IMMUNE SYSTEM

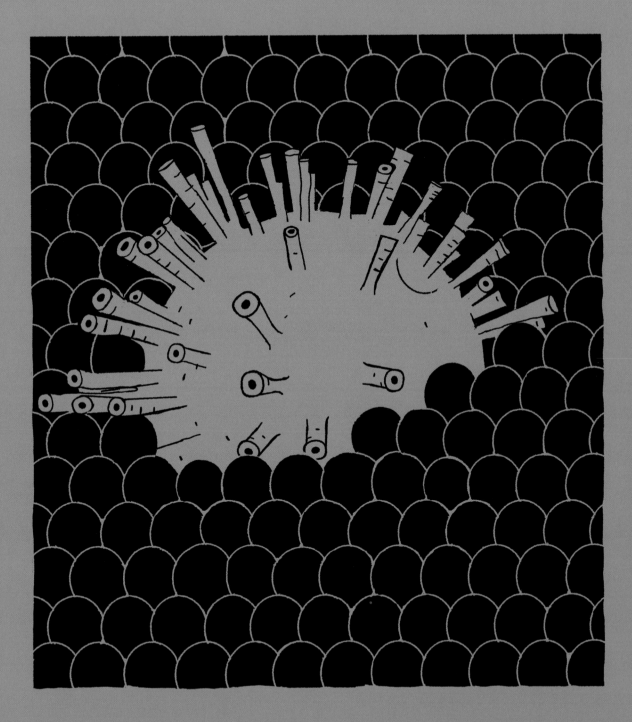

IN CONTEXT

BEFORE

c. 900 CE Al-Razi theorizes about how the body might become immune to smallpox.

1546 Girolamo Fracastoro suggests that the body gains immunity to smallpox through purification of the blood.

1796 Edward Jenner's vaccination gives people immunity to smallpox.

1861 Louis Pasteur publishes his germ theory, in which he argues that bacteria cause disease.

AFTER

2016 US-based researchers Matthew Halpert and Vanaja Konduri pin down the role of dendritic cells in working with T-helper cells.

2018 American and Japanese immunologists James P. Allison and Tasuku Honjo receive the Nobel Prize for their discovery of cancer therapy by inhibiting negative immune regulation.

> There is at bottom only one genuinely scientific treatment for all diseases and that is to stimulate the phagocytes.
> **George Bernard Shaw**
> **from Act I of his play *The Doctor's Dilemma*, 1906**

Doctors have long believed that the body has a way of protecting itself against disease. This protection came to be called immunity, but its nature remained a mystery. Since the 1880s, medical scientists such as Élie Metchnikoff, Paul Ehrlich, and Frank Macfarlane Burnet have gradually uncovered the immune system, a defense system of almost miraculous complexity.

The immune system defends the body in two main ways, using white blood cells (leukocytes) and a class of proteins called antibodies. First, there is the nonspecific "innate" system, on hand all the time to provide an immediate defense against germs and other foreign bodies. Then there is the specific "adaptive" (or acquired) system, which ramps up specifically to tackle a new threat and retains a memory of it to provide future immunity against that threat. Adaptive immunity is something only vertebrate animals have.

Once bitten, twice shy

Early physicians knew that people rarely catch smallpox twice. After one bout, they seemed immune to reinfection. Some believed it was God protecting the righteous, but there were scientific ideas, too. In the 9th century, Persian physician al-Razi suggested that smallpox pustules expel all the excess body moisture the disease would need to thrive a second time. In the 16th century, Italian doctor Girolamo Fracastoro suggested that smallpox was the final purification of toxic menstrual blood from birth and thought this might be why it seemed to attack children most.

No one knew how immunity worked, but it seemed real enough for many physicians to try inoculation—injecting diseased material into patients to stimulate immunity. British doctor Edward Jenner's breakthrough with vaccination in 1796 made the issue of immunity—to smallpox at least—beyond doubt.

Vaccination quickly spread, saving many lives, but it was still not clear how it worked. Nor could physicians work out whether the fever and inflammation that often followed infection damaged the body like a destructive fire, as some believed, or whether they were part of the body's defenses.

Germs and cells

Part of the problem was that no one even knew what caused disease. That changed in the 1870s, when Louis Pasteur and Robert Koch found that tiny microbes, or germs, are the culprits. Yet Pasteur and Koch believed the body is ultimately defenseless against them. Then, in 1882, Élie Metchnikoff, a Russian physician living in Sicily, heard that Koch had discovered the bacteria that caused tuberculosis (TB).

Metchnikoff wondered why his wife had contracted TB while he seemed immune. He knew that

---

> The physician of the future will be an immunizator.
> **Almroth Wright**
> **Inaugural address at St. Mary's Hospital, London, 1905**

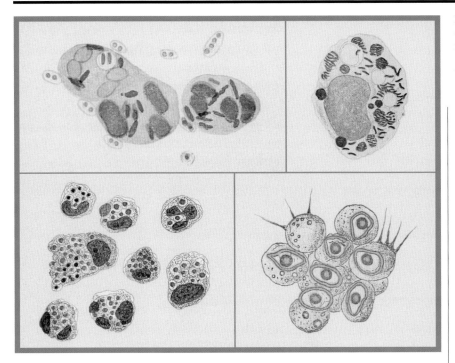

Élie Metchnikoff made these drawings of phagocytosis, the process in which a type of white blood cell called a phagocyte changes shape to engulf and destroy a pathogen.

white blood cells gather at infection sites. In fact, microorganisms were sometimes seen inside white blood cells. The prevailing theory was that white blood cells spread disease around the body, but Metchnikoff wondered whether the massing white blood cells were a sign of the body defending itself.

To test his idea, Metchnikoff pricked starfish larvae with rose thorns. Under a microscope, he saw white blood cells gathering around the thorn. He quickly developed the theory that certain white blood cells attack, engulf, and destroy germs. He called these cells "phagocytes," from the Greek for "eating cells." These white blood cells, he argued, were not spreading germs at all, but fighting the infection.

Metchnikoff went on to suggest that inflammation was part of the body's innate immune system, drawing phagocytes to the site of infection. He also distinguished between larger phagocytes, called macrophages, and smaller ones—microphages, now called neutrophils.

Battle of beliefs

Although Metchnikoff received the Nobel Prize in Physiology or Medicine in 1908, his ideas met with skepticism at first. He became caught in a war between scientists who took up his idea of cellular immunity involving phagocytes and those who insisted immunity is humoral (provided by molecules in body fluids). The word "humoral" came from the ancient idea that illness stemmed from an imbalance in four different kinds of body fluid,

Emil von Behring found that serum from infected animals such as horses contained antitoxins. The diphtheria antitoxin was used to protect humans until a vaccine was created in the 1920s.

or "humors." The battle line was drawn between the humoral camp in Germany and the cellular camp in France, where Metchnikoff was now working at the Pasteur Institute in Paris.

For a while, the German camp made the most progress. In 1890, Emil von Behring, aided by Japanese researcher Shibasaburo Kitasato, reported that serum (blood fluid) from animals infected with tetanus or diphtheria contains chemicals, or "antitoxins," that work against toxins released by bacteria. They also found that these antitoxins could be used to immunize or even cure another animal. Behring's work reinforced the idea that just as the causes of disease are specific, so are the body's defenses. He went on to play a major role in the development of vaccines.

Meanwhile, another German, Paul Ehrlich, was teasing out the importance of antigens and antibodies. Antigens are any »

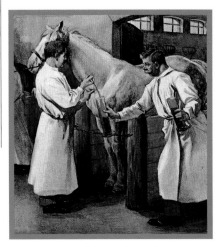

substance that provokes an immune response in the body. (These were later found to include cancer cells and foreign tissue, as well as germs.) Antibodies, or immunoglobulins, are proteins that can inactivate or weaken germs, and each one is matched to a particular antigen.

Key to the puzzle

In 1900, Ehrlich refined his "side-chain" theory, which describes how antigens and antibodies interact like lock and key. Antibodies form receptors called side-chains on the surface of white blood cells. When an antigen locks on to its matching side-chain, the cell releases floods of antibodies, which then lock on to the toxin and neutralize it.

Ehrlich suggested developing new kinds of drugs that mimicked antibodies—"magic bullets" that could hunt down and destroy particular pathogens (disease-causing microbes). This led to the creation of Salvarsan, the first drug effective against syphilis. Even more importantly, Ehrlich's theory showed how inoculation protects the body by triggering a surge of unique antibodies against the disease. This launched the ongoing search for new vaccines, which have become the key lifesaving weapon against infectious diseases.

Building on the work of fellow German Hans Buchner and Belgian scientist Jules Bordet (based at the Pasteur Institute in France), Ehrlich

also described the "complement" system—so-called because it works alongside the antibody system. When this is activated—for example, by a pathogen—a cascade of proteins is released (mainly from the liver) into the bloodstream and fluids around cells. These proteins cause invading cells to burst (lysis) and encourage phagocytes to ingest them, as well as stimulating the inflammation that draws infection-fighting white blood cells in.

It had been assumed that there was a neat division in immunity, with cells providing the crude innate first defense, while the clever adaptive immunity targeted at specific germs was chemical or "humoral." Yet the complement

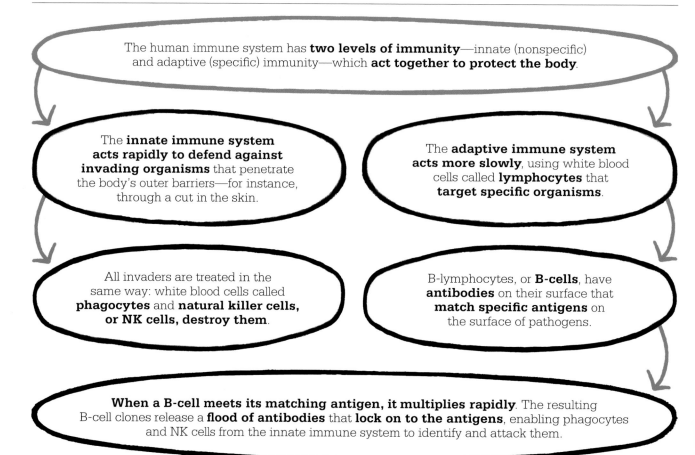

The human immune system has **two levels of immunity**—innate (nonspecific) and adaptive (specific) immunity—which **act together to protect the body**.

The **innate immune system acts rapidly to defend against invading organisms** that penetrate the body's outer barriers—for instance, through a cut in the skin.

The **adaptive immune system acts more slowly**, using white blood cells called **lymphocytes** that **target specific organisms**.

All invaders are treated in the same way: white blood cells called **phagocytes** and **natural killer cells, or NK cells, destroy them**.

B-lymphocytes, or **B-cells**, have **antibodies** on their surface that **match specific antigens** on the surface of pathogens.

When a B-cell meets its matching antigen, it multiplies rapidly. The resulting B-cell clones release a **flood of antibodies** that **lock on to the antigens**, enabling phagocytes and NK cells from the innate immune system to identify and attack them.

The white blood cells (orange) in this illustration are in attack mode, secreting antibodies (white) that bind to the invading antigens (blue), weakening them or marking them for destruction.

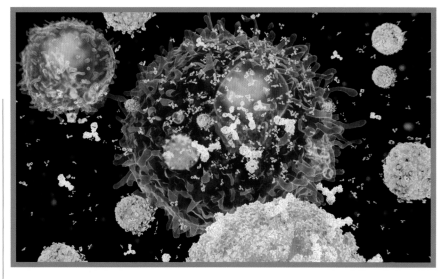

system was not only untargeted and innate but humoral, too, so there was no such neat division.

Over the next few decades, British scientist Almroth Wright cast further doubt on the cellular-humoral division. Some bacteria can naturally evade phagocytosis, but Wright showed that antibodies help phagocytes identify them.

Self-defense

The great breakthrough came in the 1940s and 1950s, when failures with transplant surgery led to the discovery that the immune system does not just fight germs; it also helps the body recognize cells that are foreign. Every body cell has its own personal identity marker, or HLA (human leukocyte antigen). British scientist Peter Medawar and Australian scientist Frank Macfarlane Burnet realized that the immune system identifies foreign cells and fights them. This was why transplants were being rejected.

Burnet went on to lay out how the body learns to identify foreigners. If a foreign substance is introduced into the embryo early on, its antigens are accepted by the body as "self," and no antibodies against it are produced later in life. In this way, the body actively identifies its own but attacks invaders ("nonself").

Burnet and others began to draw the picture of the immune system together, returning cells, not humoral chemistry, to center stage. They discovered that besides the phagocytes, which swallow invaders indiscriminately, the body is armed with an array of white blood cells that can identify and target, called lymphocytes.

Clonal selection

In 1957, Burnet introduced his groundbreaking "clonal selection" theory. This involved an array of lymphocytes now known as B-cells, because they were first discovered in the bursa organ in birds. Each B-cell, Burnet suggested, is primed to identify the antigen of a particular invader. Whenever a B-cell meets »

Frank Macfarlane Burnet

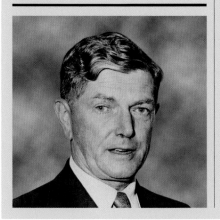

Born in Traralgon, Australia, in 1899, Frank Macfarlane Burnet took an interest in biology from a young age, collecting beetles. After graduating with a medical degree from the University of Melbourne, he studied in London, UK, then returned to Melbourne to work in medical research.

Although his experiments on viruses that attack bacteria and animals, especially influenza, led to major discoveries, Burnet is best known for his achievements in immunology—in particular, his theory of acquired immunological tolerance, for which he was awarded the Nobel Prize in 1960, and his clonal selection theory. Later in life, he lectured and wrote extensively about human biology, aging, and cancer. He died in 1985.

Key works

1940 *Biological Aspects of Infectious Disease*
1949 *The Production of Antibodies* (with Frank Fenner)
1959 *The Clonal Selection Theory of Acquired Immunity*
1969 *Cellular Immunology*

its corresponding antigen, it clones itself, multiplying rapidly. As the B-cell clones multiply, they release a flow of antibodies. These latch on to the invaders so that the body's innate defenses—including phagocytes and another type of lymphocyte called "natural killer" (NK) cells—can recognize and attack them. In 1958, Austrian-Australian immunologist Gustav Nossal and American biologist Joshua Lederberg proved Burnet right, showing that each B-cell only produces one kind of antibody.

Filling in the gaps

In 1959, British immunologist James Gowans discovered that lymphocytes can migrate around the body and that they circulate through both the blood and the lymph system. The lymph system is the body's drain, carrying away toxins and the debris from the first scuffles between phagocytes and germs. The system also includes hundreds of lymph nodes, where clusters of lymphocytes check for antigens "presented" by passing phagocytes and other kinds of cells.

The same year, French-born scientist Jacques Miller found that one group of lymphocytes migrated

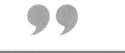

> It will be obvious that this attempt at a comprehensive discussion of antibody production is hampered in all directions by lack of knowledge.
> **Frank Macfarlane Burnet**
> *The Production of Antibodies*, 1949

away from bone marrow to mature in the thymus gland just above the heart. It was later discovered that these thymus-maturing cells, or T-cells, play a crucial role in fighting viruses, which evade B-cells.

Meanwhile, back in 1959, two chemists, Rodney Porter in the UK and Gerald Edelman in the US, discovered the Y-shaped molecular structure of antibodies. In 1975, German immunologist Georges Köhler and Argentine César Milstein described a technique for producing

"monoclonal antibodies," which (like Ehrlich's magic bullets) could be used to target specific antigens or test for the presence of them.

Despite these advances, it was still unclear how the body can create such a mind-blowing variety of antibodies, vastly outnumbering the genes that produce them. In 1976, Japanese scientist Susumu Tonegawa showed how this is done by the shuffling of genes within a cell when it is developing into an antibody-producing B-cell.

Helpers and killers

By the early 1980s, researchers knew a great deal more about how B-cells and T-cells collaborate to provide adaptive immunity. In essence, there are two responses.

Humoral immunity targets pathogens that circulate freely in the body, such as bacteria, mainly using floods of antibodies. The sequence starts with T-cells called "helpers." There is a T-helper (Th) for each antigen. When a Th meets its match, it locks on and multiplies, triggering B-cells with matching antibodies to multiply and split into plasma cells and memory cells. Plasma cells pump out a stream of antibodies, which bind to the germ

---

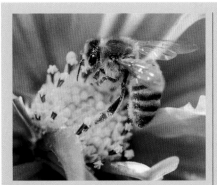

Stings from insects such as bees and wasps can cause a severe anaphylactic reaction in a small number of people.

Hypersensitivity

Sometimes, the immune system overreacts, with damaging consequences. As early as 1902, French clinician Charles Richet showed that "hypersensitivity"—an overproduction of antibodies in response to an antigen—could be harmful, leading to excessive inflammation or worse. Allergies are one reaction of this kind.

Several years later, Richet identified "anaphylaxis"—an allergic reaction so extreme it can be life-threatening. When some

people ingest nuts, for example, their innate immune system goes into overdrive, giving them symptoms such as shortness of breath and low blood pressure. Anaphylaxis can be fatal within just a few minutes, so people with severe allergies carry an adrenaline auto-injector at all times. Adrenaline is a hormone produced in response to stress, and it reverses the effects of anaphylaxis. Antihistamines or steroids that suppress the immune system are also used to treat allergies.

Immune responses

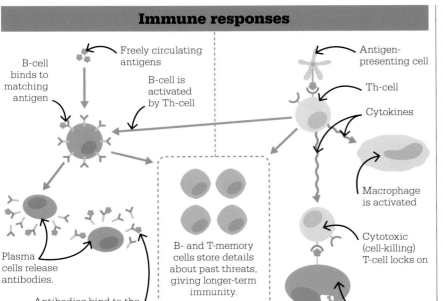

B-cell binds to matching antigen

Freely circulating antigens

B-cell is activated by Th-cell

Antigen-presenting cell

Th-cell

Cytokines

Macrophage is activated

Plasma cells release antibodies.

B- and T-memory cells store details about past threats, giving longer-term immunity.

Cytotoxic (cell-killing) T-cell locks on

Antibodies bind to the invading antigens, inactivating them.

Infected cell is destroyed

In humoral immunity, antigen-specific antibodies are produced to destroy extracellular pathogens. A B-cell binds to its matching antigen, aided by a T-helper (Th) cell. The B-cell then multiplies rapidly, producing plasma cells and memory cells.

Cell-mediated immunity targets germs within cells, such as viruses. A Th-cell is exposed to an antigen on the surface of an infected cell. Cytokines are then released, activating cytotoxic T-cells, which (along with macrophages) destroy infected cells.

and neutralize it, make it burst, or make it a target for phagocytes. Memory cells store information about the germ, so the body can react quickly to repeat infections.

Cell-mediated immunity, on the other hand, is directed against pathogens such as viruses that invade and take over cells. This is where T-cells come into their own. When a virus invades a cell, it leaves telltale antigens on the outside. When Th-cells find these antigens, they release signaling proteins called cytokines. In turn, the cytokines activate cytotoxic (cell-killing) T-cells, which bind to an infected cell's identity tag (called the major histocompatibility complex or MHC). Once locked on, cytotoxic T-cells flood the infected

cell with chemicals to kill it, virus and all. Occasionally, the T-helpers were found to overreact and produce uncontrolled floods of cytokines. These "cytokine storms" cause such severe inflammation that it can be fatal. They are a disturbing complication in viral epidemics such as the COVID-19 pandemic.

Linking the systems

In 1989, American immunologist Charles Janeway brought attention back to the innate system with his theory that certain cells, such as

After detecting an invading virus, a T-helper cell (center) releases cytokines (bottom; top left). These are interleukins, part of a family of cytokines that also includes interferons and chemokines.

macrophages (large phagocytes) and dendritic cells (tiny immune cells in the skin and linings of the airways and guts), have special receptors that enable them to detect molecular patterns produced by pathogens. These toll-like receptors (TLRs) can distinguish between "pathogen-associated molecular patterns" (PAMPs), which signify disease-bringers, and "damage-associated molecular patterns" (DAMPs), which are found on damaged or dying host cells. Macrophages and dendritic cells then "present" antigens to Th-cells—thus linking the innate and adaptive immune systems.

Prevention and cure

Since Metchnikoff's discovery of phagocytes, scientists have made vast progress in understanding the immune system. Immunologists have revealed an incredibly complex interlocking system of cells and proteins that work together to fight disease. There still remains a great deal to discover, but what has been learned so far has revealed the way in which the body defends itself against myriads of germs. It has also provided a whole new range of possibilities for both prevention, through more precise vaccination and other methods, and also cure, through drugs that work in tandem with the body's own defenses. ∎

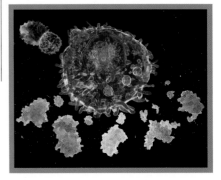

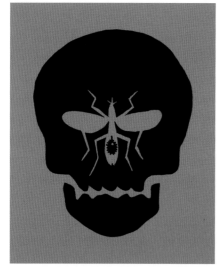

A SINGLE MOSQUITO BITE IS ALL IT TAKES

MALARIA

The causes of malaria and other insect-borne diseases were a mystery in the ancient world. For centuries, most people thought that "miasmas"—noxious vapors in the air—were to blame. The word malaria reflects this belief, as it stems from the old Italian term *mal'aria* (bad air). In Europe, miasmas were associated with the air circulating over fetid swamps and marshes, where local people were frequently infected.

In the 18th century, Italian clinician Giovanni Maria Lancisi proposed that insects might be involved in the transmission of malaria. Finally, in the 1880s, French physician Alphonse Laveran identified the specific organism responsible for malaria, carried by mosquitoes.

The mosquito vector
As early as 30 BCE, Roman scholar Marcus Terentius Varro suggested that, in marshy areas, minuscule creatures floating in the air entered the body through the mouth and nose, causing disease. The idea had little support until 1717, when Lancisi published *De Noxiis Paludum Effluviis* (*On the Noxious Effluvia of Marshes*). Like Varro, Lancisi thought that tiny organisms might cause malaria. He suggested that mosquitoes transmitted them to humans via the small incisions made when they bite. Although his theory was correct, Lancisi was unable to test and prove his ideas.

By the mid-19th century, the germ theory of disease was taking hold. Louis Pasteur in France and Joseph Lister in Britain had both demonstrated that infection is caused by living organisms.

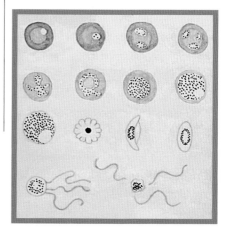

Laveran's drawing of the life stages of malaria parasites (from the lowest row upward, as they develop in blood) appeared in 1881 in the bulletin of the Société Médicale des Hôpitaux de Paris.

See also: Greek medicine 28–29 ▪ Roman medicine 38–43 ▪ Germ theory 138–145 ▪ Antibiotics 216–223 ▪ Global eradication of disease 286–287

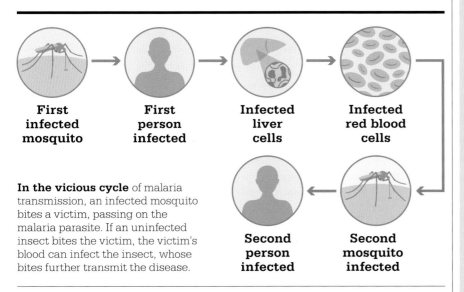

In the vicious cycle of malaria transmission, an infected mosquito bites a victim, passing on the malaria parasite. If an uninfected insect bites the victim, the victim's blood can infect the insect, whose bites further transmit the disease.

First infected mosquito → First person infected → Infected liver cells → Infected red blood cells → Second mosquito infected → Second person infected

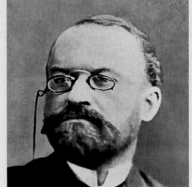

Alphonse Laveran

Born in Paris in 1845, Charles Louis Alphonse Laveran studied medicine and became a military physician, serving as a surgeon during the Franco-Prussian War of 1870. Ten years later, while working at the military hospital in Constantine, Algeria, he identified the malaria parasite.

Between 1884 and 1894, he was professor of military hygiene at the Val-de-Grâce military hospital in Paris, and later worked at the Institut Pasteur. He became a fellow of the Académie des Sciences, was awarded the Légion d'honneur, and was elected a fellow of the Royal Society. In 1907, he received the Nobel Prize in Physiology or Medicine for his discoveries of parasitic protozoans as agents of infectious disease. He died in 1922 after a brief illness.

Key works

1875 *Treatise on diseases and epidemics of the armed forces*
1881 *Parasitic nature of malaria accidents*
1884 "Treatise on Marsh Fevers"

In 1880, Laveran was examining a blood specimen from a malaria patient in Algeria, using a powerful microscope when he noticed crescent-shaped bodies moving energetically beside the red blood cells. He realized he had found the parasite that caused malaria and identified the bodies as protozoa rather than bacteria (which are smaller and, unlike protozoa, have no nucleus). When Laveran failed to find the parasite in the air, water, and soil of marshland, he began to suspect it was carried in the body of mosquitoes, which he proposed in his 1884 "Treatise on Marsh Fevers."

Scientists who believed that a bacterium caused malaria were skeptical of Laveran's new idea, so Laveran invited Pasteur to examine the organism; Pasteur was instantly convinced. In 1885, Italian zoologists Ettore Marchiafava and Angelo Celli classified the parasite in a new *Plasmodium* genus. Finally, in 1897, British physician Ronald Ross demonstrated the presence of the parasite in the stomach of an *Anopheles* species mosquito.

Scientists now know that females of 30 to 40 *Anopheles* species can carry the *Plasmodium* parasite. As the female bites to get blood to nurture her eggs, the parasite enters the victim's blood, then infects the liver and red blood cells. Uninfected mosquitoes that then bite the victim become *Plasmodium* carriers (vectors) and continue the spread of malaria.

Quest for an antidote

Malaria and other mosquito-borne diseases (such as the Zika, dengue, yellow fever, and West Nile viruses) remained deadly throughout the 20th century and still cause more than a million deaths a year. There are now effective vaccines for a few mosquito-borne diseases, and research is ongoing to develop more. The World Mosquito Program is breeding mosquitoes to carry the harmless bacteria *Wolbachia*, which affects the ability of some mosquito-borne viruses to reproduce and so reduces their transmission by mosquitoes. However, the quest for a similar means to combat malaria continues. ∎

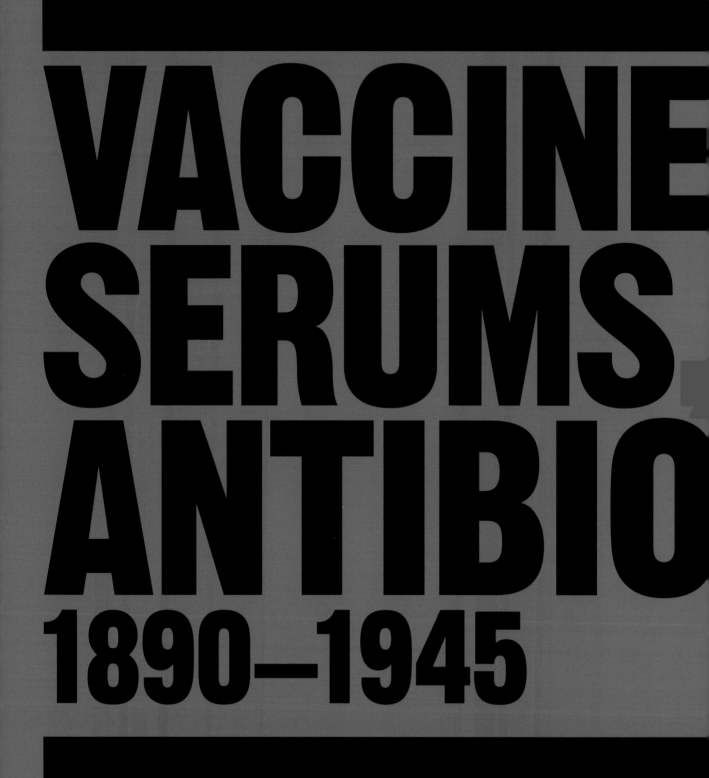

VACCINE
SERUMS
ANTIBIO
1890–1945

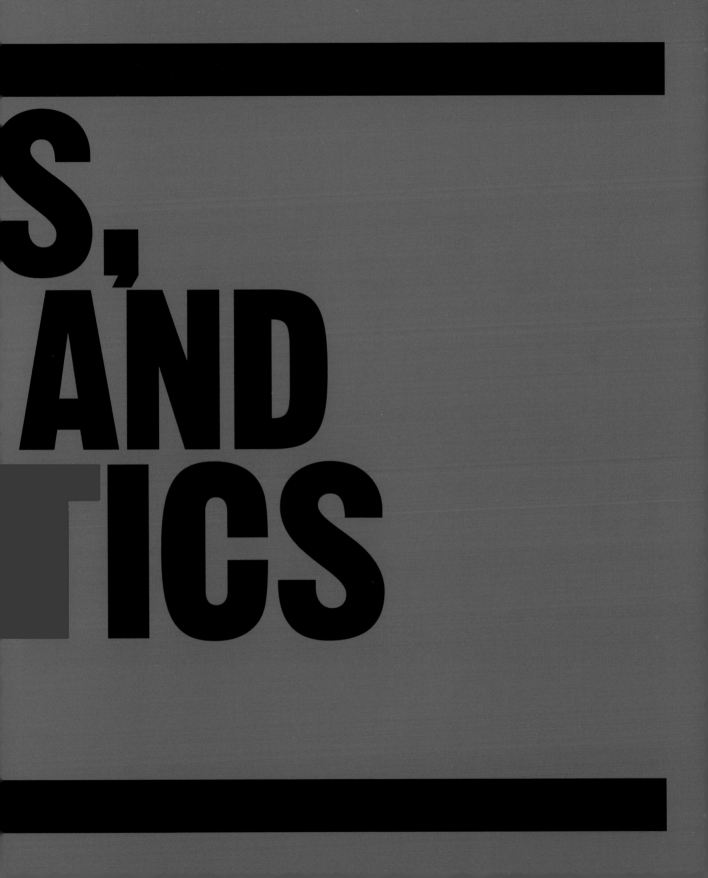

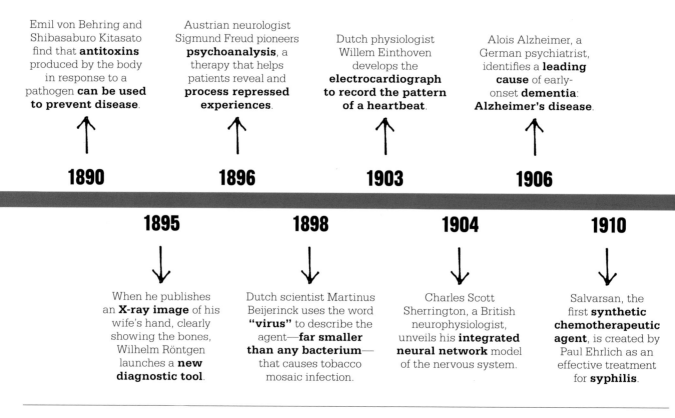

Emil von Behring and Shibasaburo Kitasato find that **antitoxins** produced by the body in response to a pathogen **can be used to prevent disease**.

Austrian neurologist Sigmund Freud pioneers **psychoanalysis**, a therapy that helps patients reveal and **process repressed experiences**.

Dutch physiologist Willem Einthoven develops the **electrocardiograph to record the pattern of a heartbeat**.

Alois Alzheimer, a German psychiatrist, identifies a **leading cause** of early-onset **dementia: Alzheimer's disease**.

1890　　**1896**　　**1903**　　**1906**

1895　　**1898**　　**1904**　　**1910**

When he publishes an **X-ray image** of his wife's hand, clearly showing the bones, Wilhelm Röntgen launches a **new diagnostic tool**.

Dutch scientist Martinus Beijerinck uses the word **"virus"** to describe the agent—**far smaller than any bacterium**—that causes tobacco mosaic infection.

Charles Scott Sherrington, a British neurophysiologist, unveils his **integrated neural network** model of the nervous system.

Salvarsan, the first **synthetic chemotherapeutic agent**, is created by Paul Ehrlich as an effective treatment for **syphilis**.

In the last decade of the 19th century, infectious diseases such as the flu and tuberculosis killed millions every year. In the US, life expectancy was just 44 years in 1890. Despite earlier advances in microscopy and anesthesia, and an understanding of germ theory and the cellular basis of disease, there remained much to discover about how the body works and what causes it to go wrong. In addition, the pathogens responsible for many diseases were still unknown. By 1945, physicians had acquired new tools to prevent and treat disease.

War on pathogens
German physiologist Emil von Behring and Japanese physician Shibasaburo Kitasato made a breakthrough in 1890 in the hunt for new ways to fight pathogens.

They found that the blood serum of animals infected with diphtheria contains a chemical, or "antitoxin," that works against bacterial toxins. By injecting the antitoxin into another animal, they could cure the disease. "Serotherapy" became a lifesaver for many people who had contracted diphtheria, although the search continued for a vaccine to prevent infection in the first place.

Behring and Kitasato's work inspired German scientist Paul Ehrlich to find a "magic bullet" to fight disease. Ehrlich noticed that some chemical dyes attach only to certain pathogenic cells and theorized that antitoxins work in the same way to target specific pathogens. After years of research, he discovered that the synthetic compound arsphenamine targeted and killed the bacteria responsible

for syphilis and launched the first chemotherapeutic drug (Salvarsan) in 1910 to treat the disease.

Prevention and cure
Gradually, vaccines were found for the deadly diseases of cholera, tetanus, whooping cough, bubonic plague, and yellow fever. In 1921, French scientists Albert Calmette and Camille Guérin developed the first live attenuated (weakened) vaccine against tuberculosis (TB)—the BCG vaccine. Another live attenuated vaccine soon followed—this time, against diphtheria.

In 1928, Scottish bacteriologist Alexander Fleming accidentally discovered that *Penicillium* fungus kills *Staphylococcus* bacteria, which cause many infections. As a result, penicillin became the first naturally occurring antibiotic to be used

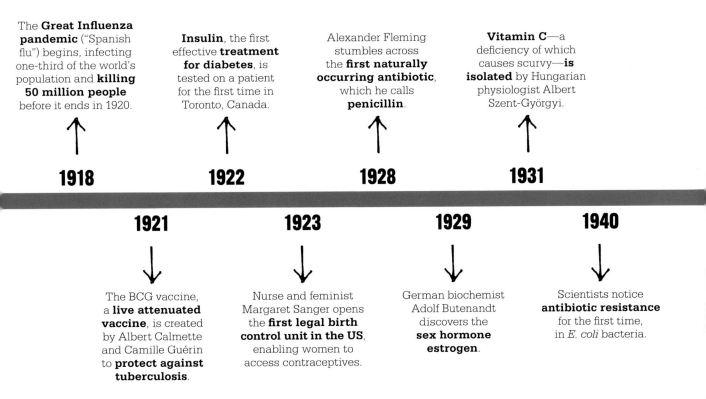

The **Great Influenza pandemic** ("Spanish flu") begins, infecting one-third of the world's population and **killing 50 million people** before it ends in 1920.

Insulin, the first effective **treatment for diabetes**, is tested on a patient for the first time in Toronto, Canada.

Alexander Fleming stumbles across the **first naturally occurring antibiotic**, which he calls **penicillin**.

Vitamin C—a deficiency of which causes scurvy—**is isolated** by Hungarian physiologist Albert Szent-Györgyi.

1918   **1922**   **1928**   **1931**

1921   **1923**   **1929**   **1940**

The BCG vaccine, a **live attenuated vaccine**, is created by Albert Calmette and Camille Guérin to **protect against tuberculosis**.

Nurse and feminist Margaret Sanger opens the **first legal birth control unit in the US**, enabling women to access contraceptives.

German biochemist Adolf Butenandt discovers the **sex hormone estrogen**.

Scientists notice **antibiotic resistance** for the first time, in *E. coli* bacteria.

therapeutically. In 1945, 6.8 trillion units were produced in the US. It was the first of many antibiotics, which have saved millions of lives.

Vaccines and antibiotics aside, the fight against pathogens was often untargeted, especially in the case of cancer. The X-ray machine, invented by German physicist Wilhelm Röntgen in 1895, was a crucial tool in the diagnosis and treatment of trauma, and X-rays were also used by many doctors to attack cancer tumors—but this radiation therapy killed healthy as well as cancerous cells. It was not until 1942 that American pharmacologists Louis Goodman and Alfred Gilman produced the first chemical treatment for cancer—nitrogen mustard injected into the blood to kill cancerous cells. The next year, Greek American physician George

Papanicolaou published the results of his research into screening for cervical cancer. By the 1950s, the "Pap smear" test was being used widely in the US. The battle against cancer was at last underway.

Understanding the body

At the start of the 20th century, scientists believed that organs communicated with each other using electrical signals carried by nerves. However, in 1902, British physiologists Ernest Starling and William Bayliss demonstrated that some communication was chemical, in the form of secretions from the pancreas into the bloodstream. The discipline of endocrinology was born, and these chemicals, or hormones, and the endocrine glands that produce them were gradually identified. One hormone, insulin,

was found to regulate blood sugar levels, and in 1922, a patient with diabetes was treated with insulin for the first time.

Physicians had long known the cause of scurvy, the deadliest deficiency disease. In 1912, Polish-born biochemist Casimir Funk described the preventative role of vitamins. By the late 1940s, all the essential vitamins were known.

New ways of "reading" the body, such as the electrocardiograph and electroencephalogram, also helped clinicians make faster diagnoses and save more lives. By 1945, life expectancy in the US had leapt to 65 years. But medicine faced new challenges. Bacterial resistance to antibiotics had been detected, and changing lifestyles created different problems, including widespread obesity and new forms of cancer. ∎

SOLVING THE PUZZLE OF CANCER

CANCER THERAPY

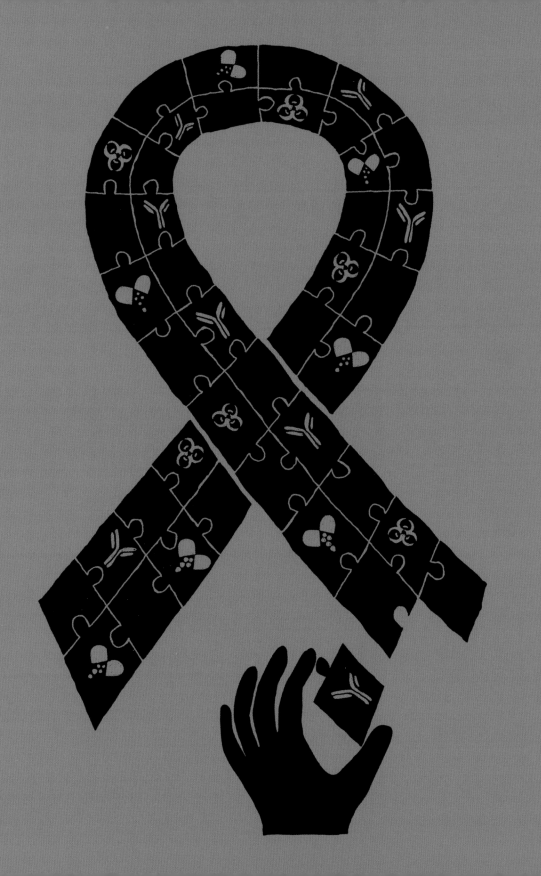

IN CONTEXT

BEFORE

c. 17th century BCE Egypt's Edwin Smith papyrus details the cauterization of cancers.

c. 1000 CE Al-Zahrawi removes a breast tumor surgically.

1871 Campbell de Morgan discovers how cancers spread.

AFTER

1932 Scientists discover a way to measure radiation therapy doses accurately.

1947 Sidney Farber uses aminopterin to halt the spread of leukemia in children.

1975 César Milstein and Georges Köhler find a way to stimulate the production of immune system antibodies.

1976 Harald zur Hausen proposes that cervical cancer is caused by a virus.

2002 Cancer immunologists find a way to "arm" T-cells to seek and destroy cancer cells.

> Nature often gives us hints to her profoundest secrets, and … may lead us on to the solution of this difficult problem.
> **William Coley**
> *Contribution to the knowledge of sarcoma, 1891*

In 1890, American surgeon William Coley was deeply affected by the experience of treating a young woman with a malignant tumor in her hand. With no effective therapies available, he was forced to amputate her forearm, but within a few weeks she died because the cancer had already spread to other parts of her body.

Eager to find an alternative treatment, Coley searched hospital records and found an intriguing case. A patient treated for a neck tumor several years before had suffered a severe postoperative skin infection that had almost killed him—a common occurrence before the invention of antibiotics. When Coley traced the patient, he found the man no longer had any evidence of cancer. Coley found similar cases in the medical records and surmised (wrongly) that bacterial infections can release toxins that attack malignant tissue.

In 1891, when Coley injected live *Streptococcus* bacteria into a patient who had only weeks to live, the patient made a full recovery and lived for eight years. Coley continued experimenting but was forced to switch from live to dead bacteria after several patients died from the infection he had given them. He persisted for 30 years, treating more than 1,000 people, and achieved a high rate of lasting remissions. Through his work, Coley discovered a link between administering what became known as "Coley's toxins" and a reduction in tumor size.

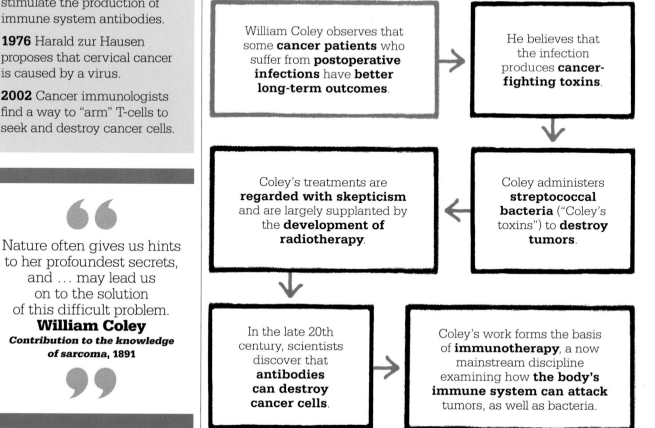

William Coley observes that some **cancer patients** who suffer from **postoperative infections** have **better long-term outcomes**.

He believes that the infection produces **cancer-fighting toxins**.

Coley administers **streptococcal bacteria** ("Coley's toxins") to **destroy tumors**.

Coley's treatments are **regarded with skepticism** and are largely supplanted by the **development of radiotherapy**.

In the late 20th century, scientists discover that **antibodies can destroy cancer cells**.

Coley's work forms the basis of **immunotherapy**, a now mainstream discipline examining how **the body's immune system can attack** tumors, as well as bacteria.

While Coley was convinced his treatment was valid, the medical establishment disagreed. His methods were questioned by the American Cancer Society, and in 1894, the American Medical Association described them as an "alleged remedy." When radiation therapy was discovered around the same time, Coley's therapy was largely dropped and did not become a standard cancer treatment.

However, Coley's work left a legacy. Modern cancer research shows that some tumors are sensitive to an enhanced immunity, so when a body's immune system attacks invasive bacteria, it can also attack tumors. This cancer immunotherapy, which began to be used in the late 1990s, was foreshadowed by Coley's work.

Early cancer treatments

The catastrophic effects of cancer have been known since at least ancient Egyptian times. Breast cancer was described in the Edwin Smith papyrus, one of the oldest medical texts, dating from c. 17th

century BCE. Later, the ancient Greek physician Hippocrates cited several varieties of cancer in the 5th century BCE, and Roman medical writer Aulus Celsus described the excision of breast tumors with a knife in the 1st century CE. Al-Zahrawi, the great surgeon of Islam's Golden Age, detailed the removal of breast tumors in his medical encyclopedia, the *Kitab al-Tasrif*, around 1000 CE.

The Edwin Smith papyrus—the oldest known scientific text that promotes rational observation of injury and disease—gives evidence of cancer patients as early as c. 17th century BCE.

The 17th century saw the invention of a practical microscope, which enabled physicians to examine the human body at a cellular level. The advent of general anesthesia in 1846 was a further breakthrough, allowing for far more radical and invasive surgery to search for and remove more tumors.

In 1894, American surgeon William Halsted pioneered radical tissue removal, which many others emulated—but in their efforts to remove every secondary tumor, surgeons often cut out parts of organs, muscle, and bone. Patients were left disfigured, and the cancer had often already spread unseen. Survival from cancer is now understood to be more closely related to how much the cancer has spread before surgery than how much tissue is removed during the surgical procedure. »

William Coley

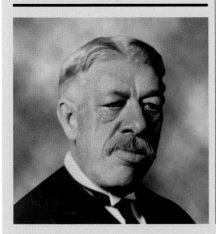

Often described as the "Father of cancer immunology," William Coley was born in Connecticut in 1862. He graduated from the Harvard Medical School in 1888 and worked as a surgical intern at New York Hospital.

Coley realized the limitations of surgery as a cancer treatment and became convinced that an alternative involved stimulating the body's immune system to fight cancer. His bacteria-based "Coley's toxins" were used to treat various forms of cancer, in the US and overseas, but were widely criticized and gradually

faded from view. Coley died in 1936, but his clinical contribution is remembered in the annual William B. Coley Award, presented by the US Cancer Research Institute to major contributors to tumor immunology research.

Key works

1891 *Contribution to the knowledge of sarcoma*
1893 "The treatment of malignant tumors by repeated inoculations of erysipelas"

In the late 19th century, British surgeon Campbell de Morgan demonstrated the first genuine understanding of how cancer works. He explained the process of metastasis—the spread of cancer from a primary tumor through lymph nodes to other sites in the body. Crucially, de Morgan noted the practical relevance of this: when cancer is discovered, it should be treated immediately, before the tumor spreads any further.

Radiation therapy

X-rays were discovered in 1895, and just a year later, American surgeon Emil Grubbe used them to treat a breast cancer patient. Although it was not understood at the time, radiation works by disabling the DNA that allows cells to divide. In the first decade of the 20th century, radiation therapy (or radiotherapy) was used mainly to treat skin cancers. In 1900, Swedish physicist Thor Stenbeck used small daily doses of radiation to cure a skin

A patient receives cobalt-60 radiotherapy to treat cancer. Cobalt-60 was developed during the 1950s and widely used to deliver radiotherapy externally via a beam of gamma rays.

cancer, and this procedure was adopted by others. Unfortunately, radiation also kills the genetic material of healthy cells—a major problem before accurate targeting became possible. It can also *cause* cancer, as many early radiologists found to their cost. Many would test the strength of the radiation on their own arms before treating a patient without realizing the damage it was doing to them. Overall, early radiation treatment had inconsistent results, and the side effects on healthy tissues were often worse than the benefits.

Radiation targeting techniques increased during the 20th century. Modern radiotherapy may be delivered externally or internally—the former by a beam directed at a tumor and the latter either by a source implanted near the tumor or by a liquid source injected into the bloodstream. There are several varieties of external delivery. Conformal radiation therapy (CRT) uses computerized tomography (CT) imaging to precisely map a tumor in 3D. The tumor is then blasted by radiation from several angles, and the direction and intensity of the rays can be adjusted. 3D-CRT was developed to customize

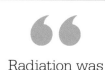

> Radiation was a powerful invisible knife, but still a knife. And a knife, no matter how deft or penetrating, could only reach so far in the battle against cancer.
> **Siddhartha Mukherjee**
> **Indian American oncologist (1970–)**

the delivery of individual radiation beams to the shape of each tumor. Another variety is conformal proton beam radiation therapy, which uses positively charged subatomic particles called protons instead of X-rays. Whereas even targeted X-rays can damage healthy tissues, protons deliver less of a radiation dose to these surrounding tissues while still attacking the tumor.

Chemotherapy

In late 1942, American research pharmacologists Louis Goodman and Alfred Gilman experimented with the medicinal effects of nitrogen mustard. This agent of chemical warfare was used to make mustard gas, which had been deployed to deadly effect in World War I. It is a cytotoxic compound, meaning that it is harmful to cells. Goodman and Gilman knew that it killed lymphocytes (a type of white blood cell) and administered it via intravenous injections to terminally ill blood cancer patients who hadn't responded to radiotherapy. The treatment temporarily eliminated

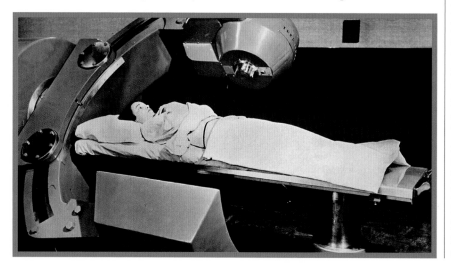

cancerous lymphocytes and, while they later returned, this therapy represented a major breakthrough in treating cancer. Developed through trial and error, the age of chemotherapy had dawned.

In the 1940s, aware that folic acid could have positive effects on some anemia sufferers, American pathologist Sidney Farber tried administering it to child leukemia patients. When it worsened their condition, he changed tack. Farber realized that to divide rapidly, cancer cells depend on folic acid—if deprived of it, they would die. In one of the first examples of drug design (rather than accidental discovery), Farber created two synthetic compounds, aminopterin and amethopterin (later called methotrexate), both analogs of folic acid.

An analog chemical has a structure that is similar to another but differs sufficiently to interfere with cell function. In 1947, Farber used aminopterin to successfully stop the synthesis of DNA in cancer cells, which was necessary for their growth and proliferation. This was the first step to finding a successful treatment for childhood leukemia. While aminopterin was abandoned in 1956, methotrexate

> 66
> My plans
> for the future are
> to continue seeking
> a cure for cancer.
> **Jane Wright**
> **Acceptance speech for**
> **the Merit Award, 1952**
> 99

Metastasis is the process by which cancer cells spread from an original site of development to form additional tumors around the body. The new tumors that form are still the same type of cancer as the original, regardless of where in the body they reform.

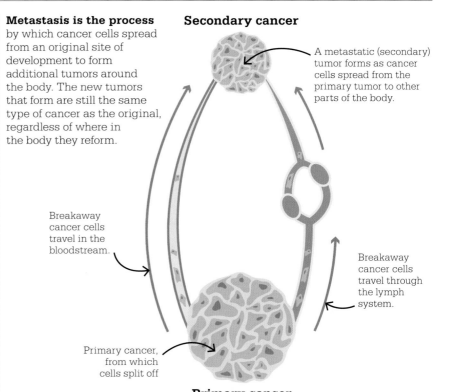

Secondary cancer

A metastatic (secondary) tumor forms as cancer cells spread from the primary tumor to other parts of the body.

Breakaway cancer cells travel in the bloodstream.

Breakaway cancer cells travel through the lymph system.

Primary cancer, from which cells split off

Primary cancer

remains a staple of chemotherapy. In the early 1950s, chemotherapy was considered an experimental method of tackling cancer, while surgery and radiation remained the core; this was soon to change. African American oncologist Jane Wright, based at New York's Harlem Hospital Cancer Research Foundation, helped establish chemotherapy as a mainstream cancer treatment. In 1951, Wright led research that demonstrated how chemotherapy could destroy solid tumors (abnormal masses of tissue). She successfully treated breast cancer patients with methotrexate and experimented with adjustments to the treatment regime according to an individual patient's symptoms. In a move toward personalized therapy, she and her colleagues cultured tumor tissue taken from patients and,

when grown, treated it with a variety of chemotherapeutic agents. Her team then assessed the results and decided on the most effective course of treatment for each patient.

Metastatic cancer

Whereas surgical removal and radiotherapy have to be targeted at specific areas of the body, chemotherapeutic agents are carried to cells in many areas of the body. This type of therapy is useful if the cancer has spread from a primary tumor. In the early 1950s, however, there was no effective treatment for metastatic (spreading) cancers. Successful as methotrexate had been against leukemia, it was not known to be effective against solid tumors.

In 1956, American researchers Min Li and Roy Hertz made critical breakthroughs. Li showed that methotrexate was able to destroy » metastatic melanomas (skin tumors), and Hertz used it to cure metastatic choriocarcinoma (cancer of the placenta). The effect of these discoveries was dramatic: before, choriocarcinoma had nearly always been fatal; by 1962, 80 percent of cases in the US were cured.

The American team of James Holland, Emil (Tom) Frei, and Emil Freireich knew that in the treatment of tuberculosis several antibiotics were used concurrently to reduce the risk of the bacteria developing resistance. In 1965, the team rationalized that cancer cells could also mutate to become resistant to a single agent, but if more than one agent was used, this would be less likely. By using a cocktail of up to four drugs, including methotrexate, they successfully treated cases of acute lymphocytic leukemia and Hodgkin's lymphoma—previously considered incurable. This technique became known as combination chemotherapy and is now the norm.

Vaccination
In 1976, German virologist Harald zur Hausen proposed that viruses played a role in cervical cancer, and within a decade, the human

Targeted therapies have been developed that substitute subtle intervention for brute force, aiming to disable or block processes that enable cancer cells to grow, divide, and spread.
Nigel Hawkes
British health journalist, 2015

papillovirus (HPV) viral infection had been identified as responsible for inducing cervical cancer. In the late 1980s, Australian immunologist Ian Frazer and Chinese virologist Jian Zhou began research for a vaccine. After 25 years, they were successful in developing the HPV vaccine, which first became available in 2006 and is now widely used to protect against cervical and anal cancers and some kinds of mouth and throat cancer.

By the early 21st century, a combination of radiotherapy, surgery, chemotherapy, and vaccination had produced a dramatic increase in survival rates for many cancers, especially in the developed world. This was true particularly for cancers of the breast, lung, bowel, and prostate. In the US, death rates for breast cancer fell by 39 percent between 1989 and 2015, with survival rates five years after treatment of around 90 percent there and 85 percent in Western Europe.

Success did not apply to all cancers, however. For pancreatic, liver, and a number of lung cancers, survival rates remain very low; in 2015, five-year survival rates for pancreatic cancer were still below 15 percent. Typically, treatment may involve surgery, followed by daily radiotherapy, then regular combination chemotherapy over a period of months.

Immunology
Cancer immunotherapy (immune-oncology) loosely echoes the radical therapy developed by William Coley in the late 19th century, in which he injected bacteria into cancer patients. Modern immunotherapy

---

Jane Wright

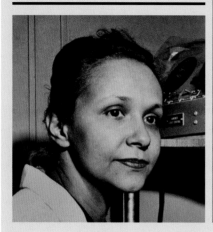

Born in 1919 in Connecticut, Jane Wright followed her father into medicine and graduated from New York Medical College in 1945. She then worked at the Harlem Hospital in chemotherapy research.

A believer in systematic clinical trials and a pioneer of personalized chemotherapy treatment, Wright became head of her father's Cancer Research Foundation at Harlem Hospital aged 33. She co-founded the American Society of Clinical Oncology in 1964, and joined a commission set up by President Lyndon B. Johnson to advise on cancer, heart disease, and

stroke policy. As a pioneering researcher and surgeon, Wright led international delegations of oncologists in Europe, Asia, and Africa and treated cancer patients in Ghana and Kenya. She died in 2013.

Key works

1957 "Investigation of the Relationship between Clinical and Tissue Response to Chemotherapeutic Agents on Human Cancer"
1984 "Cancer Chemotherapy: Past, Present, and Future"

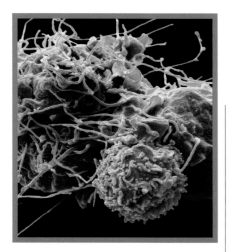

focuses on "educating" and boosting a body's immune system so that it can recognize and attack cancer cells. Natural killer cells (a type of white blood cell) are harnessed to identify and target infected cells.

In 1975, two biochemists—César Milstein (from Argentina) and Georges Köhler (Germany)—laid the foundations for using antibodies as a means to destroy cancer cells. Antibodies are protein molecules made by B-cells, which are a type of lymphocyte. They bind to molecules (antigens) on the surface of targeted cells, such as bacteria, and signal to the immune system to destroy them. Milstein and Köhler found a way to stimulate B-cells to produce unlimited numbers of one specific type of antibody (monoclonal antibodies). The next step was to develop them to target cancer cells, a technique now used in the diagnosis and treatment of some cancers.

The quest for immunotherapy with a greater reach has continued into the early 21st century. Much contemporary research focuses on T-cells, another type of lymphocyte. The role of killer T-cells is to travel around the body finding and destroying defective cells. When someone comes in contact with an

Natural killer cells are lymphocytes that recognize infected body cells and attack but have no specific immunity. This image shows a natural killer cell (pink) attacking a cancerous cell.

infection, the body makes T-cells to fight that specific disease. After T-cells have performed their search-and-destroy mission, the body keeps a few of them in reserve in case the same infection reoccurs. However, even though T-cells are good at fighting infections, they find it hard to identify cancer cells as "enemies."

During the 1980s, American immunologist James P. Allison and his Japanese counterpart Tasuku Honjo had discovered the chemical mechanism T-cells use to recognize "hostile" infection cells and realized their potential to identify cancer

cells. Later, Allison sought ways to "rearm" T-cells to destroy cancer cells. In 2002, researchers used CAR (chimeric antigen receptor) T-cells to destroy prostate cancer cells in a laboratory experiment. After successful clinical trials, CAR T-cells are now used to fight certain kinds of leukemia and lymphoma cancers. In this form of therapy, T-cells are taken from a patient's bloodstream, and their receptors are modified so they can recognize a specific protein on cancer cells. Then the CAR T-cells are put back into the patient's bloodstream. Similar procedures are being researched for solid tumors, too. Although still at a relatively early stage of development, this huge innovation represents the potential for a new type of cancer therapy. ∎

CAR T-cell therapy is a complex and specialty treatment in which a patient's T-cells (immune cells) are extracted from the body and genetically altered. Once modified into CAR T-cells, they are able to actively target and fight cancer cells in the body.

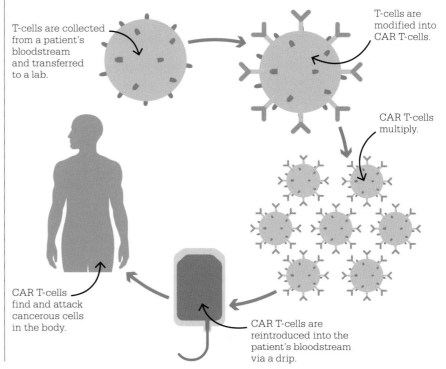

T-cells are collected from a patient's bloodstream and transferred to a lab.

T-cells are modified into CAR T-cells.

CAR T-cells multiply.

CAR T-cells find and attack cancerous cells in the body.

CAR T-cells are reintroduced into the patient's bloodstream via a drip.

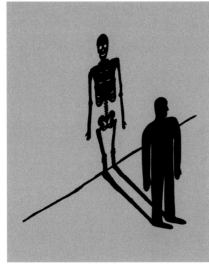

THE DARKER SHADOW OF THE BONES

X-RAYS

IN CONTEXT

BEFORE
1800 German-born British astronomer William Herschel discovers infrared light from the heat energy it carries.

1801 In Germany, physicist Johann Wilhelm Ritter detects ultraviolet light by exploring the purple end of the spectrum.

AFTER
1905 American X-ray pioneer Elizabeth Fleischman dies of cancer—the result of overexposure to radiation.

1971 Radiographers at a London hospital conduct the first computed tomography (CT) scan.

1984 The US Food and Drug Administration (FDA) approves the use of a whole-body magnetic resonance imaging (MRI) scanner.

2018 Scientists in New Zealand conduct the first 3D color X-ray on a human.

I n December 1895, German physicist Wilhelm Röntgen published a paper announcing his discovery of "a new kind of rays." He had produced the first X-ray images, including one of his wife's hand. Physicians around the world soon realized the potential of X-rays for clinical diagnosis, and in 1901, Röntgen received the first Nobel Prize in Physics for his work.

X-rays are a form of invisible electromagnetic radiation. When they pass through the body, different types of tissue absorb the radiation's energy at varying rates. A device placed on the opposite side of the body detects the differences and turns them into a photographic image. X-rays are used to diagnose conditions such as bone fractures, tooth problems, scoliosis (spine curvature), and bone tumors.

Early risks

The dangers of radiation were not fully understood in the early days of X-rays. Several researchers and physicians suffered burns and hair loss, and at least one died. Today,

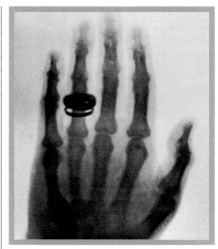

Röntgen's X-ray of his wife's hand (and wedding ring) prompted her to say she had seen her death. About 3.6 billion X-ray scans are now performed annually.

patients are only minimally exposed to low radiation levels, making X-ray scanning virtually risk-free for most people. In the mid-1970s, hospitals began to introduce computed tomography (CT), which uses X-rays to provide 3D images by rotating the X-ray source and detector around the body as it passes through a tube. ∎

See also: The stethoscope 103 ▪ Histology 122–123 ▪ Ultrasound 244 ▪ Orthopedic surgery 260–265 ▪ MRI and medical scanning 278–281

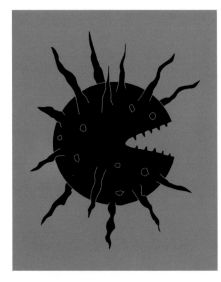

VIRUSES ARE ALPHA PREDATORS

VIROLOGY

O f the trillions of viruses that exist in the world, around 220 are known to cause disease in humans. They are up to a thousand times smaller than bacteria and consist of DNA or RNA enclosed in a protein coat. Viruses are inert until they infect other organisms and can replicate only when they take over the host's cells.

Isolated from tobacco sap

Dutch microbiologist Martinus Beijerinck first used the word "virus" in his 1898 study of tobacco mosaic infection. Six years earlier, Russian botanist Dmitri Ivanovsky, who also studied the disease, had filtered sap from infected tobacco leaves through porcelain in a bid to isolate the parasite but found that the filtered sap remained infectious. He had concluded that the sap must contain bacteria smaller than any known or a soluble bacterial toxin.

In 1897, Beijerinck conducted similar experiments, adding a second filter of gelatin. The filtered sap was still infected, yet he could not culture it; it spread only when injected into leaves. He concluded that it was not a microbe but a new liquid pathogen, which he called "virus"—Latin for "poisonous fluid."

Viruses were soon implicated in human diseases; the first was yellow fever virus, discovered in 1901. In the US, scientist Francis Holmes showed that viruses were discrete particles rather than fluids in 1929, and virologist Wendell Stanley crystallized tobacco mosaic virus from infected leaves in 1935. ∎

> The true nature of viruses was a complete mystery.
> **Wendell Meredith Stanley**
> Nobel Lecture, 1946

See also: Vaccination 94–101 ▪ Germ theory 138–145 ▪ Bacteriophages and phage therapy 204–205 ▪ HIV and autoimmune diseases 294–297 ▪ Pandemics 306–313

DREAMS
ARE THE ROYAL ROAD TO THE UNCONSCIOUS

PSYCHOANALYSIS

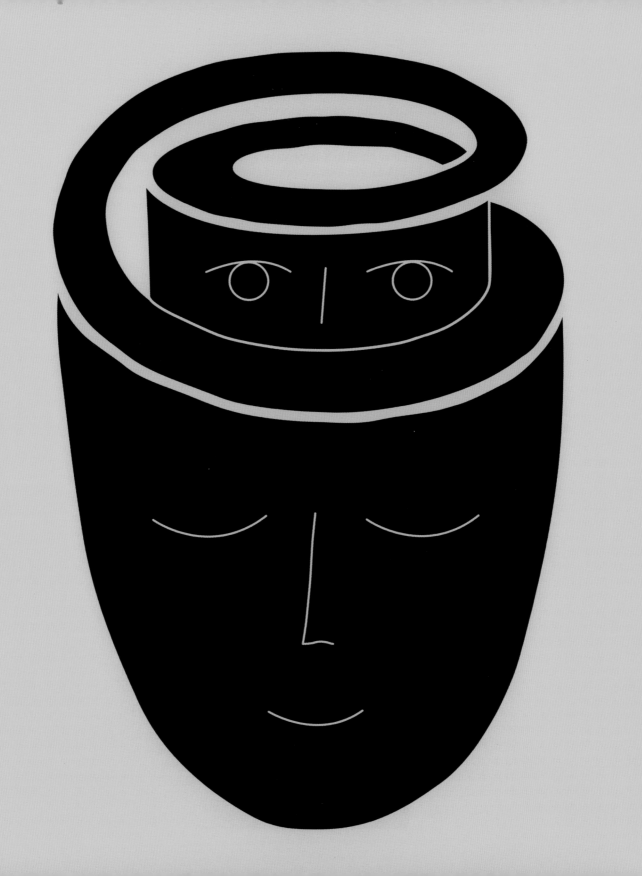

IN CONTEXT

BEFORE

c. 1012 Islamic physician Ibn Sina mentions the unconscious in *The Canon of Medicine* and recognizes that inner feelings can trigger physical effects.

1758 British physician William Battie publishes his *Treatise on Madness*, which advocates sensitive treatment for people suffering from mental illnesses.

1817 In his *Encyclopedia of the Philosophical Sciences*, German philosopher Georg Wilhelm Friedrich Hegel describes the unconscious as a "nightlike abyss."

AFTER

1939 Austrian psychoanalyst Heinz Hartmann, who was analyzed by Freud, publishes *Ego Psychology and the Problem of Adaptation.* Its ideas spread in the US, dominating psychoanalysis there for three decades.

1942–1944 Psychoanalysts Melanie Klein and Anna Freud clash over differing theories about child development in "Controversial Discussions"— a series of meetings of the British Psychoanalytical Society in London.

1971 In *The Analysis of the Self*, Austrian American psychoanalyst Heinz Kohut rejects Freudian ideas about the role of sexual drive and recognizes empathy as a key force in human development— a view that underpins modern psychoanalysis.

Psychology—a term derived from the Greek *psychologia,* meaning "study of the soul"— was in its infancy in the 1870s, when Austrian neurologist Sigmund Freud studied medicine in Vienna. A few notable European physicians, such as Wilhelm Wundt in Germany, had begun to work in the new area of experimental psychology and were studying the senses and nerves in a bid to discover how the brain processes information. Freud, however, grew more interested in exploring the nonphysical roots of mental disorders, a field he later called psychoanalysis.

French neurologist Jean-Martin Charcot, who used hypnosis to treat a condition then known as hysteria, was a key early influence. In 1885, Freud spent 19 weeks in Paris working under Charcot, who introduced him to the idea that the source of mental disorders lay in the mind—the domain of thought and consciousness—rather than in the physical brain.

The case of Anna O

Returning to Vienna, Freud began a partnership with Austrian physician Josef Breuer, who became his mentor. He was particularly fascinated by the case of Anna O, a pseudonym for Bertha Pappenheim. She suffered from hysteria, displaying symptoms including paralysis, convulsions, and hallucinations that had baffled other doctors. After a series of sessions with Breuer during which she freely expressed any thought that came into her mind, she had begun to improve. Breuer termed this "the talking cure."

It transpired that Anna O's symptoms had emerged during her father's long, terminal illness. The anxiety this provoked had, among her other symptoms, prompted an aversion to liquids—seemingly the result of a repressed childhood memory of a dog drinking from her glass. It was evident that her talks with Breuer had revealed previously hidden emotions and painful memories and that voicing them had effected her cure.

Freud wrote about Anna O in his 1895 *Studies on Hysteria*, in which he proposed that repressed conflicts manifest themselves physically. This, in turn, led him

Jean-Martin Charcot lectures on hypnosis at the Salpêtrière Hospital, Paris, as an assistant doctor holds a hysterical patient, in this copy of an 1887 painting by André Brouillet.

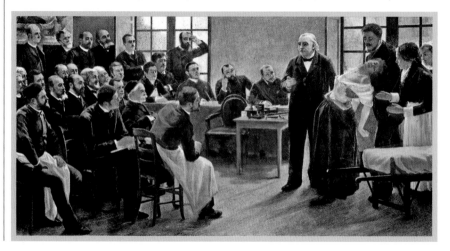

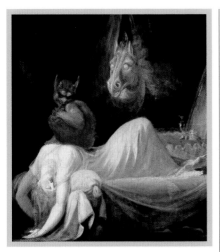

The Nightmare, painted by Swiss artist Henry Fuseli around 1790, portrays the suffocating anxiety of a terrifying dream. Freud is said to have had an engraving of it in his Vienna waiting room.

Experiences **too painful** for the **conscious mind** to bear are **repressed** in the **unconscious** mind.

⬇

Because the mind has **not resolved** the experiences, they cause **psychic tension**—conflict between the **conscious** and **unconscious** mind.

⬇

The **conflict** manifests itself as **mental illness**, such as **anxiety**, **depression**, or **neuroses**.

⬇

To successfully **treat** such problems, the **unresolved issues** must be **exposed**.

⬇

Psychoanalysis **probes the unconscious**, revealing and releasing **repressed experiences** and encouraging the patient's **conscious** mind to **manage them**.

to suggest there were three levels of the human mind: the conscious, preconscious, and unconscious. To describe the three levels, the analogy of an iceberg is often used. The tip of the iceberg, visible on the water's surface, represents the conscious mind—the thoughts and feelings that a patient is aware of and understands. Residing just beneath the conscious mind is the preconscious mind, which contains memories and knowledge that a person can easily access. At the deepest level of the iceberg, and occupying the largest area, lies the unconscious mind. For Freud, this area was a sealed chamber of repressed emotions, primitive desires, violent impulses, and fears.

Delving into dreams

In 1896, after his father died, Freud had a series of disturbing dreams, which he wrote down and studied as he began his self-analysis. In one dream, he received a hospital bill for someone who had been in the family home 40 years earlier, before his own birth. In the dream, his father's ghost admitted to getting drunk and being detained. Freud believed the dream indicated there was something that his unconscious mind would not allow him to see in his father's past, such as a sexual abuse or other hidden vices. His relationship with his father had been difficult. Freud told a friend, German physician Wilhelm Fliess, that his self-analysis and dreams had revealed a jealousy of his father and love for his mother—something he later described as an Oedipus complex, from the Greek myth of Oedipus, king of Thebes, who killed his father and unwittingly married his mother.

In his landmark 1899 text, *The Interpretation of Dreams*, Freud outlined his theory that repressed emotions or urges (often of a sexual nature) are expressed or acted out in dreams and nightmares in a form of wish fulfillment. Dreams, he considered, were the outlet of »

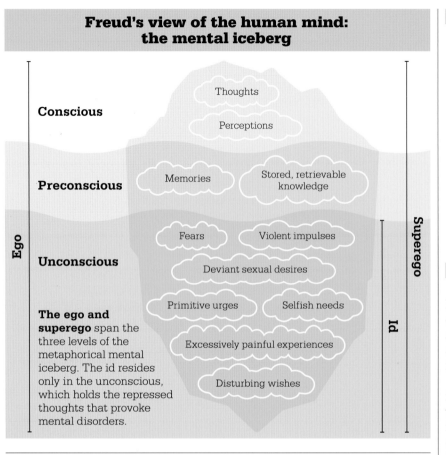

Freud's view of the human mind: the mental iceberg

Conscious

Thoughts

Perceptions

Preconscious

Memories

Stored, retrievable knowledge

Ego

Unconscious

Fears

Violent impulses

Deviant sexual desires

Primitive urges

Selfish needs

Excessively painful experiences

Disturbing wishes

Superego

Id

The ego and superego span the three levels of the metaphorical mental iceberg. The id resides only in the unconscious, which holds the repressed thoughts that provoke mental disorders.

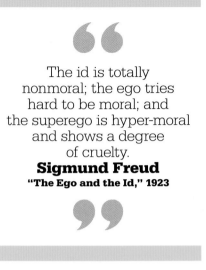

> The id is totally nonmoral; the ego tries hard to be moral; and the superego is hyper-moral and shows a degree of cruelty.
> **Sigmund Freud**
> **"The Ego and the Id," 1923**

emotions too powerful and painful for the conscious mind to tolerate. He became increasingly convinced that it was traumatic events in childhood that led to mental health issues in adults, as such memories were invariably repressed.

As patients could not explain or understand feelings or behavior caused by factors outside their realm of consciousness, the only route to a cure lay in probing the unconscious, and dreams were a potent route to this unknown area.

Id, ego, and superego

By the 1920s, Freud had extended the model of the unconscious, conscious, and preconscious minds to contain what he believed were the essential parts of the

human personality—the id, ego, and superego—which developed at different points of childhood. In the iceberg metaphor, the id—the most primitive, instinctive component—is submerged in the unconscious and consists of inherited traits, deep fears, and aggressive and sexual urges. It drives much of what goes on in the mind, but the conscious mind is unaware of it, although inadvertent words or behavior—what we now term "Freudian slips"—can reveal its hidden impulses.

The ego, according to Freud, is the self, perceiving and interacting with the outside world while also mediating conflicts in the mind's inner world. It develops during infancy and spans the conscious, preconscious, and unconscious.

During early childhood, as the ego develops, the superego, similarly straddling all three levels, becomes apparent, controlling impulses and imposing moral standards.

Freud proposed that one element is always at odds with the other two elements, which then causes inner conflict. Typically, when the goals of the id and superego come into conflict, the ego has to step in to mediate. When this happens, the ego deploys defense mechanisms, such as denial and repression.

Instincts and fixations

Freud grouped all human instincts into two opposing groups—Eros, the life instinct for personal and species survival, and Thanatos, the death instinct. Eros instincts include sex, thirst, and hunger, while Thanatos is destructive. Because the Eros instinct is for survival, it thwarts the Thanatos urge to self-destruct. As a result, Thanatos is often expressed as aggression or cruelty toward others.

Thanatos is also in conflict with libido, the psychosexual energy that fuels Eros. Freud believed that sexual impulses are a key factor in

> What we learn about the child and the adult through psychoanalysis shows that all the sufferings of later life are for the most part repetitions of these earlier ones.
> **Melanie Klein**
> *Love, Guilt, and Reparation, 1921–1945*

child development. He identified five crucial stages in infancy when sexuality develops—oral, anal, phallic, latent, and genital—as children become fixated initially with an area of their mother's body and then with other areas of their own bodies. Those who failed to successfully complete any one of these stages, Freud believed, would as adults become fixated on that stage, prompting a range of destructive behaviors.

To probe a patient's problem, Freud used tools such as Rorschach inkblots (in which he analyzed a patient's perception of inkblot patterns) and free association of words, as well as dream analysis. The patient lay on a sofa, while Freud sat taking notes behind.

Modified but still potent

Freud was a dominant figure in the field of psychiatry throughout his life and is rightly hailed as the father of psychoanalysis. He had detractors, however, and many of his theories are now thought antiquated. Critics have argued that his ideas have no scientific basis, that psychoanalysis is too long and expensive, and that

the nature of the sessions can create an unhealthy imbalance of power between therapist and patient. Freud himself noted problems with that relationship—a patient projects feelings about his or her parents onto a therapist, later termed the "transference phenomenon."

Over time, Freud's theories have been modified, and psychoanalysis today embraces more than 20 different schools of thought, largely taught in institutes separate from those of other medical disciplines. This is one point of contention with its detractors, who criticize psychoanalysis for basing theories on clinical experience rather than replicable scientific evidence. One attempt to address this is the new field of neuropsychoanalysis, which combines brain imaging with psychoanalysis; however, some psychiatrists are not yet convinced.

While its practice has declined, the study of psychoanalysis still attracts a large number of clinical psychologists, and psychiatrists acknowledge the legacy of Freud's central belief in the importance of patients' life histories and the value of listening to what patients say. ■

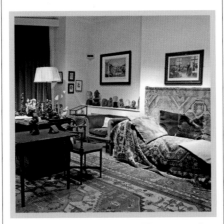

The Freud Museum in Hampstead, London, is housed in Freud's last home. It includes his original psychoanalytic couch, preserved in the study where he treated his patients.

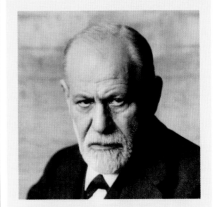

Sigmund Freud

Born in 1856 to Jewish parents in Freiberg, Moravia, Sigismund (later Sigmund) Freud was raised in Leipzig and Vienna. After studying medicine at the University of Vienna, he spent a formative period in Paris. On his return to Vienna, he worked with Josef Breuer on the treatment of hysteria and set up a private practice to treat patients with nervous disorders. In 1886, he married Martha Bernays; the couple had six children.

In 1897, Freud began an intense self-analysis, the basis of his book on dreams. He was appointed Vienna University's professor of neuropathology in 1902 and founded the International Psychoanalytic Association in 1910. In 1938, Freud, his wife, and other family members fled Austria (newly annexed by Nazi Germany) and settled in London. Suffering terminal cancer, Freud died in 1939.

Key works

1899–1900 *The Interpretation of Dreams*
1904 *The Psychopathology of Everyday Life*
1923 "The Ego and the Id"

IT MUST BE A CHEMICAL REFLEX

HORMONES AND ENDOCRINOLOGY

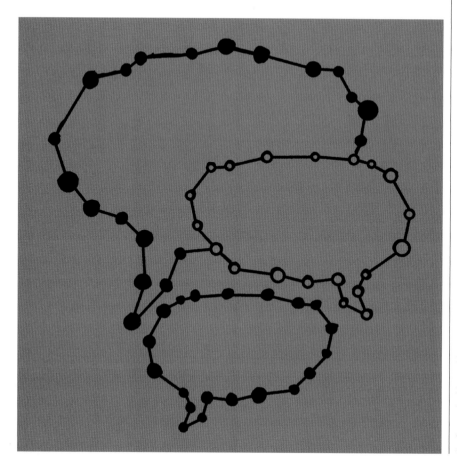

Endocrinology is the branch of medicine that deals with hormones—the body's chemical messengers. Hormones are made by specialized cells mostly found in the endocrine glands: the hypothalamus, testes, and ovaries and the thyroid, parathyroid, pituitary, adrenal, and pineal glands. Traveling through the body mainly in the bloodstream, hormones from one endocrine gland can stimulate another gland to adjust the levels of hormones it is producing or can carry instructions to cells in organs and tissues. In this way, hormones regulate almost every organ, process, and function in our bodies, including muscle and bone growth, fertility, appetite, metabolism, and heart rate.

Until 1902, it was believed that organs only communicated with each other using electrical signals

See also: Physiology 152–153 ▪ The nervous system 190–195 ▪ Diabetes and its treatment 210–213 ▪ Steroids and cortisone 236–239 ▪ Hormonal contraception 258

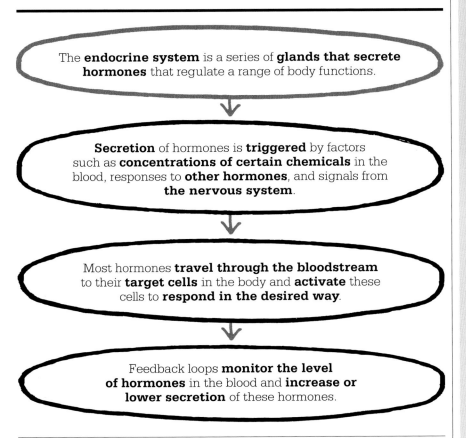

The **endocrine system** is a series of **glands that secrete hormones** that regulate a range of body functions.

Secretion of hormones is **triggered** by factors such as **concentrations of certain chemicals** in the blood, responses to **other hormones**, and signals from **the nervous system**.

Most hormones **travel through the bloodstream** to their **target cells** in the body and **activate** these cells to **respond in the desired way**.

Feedback loops **monitor the level of hormones** in the blood and **increase or lower secretion** of these hormones.

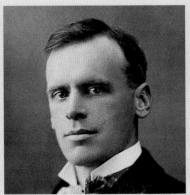

Ernest Starling

Born in 1866 in London, UK, Starling studied medicine at Guy's Hospital Medical School and became a demonstrator in physiology in 1887. In 1890, he began a lifelong association with fellow physiologist William Bayliss at University College, London. They made a good team: Starling was said to be visionary and impatient, while Bayliss was cautious and methodical. Bayliss married Starling's sister Gertrude in 1893. In addition to his work with Bayliss on the function of the endocrine system, Starling made significant contributions to the understanding of the mechanism that regulates heart function.

Starling was elected a fellow of the Royal Society in 1899. Committed to improving medical education, he assisted the 1910 Royal Commission on university education. He died in 1927, while on a Caribbean cruise, and was buried in Kingston, Jamaica.

Key works

1902 "The Mechanism of Pancreatic Secretion"
1905 "On the Chemical Correlation of the Functions of the Body"

---

conducted by nerves. That year, British physiologist Ernest Starling and his brother-in-law William Bayliss, working at University College London (UCL), performed an experiment that proved beyond doubt that organs communicate using chemical messengers, as well as via the nervous system. Their discovery kick-started the field of endocrinology.

Early indications

Pioneering experiments in the 19th century suggested the existence of hormones and hinted at their roles. Claude Bernard's studies of liver function in 1848 first established the concept of "internal secretion," or the ability of an organ to make a substance and release it directly into the bloodstream. In 1849, intrigued by the behavioral and physical changes that castration induced, German physiologist Arnold Berthold removed the testes from four male chicks and noted that they failed to develop male sexual characteristics such as combs and wattles or interest in hens. He then transplanted testes from a rooster into the abdomens of two castrated birds and found that they developed male characteristics as normal.

The prevailing theory was that sexual development was controlled by the nervous system, but when Berthold dissected his chickens, the transplanted testes had established a new blood supply but no neural »

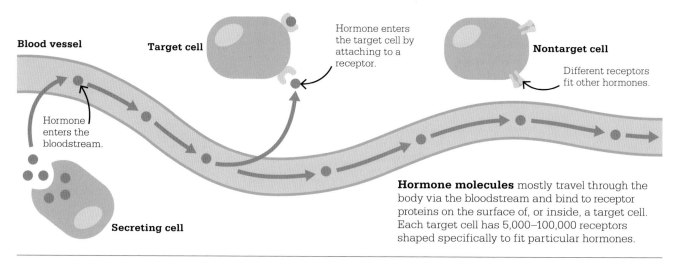

Blood vessel

Target cell

Hormone enters the target cell by attaching to a receptor.

Nontarget cell

Different receptors fit other hormones.

Hormone enters the bloodstream.

Secreting cell

Hormone molecules mostly travel through the body via the bloodstream and bind to receptor proteins on the surface of, or inside, a target cell. Each target cell has 5,000–100,000 receptors shaped specifically to fit particular hormones.

connections. Whatever triggered sexual development had to be traveling via the bloodstream. Despite Berthold's research, belief in nerves as the only conduit of messages in the body persisted.

In 1889, French neurologist Charles-Édouard Brown-Séquard, then aged 72, reported to the Academy of Sciences in Paris that he had injected himself with a concoction of veins, semen, and other fluids from the testicles of dogs and guinea pigs. Brown-Séquard noted a marked improvement in his

… the discovery of the nature of these [chemical] substances will enable us … to acquire absolute control over the workings of the human body.
Ernest Starling
Croonian Lecture, 1905

strength, stamina, and ability to concentrate. He attributed this to an action on the nervous system and suggested that similar extracts could be used to rejuvenate men.

The following year, Brown-Séquard reported that Augusta Brown, an American doctor working in Paris, had injected several women with the filtered juice of guinea pigs' ovaries, which appeared to show benefits for hysteria, uterine disorders, and aging. This claim could not be validated, but it fueled interest in the idea that internal secretions produced by organs might have significant functions and therapeutic applications.

Chemical signaling
At UCL in the late 1890s, Starling and Bayliss were researching the physiology of the small intestine. After becoming the first scientists to describe peristalsis (the muscular contractions that propel digested food along the intestine), they began investigating whether the nervous system influenced digestion.

Starling and Bayliss knew that the pancreas secreted digestive fluids after food passed from the stomach to the intestines. In 1888, Russian physiologist Ivan Pavlov

had posited that these pancreatic secretions were controlled by nerve signals that traveled from the small intestine to the brain and then back to the pancreas. In 1902, aiming to test these claims, Starling and Bayliss carefully cut away all the nerves linked to the pancreas in an anesthetized dog. When they introduced acid into the small intestine, the pancreas still secreted digestive fluids. This implied that the secretions were not controlled by nerve signals.

To prove their hypothesis that a factor released from the intestine into the bloodstream triggered the pancreas to secrete digestive fluids, Starling and Bayliss injected a solution of intestinal material and acid into a vein. Within a few seconds, they detected secretions from the pancreas. This proved that the triggering link between the small intestine and the pancreas was a chemical messenger and was not carried by the nervous system.

The first hormone
In a lecture at the Royal College of Physicians in 1905, Starling used a new term "hormone," from the Greek word *ormao* ("to excite or arouse"), to describe the substance found.

He named this hormone "secretin." The 1902 experiment showed that the small intestine releases secretin into the bloodstream when gastric acid fluid arrives in the intestine from the stomach. Secretin then stimulates the pancreas to secrete bicarbonate, which neutralizes the acid fluid in the intestine.

The discovery of secretin soon prompted the identification of other hormones. Insulin, released by the pancreas to regulate blood sugar levels, was isolated by Canadian scientist Frederick Banting and Scottish physiologist John Macleod in 1921. The sex hormone estrogen was identified in 1929 by German biochemist Adolf Butenandt, and also independently by American biochemist Edward Doisy, followed by progesterone in 1934, and both testosterone and estradiol in 1935. In all, scientists have identified more than 50 human hormones to date.

New therapies
After isolating secretin, Starling and Bayliss discovered that it was a universal stimulant: secretin from one species stimulated the pancreas of any other species. This suggested that it might be possible to use animal-derived hormones as

> We don't want to alarm women, but we don't want to give them false reassurance.
> **Gillian Reeves**
> **British cancer epidemiologist, on the risks of HRT, 2019**

therapies for previously untreatable endocrine disorders. Pharmaceutical companies were quick to explore these new opportunities as more hormones were identified.

Just two years after Banting and Macleod's isolation of insulin, the American pharmaceutical company Eli Lilly began manufacturing Iletin, the first commercially available insulin product for treating diabetes. By the mid-1930s, oral and injectable estrogens were also available for treating menstrual irregularities and the symptoms of menopause.

Demand for hormone therapies synthesized from animal products, which were expensive and only available in limited quantities, quickly outstripped supply. Scientists began to investigate biochemical processes that could enable hormone synthesis on a larger scale.

In 1926, British biochemist Charles Harington achieved the first chemical synthesis of a hormone, thyroxine (originally isolated by American chemist Edward Kendall in 1914). This significant step toward mass-producing hormones also helped improve the efficacy of hormones such as insulin. The first insulin preparations, derived from horse pancreas, varied greatly in strength and required several daily injections. By the 1930s, the addition of zinc prolonged the action of insulin to around 24 hours.

Modern developments
Progress in hormone synthesis also allowed for wider applications. The contraceptive pill, containing synthetic progesterone and synthetic estrogen, was introduced in 1960, and marked a turning point in the availability and marketing of manufactured hormone products for general use. The use of synthetic estrogen for hormone replacement therapy (HRT) also gained mass

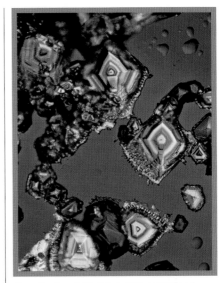

A polarized light micrograph of the female sex hormone progesterone. Secreted by the ovaries following the release of an egg, it prepares the inner lining of the womb for pregnancy.

popularity in the 1960s, as women seized the opportunity to counter debilitating menopausal symptoms such as hot flashes and osteoporosis.

During the late 1970s, advances in biotechnology enabled genetically engineered human hormones. New gene-splicing techniques meant that common bacteria (usually *Escherichia coli*) could be genetically modified to produce hormones, such as insulin, in the laboratory.

As research continues adding to our knowledge of hormones, recent studies have begun to question the safety of some hormone treatments, recording evidence of side effects ranging from fatigue to cancer. In 2002, for example, studies linking HRT to an increased risk of breast cancer and stroke showed that the risks versus the benefits of altering hormone levels must be carefully calculated. The adverse effects of some drugs on the body's delicate balance of hormones is also an ongoing area of research. ■

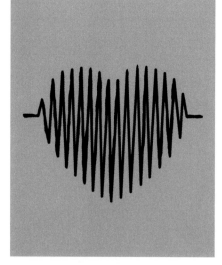

THE ACTION CURRENTS OF THE HEART

ELECTROCARDIOGRAPHY

IN CONTEXT

BEFORE

1780s Italian physicist Luigi Galvani stimulates electrical responses in animal muscles, calling it "animal electricity."

1887 To measure the heart's electrical activity, Augustus D. Waller uses a machine based on the capillary electrometer developed by French physicist Gabriel Lippmann.

AFTER

1909 With the aid of an early electrocardiograph, British physician Thomas Lewis discovers atrial fibrillation—a condition that causes an irregular heart rate.

1932 New York cardiologist Albert Hyman invents a device to restart a stopped heart and calls it an artificial pacemaker.

1958 In Sweden, cardiac surgeon Åke Senning implants the first cardiac pacemaker, designed by engineer and former doctor Rune Elmqvist.

In the ancient world, physicians listened to the body for signs of disease. The heart had a recognizable pulse, which, 2 millennia later, could be clearly heard through the stethoscope invented in France by René Laënnec in 1816. In 1903, Dutch physiologist Willem Einthoven took heart monitoring a crucial step forward when he introduced the first viable electrocardiograph.

Electrocardiographs record the pattern of a patient's heartbeat by detecting (via electrodes on the body) the varying electrical signals the heart produces—a procedure called an electrocardiogram (ECG).

Animal experiments carried out by Italian physicist Carlo Matteucci in 1842 had shown that an electrical current accompanies each beat of the heart. In the following decades, scientists sought ways to record the

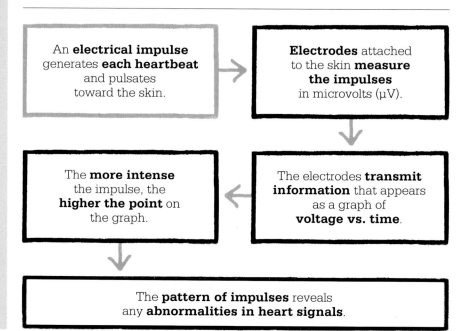

An **electrical impulse** generates **each heartbeat** and pulsates toward the skin.

Electrodes attached to the skin **measure the impulses** in microvolts (µV).

The **more intense** the impulse, the **higher the point** on the graph.

The electrodes **transmit information** that appears as a graph of **voltage vs. time**.

The **pattern of impulses** reveals any **abnormalities in heart signals**.

See also: Traditional Chinese medicine 30–35 ▪ Blood circulation 68–73 ▪ The stethoscope 103 ▪ Transplant surgery 246–253 ▪ Pacemakers 255

This 1911 electrocardiograph took five people to operate it. Instead of wearing electrode pads, patients dipped their arms and left leg into saline, an electrical conductor.

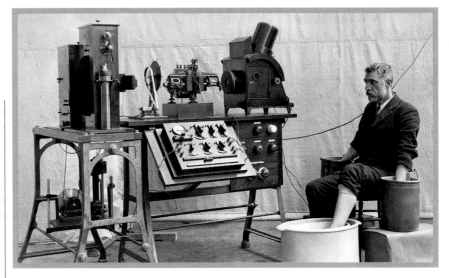

human heart's electrical activity. Einthoven became interested after seeing British physiologist Augustus D. Waller demonstrate a device that detected the heart's electrical surges from the way they made mercury move inside a tiny glass tube.

Refining the machines
By 1903, Einthoven had developed a sensitive string galvanometer. When electrical current from the heart passed through a fine wire or string set between two electromagnets, the string moved, and the shadow cast by its movements was recorded on moving photographic paper. Einthoven's model produced more accurate readings than Waller's and reduced the electrode points from five to three to give readings from the left and right arm and left leg, creating what was later known as Einthoven's triangle.

The early electrocardiographs were large and cumbersome, but over the years, the machines were modified and shrank in size. Today's portable devices can be used to monitor a patient's heart digitally over days or weeks. The number of electrodes used for a standard ECG has risen to 10—six on the chest and one on each limb—giving 12 measurements ("leads") of the heart's activity from different combinations of electrodes.

Since Einthoven developed his first machine, the ECG has been in constant use. While many new treatments have emerged—such as beta-blockers (drugs to slow down the heart rate), pacemakers (devices to regulate the heart's contractions), heart transplants, and bypass and valve replacement surgeries—the ECG still plays a key role in the early diagnosis of heart disease, which is the world's leading cause of death. ▪

Willem Einthoven

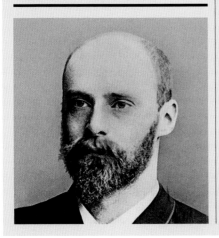

Born in 1860, Willem Einthoven spent his early years on the island of Java in the Dutch East Indies (now Indonesia). When he was 6, his father died, and in 1870, the family went to live in Utrecht in the Netherlands.

Einthoven trained as a doctor in Utrecht, and in 1886 was made professor of physiology at the University of Leiden. He initially studied optical illusions and the eye's electrical response to light, but his interest turned to building a machine to monitor the heart's electrical activity. After introducing his electrocardiograph, he went on to describe how various heart disorders appear on an ECG, and corresponded regularly with British physician Thomas Lewis, who worked on the device's clinical application. In 1924, Einthoven was awarded the Nobel Prize in Physiology or Medicine and died three years later, in 1927.

Key works

1906 "The Telecardiogram"
1912 "The different forms of the human electrocardiogram and their significance"

STRINGS OF FLASHING AND TRAVELING SPARKS

THE NERVOUS SYSTEM

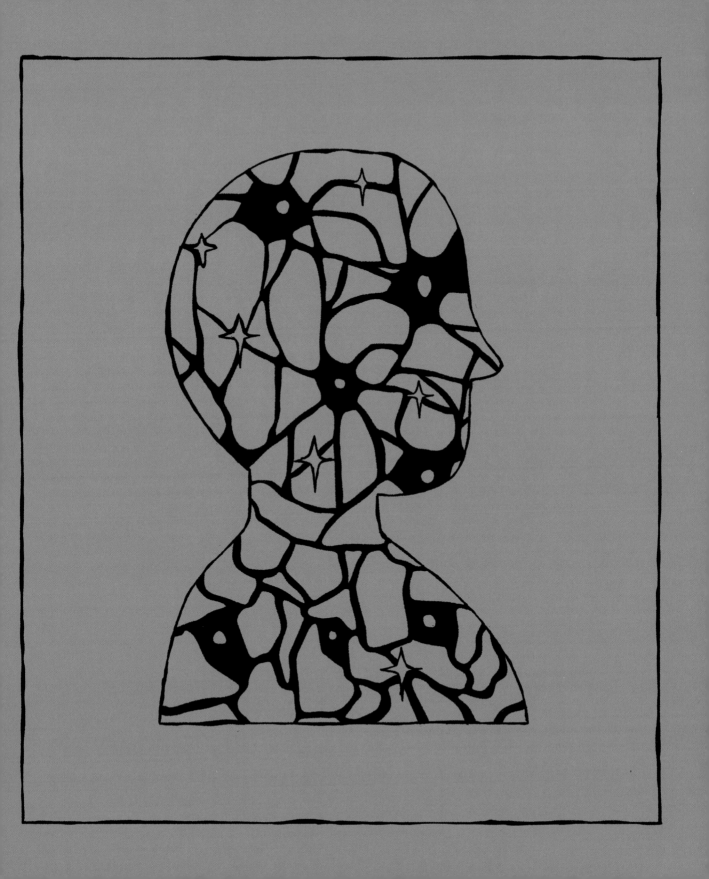

IN CONTEXT

BEFORE
c. 1600 BCE The Edwin Smith papyrus describes the impact of spinal injury on the body.

1791 Luigi Galvani shows that a frog's leg responds to electrical stimulus.

1863 Otto Deiters describes the axon and dendrites of a nerve cell.

1872 Jean-Martin Charcot publishes his pioneering work *Lectures on the Diseases of the Nervous System*.

AFTER
1914 Henry Dale finds the neurotransmitter responsible for chemical communication between nerve cells.

1967 Levodopa becomes the first effective drug treatment for a neurodegenerative condition (Parkinson's disease).

1993 A disease-associated gene (for Huntington's disease) is mapped to a human chromosome for the first time.

In a series of lectures at Yale University in 1904, British neurophysiologist Charles Scott Sherrington gave the first extensive exposition of the human nervous system. Published two years later in *The Integrative Action of the Nervous System*, this research resolved several issues about how the nervous system functions and directly influenced the development of brain surgery and treatment for neurological disorders.

Muscle messaging

Three of Sherrington's ideas were particularly groundbreaking. He explained that muscles do not simply *receive* instructions from the nerves that travel to them from the spinal cord (which conducts messages to and from the brain); they also *send* information back to the brain about muscle position and tone. The body needs this information, which he called proprioception, to control movement and posture.

Back in 1626, French philosopher and scientist René Descartes had observed reciprocal innervation—the way the activation of one muscle influences the activity of others—but Sherrington's studies in the 1890s clarified how the process works.

"Sherrington's law" established that for every activation of a muscle, there is a corresponding relaxation of the opposing muscle. When, for example, you flex your arm at the elbow, the bicep muscle is activated (contracting the arm), but the tricep muscle is inhibited (relaxing to allow the movement).

In 1897, Sherrington coined the term "synapse" for the meeting point between two nerve cells (neurons). Although he could not observe synapses (microscopes were not advanced enough), he believed these junctions existed because reflexes (involuntary motor responses) were not as fast as they should be if they involved the simple conduction of impulses along continuous nerve fibers. He explained how a neuron communicates via electric signals, which pass along threadlike fibers (axons) protruding from the neuron and are transmitted to neighboring cells by chemical messengers (called neurotransmitters) across a synapse.

Ancient observations

As far back as ancient Egypt, the Edwin Smith papyrus notes how brain injuries are associated with changes in the functioning of other body parts and describes the brain's

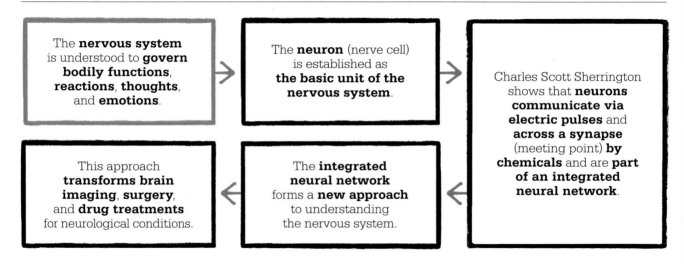

The **nervous system** is understood to **govern bodily functions, reactions, thoughts,** and **emotions**.

The **neuron** (nerve cell) is established as **the basic unit of the nervous system**.

Charles Scott Sherrington shows that **neurons communicate via electric pulses** and **across a synapse** (meeting point) **by chemicals** and are **part of an integrated neural network**.

This approach **transforms brain imaging, surgery,** and **drug treatments** for neurological conditions.

The **integrated neural network** forms a **new approach** to understanding the nervous system.

exterior folds and the colorless fluid surrounding it—the cerebrospinal fluid (CSF) that provides physical and immune protection.

Using a mixture of observation and philosophy, the ancient Greeks were the first to attempt a detailed description of the nervous system. Hippocrates pioneered the concept of the brain as the seat of cognition, thought, sensations, and emotion in the 4th century BCE. In the 3rd century BCE, Herophilus understood the brain and spinal cord's combined role in what we now call the central nervous system (CNS). This gathers information from the rest of the body and our external environment and controls movement, sensations, thought, memory, and speech. He identified six of the cranial nerves, as well as the peripheral nerves that link the brain and spinal cord to the rest of the body's organs, muscles, limbs, and skin.

By dissecting animals' brains in the 2nd century CE, Roman physician Galen of Pergamum established that the nerves directing motor functions and those linked to the senses are controlled by different parts of the

> ❝ The brain is a world consisting of a number of unexplored continents and great stretches of unknown territory. ❞
> **Santiago Ramón y Cajal**
> **Spanish neuroscientist (1852–1934)**

CNS. This pointed to the existence of the autonomic nervous system, which connects the CNS with the heart, lungs, stomach, bladder, and sex organs and which operates without us thinking about it to regulate involuntary functions, such as breathing and heartbeat.

Increasing knowledge

There is evidence of early attempts to treat neurological disorders. In Muslim Spain around 1000 CE, for example, al-Zahrawi operated on patients with hydrocephalus (excess cerebrospinal fluid in the brain) and with head and spinal injuries, but there was little progress in neural understanding until the 16th-century revival in human dissection.

In 1543, Flemish anatomist Andreas Vesalius published *De Humani Corporis Fabrica* (*On the Structure of the Human Body*), »

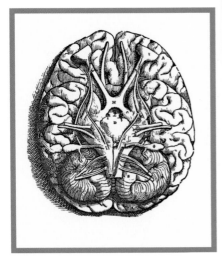

De Humani Corporis Fabrica depicted the different brain regions and the cranial nerves (seen here from below), which originate from the cerebrum and the brainstem.

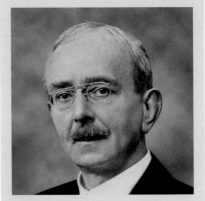

Charles Scott Sherrington

Born in London, UK, in 1857, Charles Scott Sherrington studied medicine at Cambridge University and was inspired to begin serious neurological research after attending a lecture on nerve function at a medical conference in 1881. A year spent at Berlin University, under the tutelage of German microbiologist Robert Koch, gave him a good grounding in physiology and histology.

Between 1892 and 1913, Sherrington conducted his seminal research into reflex reactions, the nerve supply of muscles, and how neurons communicate while teaching at the universities of London and Liverpool. In 1932, when he was a tutor at Oxford University, he shared the Nobel Prize in Physiology or Medicine with Edgar Adrian for their work on the function of neurons. Three of Sherrington's Oxford students went on to become Nobel laureates. He retired from Oxford in 1936, and died of heart failure in 1952.

Key works

1906 *The Integrative Action of the Nervous System*
1940 *Man on His Nature*

which included thorough descriptions of the human brain based on his dissection of cadavers. This book transformed anatomical knowledge and medical practice. Its neurological information was later supplemented by English physician Thomas Willis, who elucidated the brain and cranial and spinal nerves, providing explanations of their function, in the early 17th century.

In 1791, Italian physicist and physician Luigi Galvani published his description of an important breakthrough: his observation that a dead frog's legs twitch when in contact with a spark. His discovery of bioelectricity was the first indication that nerves function by electrical impulses and that the electrical stimulation of nerves produces muscle contraction.

Understanding disease

The growing understanding of brain structure and nervous system function gave scientists new means of studying neurological and psychological diseases. In 1817, British surgeon James Parkinson described the symptoms of six people suffering "the shaking palsy" (later renamed Parkinson's disease). Although he wrongly believed the disease was caused

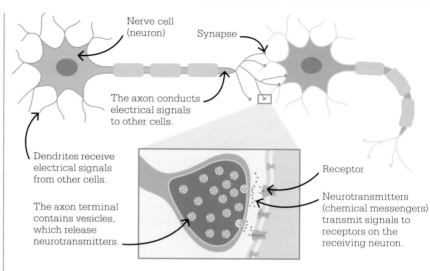

Nerve cell (neuron)

Synapse

The axon conducts electrical signals to other cells.

Dendrites receive electrical signals from other cells.

The axon terminal contains vesicles, which release neurotransmitters.

Receptor

Neurotransmitters (chemical messengers) transmit signals to receptors on the receiving neuron.

Nerve signals travel along neurons in electrical form but pass between them—or from neurons to cells in muscles and glands— across synaptic junctions in chemical form. Neurological disorders may occur if this communication between cells is disrupted through viral infections, drug use, aging, or genetic factors.

> The brain seems a thoroughfare for nerve-action passing its way to the motor animal.
> **Charles Sherrington**
> *The Brain and its Mechanism, 1933*

by lesions in the cervical spinal cord, his systematic and analytical approach was significant.

Parkinson's was one of several diseases studied between 1868 and 1891 by French clinical neurologist Jean-Martin Charcot. He also described multiple sclerosis (MS), which damages the insulating sheath of nerve cells in the brain and spinal cord, and noted three signs of MS, subsequently known as Charcot's triad. Modern psychiatry also owes much to Charcot, who is probably best known for his use of hypnosis to study the symptoms of hysteria while teaching at the Salpêtrière School in Paris.

Age of the microscope

In the early 19th century, better-quality achromatic microscopes created the new field of histology— the microscopic study of cells and tissues—which led to a number of neurological revelations. Czech anatomist Johann Purkinje was the first to describe a neuron in 1837.

He went on to detail particularly large neurons (now called Purkinje cells) with branching, threadlike extensions in the cerebellum. In 1863, German anatomist Otto Deiters described these extensions (later known as dendrites), which conduct messages to neurons, and also identified the cell's axons—thin fibers that conduct messages away from neurons.

The first anatomical proof that different parts of the brain performed specific functions was presented in the early 1860s by French anatomist Paul Broca. He discovered that aphasia (the inability to understand and formulate language) was linked to lesions in part of the frontal lobe of the brain (later named Broca's area) after conducting autopsies on recently deceased patients.

During the 1870s, Italian biologist and pioneering neuroanatomist Camillo Golgi produced detailed descriptions of the spinal cord and the brain's olfactory lobe, cerebellum, and hippocampus. In 1873, he

Major neurotransmitters in the body

Neurotransmitter	Role in the body
Acetylcholine	All body movements are controlled by this neurotransmitter, which activates muscles. In the brain, it plays a role in memory, learning, and attention.
Dopamine	Linked to the brain reward system, this neurotransmitter produces feelings of pleasure, affecting mood and motivation. It also influences movement and speech.
Gamma-aminobutyric acid (GABA)	This neurotransmitter blocks or inhibits brain signals, decreasing activity in the nervous system to allow processes such as sleep or the regulation of anxiety.
Glutamate	The predominant neurotransmitter in the brain and central nervous system, glutamate stimulates brain activity and is critical for learning and memory.
Glycine	Used mainly by neurons in the brainstem and spinal cord, glycine helps the body process motor and sensory information.
Noradrenaline (or norepinephrine)	Part of the body's flight-or-fight response, this neurotransmitter is released into the bloodstream as a stress hormone. It regulates normal brain processes, including emotions, learning, and attention.
Serotonin	This neurotransmitter regulates many body processes and influences mood, appetite, and memory function. It also plays a role in managing our response to pain.

invented a new staining technique using silver nitrate, which showed the intricate structure of neural cells on a microscope slide much more clearly. This was the second great technological enabler.

Golgi went on to propose that the brain is made up of a single network (or reticulum) of nerve fibers through which signals pass unimpeded. This reticular theory was challenged at the time by Spanish neuroscientist Santiago Ramón y Cajal, who argued that the nervous system is a collection of many individual but interconnected cells. Cajal's view came to be known as the "neuron doctrine." Supported by Sherrington, this theory was proved to be correct in the 1950s, when new electron microscopes were able to show the connections between cells.

Later advances

New discoveries continued during the 20th century, many based on Sherrington's landmark description of neural pathways. In 1914, British physiologist Henry Dale noted the effect of acetylcholine on nerve cells.

German pharmacologist Otto Loewi confirmed its role as a chemical neurotransmitter in 1926. So far, more than 200 neurotransmitters have been identified.

In 1924, German psychiatrist Hans Berger performed the first human electroencephalogram (EEG). Able to record brain activity by detecting the electrical signals fired by neurons, EEG tests allowed British physiologist Edgar Adrian to conduct detailed studies of brain function in the 1930s.

In 1952, two British scientists, Alan Hodgkin and Andrew Huxley, published their research on the nervous system of squid. This work, now known as the Hodgkin-Huxley model, showed how electrical signals are generated in nerve cells.

By this time, the third great technological leap forward had occurred—the invention of the

Magnetic resonance imaging (MRI) is often used to provide detailed images of the brain for diagnostic purposes, such as detecting dementia, tumors, injury, stroke, or developmental issues.

electron microscope. This enabled scientists to examine much smaller elements of the nervous system, including the synapses described but never seen by Sherrington.

New technologies, such as magnetic resonance imaging (MRI) and computed tomography (CT) scanning, continue to widen the applications of Sherrington's initial findings. They currently fuel research on behavior, brain function, the efficacy of drugs for neurological conditions, brain surgery, and the causes and effects of diseases such as epilepsy and Alzheimer's. ∎

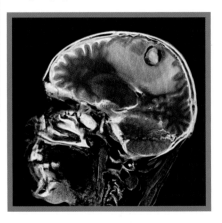

A PECULIAR DISEASE OF THE CEREBRAL CORTEX
ALZHEIMER'S DISEASE

IN CONTEXT

BEFORE

6th century BCE The Greek philosopher Pythagoras of Samos describes mental and physical decay in old age.

1797 Philippe Pinel uses the term "dementia," derived from the Latin for "out of the mind" to describe a gradual decline in brain function.

1835 British physician James Cowles Prichard uses the term "senile dementia" to describe a state characterized by "forgetfulness of recent impressions" in the elderly.

AFTER

1984 American biochemists George Glenner and Caine Wong isolate beta-amyloid, the protein that forms plaque in the brains of Alzheimer patients.

1993 Tacrine is the first cholinesterase inhibitor drug for Alzheimer's, but it is withdrawn from general use in 2013 due to safety concerns.

Dementia is not a disease, but a blanket term used to describe a number of conditions associated with a decline in brain function, such as memory impairment, loss of physical and social skills, and a decline in intellectual ability. It has many causes, including chronic alcohol abuse, strokes (often leading to vascular dementia in which the brain's blood vessels are damaged), Creutzfeldt-Jakob disease (a fatal brain disorder), and Alzheimer's disease—an irreversible and ultimately fatal neurogenerative disease that accounts for two-thirds of dementia cases.

Early-onset dementia

Like other causes of dementia, Alzheimer's disease generally affects the elderly, but it is also the most common form of early-onset dementia found in those aged under 65. The disease was identified as a distinct cause of dementia by Alois Alzheimer, a German psychiatrist.

In 1906, he gave a lecture on "a peculiar disease of the cerebral cortex" based on a study of Auguste Deter, a patient at a Frankfurt asylum. Alzheimer had begun observing Deter in 1901 (when she was 51) on account of her problems with memory and language, as well as disorientation and hallucinations. Her symptoms had matched those of dementia, but Alzheimer had diagnosed "presenile dementia" because of her relatively young age.

After Deter's death in 1906, Alzheimer had sought and received permission to perform an autopsy on

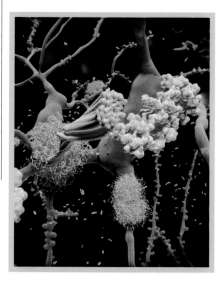

Plaque formed from the beta-amyloid protein in the brain is characteristic of Alzheimer's disease. Clumps of plaque (orange in this illustration) block the synapses between nerve cells (blue).

See also: Humane mental health care 92–93 ▪ Inheritance and hereditary conditions 146–147 ▪ The nervous system 190–195 ▪ MRI and medical scanning 278–281 ▪ Genetics and medicine 288–293 ▪ Stem cell research 302–303

How Alzheimer's progresses

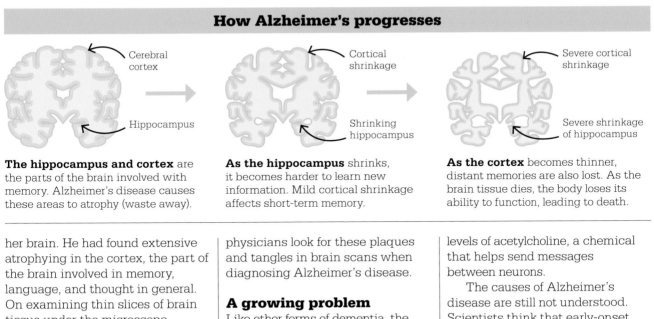

Cerebral cortex

Hippocampus

Cortical shrinkage

Shrinking hippocampus

Severe cortical shrinkage

Severe shrinkage of hippocampus

The hippocampus and cortex are the parts of the brain involved with memory. Alzheimer's disease causes these areas to atrophy (waste away).

As the hippocampus shrinks, it becomes harder to learn new information. Mild cortical shrinkage affects short-term memory.

As the cortex becomes thinner, distant memories are also lost. As the brain tissue dies, the body loses its ability to function, leading to death.

her brain. He had found extensive atrophying in the cortex, the part of the brain involved in memory, language, and thought in general. On examining thin slices of brain tissue under the microscope, Alzheimer found insoluble protein deposits, or plaques, and twisted protein threads (neurofibrillary tangles) that impede the electrical impulses between neurons (nerve cells). He was not the first person to note these signs, but this was the first time they had been seen in someone as young as Deter. Today,

physicians look for these plaques and tangles in brain scans when diagnosing Alzheimer's disease.

A growing problem

Like other forms of dementia, the incidence of Alzheimer's has risen with increased life expectancy. Worldwide, there are approximately 50 million people with dementia, including 1 in 10 Americans over the age of 65. There is currently no cure for Alzheimer's, although cholinesterase inhibitor drugs can alleviate symptoms by boosting the

levels of acetylcholine, a chemical that helps send messages between neurons.

The causes of Alzheimer's disease are still not understood. Scientists think that early-onset forms may be the result of a genetic mutation, while late-onset may arise from a combination of genetic, lifestyle, and environmental factors that trigger changes to the brain over decades. A healthy diet, exercise, and mental stimulation may reduce the risk of getting Alzheimer's, but there is little proof. ▪

Alois Alzheimer

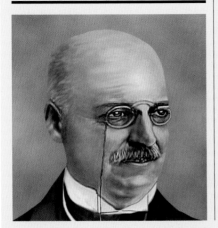

Born in Markbreit, a small village in Bavaria, Germany, in 1864, Alois Alzheimer excelled in science at school. He went on to study medicine in Berlin, Tübingen, and Würzburg. After graduating in 1887, he joined the staff at the state asylum in Frankfurt, where he studied psychiatry and neuropathology and began to research the cortex of the brain.

In 1903, Alzheimer became assistant to Emil Kraepelin, a psychiatrist at the Munich medical school. After Alzheimer described Auguste Deter's form of dementia in 1906 and published his lecture

the following year, Kraepelin named the disease after Alzheimer in the 1910 edition of his textbook *Compendium of Psychiatry*.

In 1913, on his way to take up the post of chair of the department of psychology at the Friedrich-Wilhelm University, in Berlin, Alzheimer caught an infection from which he never fully recovered. He died in 1915, at the age of 51.

Key work

1907 "About a Peculiar Disease of the Cerebral Cortex"

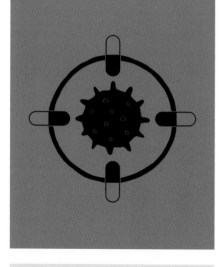

MAGIC BULLETS
TARGETED DRUG DELIVERY

IN CONTEXT

BEFORE
1530 Paracelsus pioneers the use of mercury as a treatment for syphilis.

1856 William Henry Perkin discovers mauveine, the first synthetic organic dye.

1882 Élie Metchnikoff discovers macrophages.

1890 Emil von Behring and Shibasaburo Kitasato discover the first antitoxin.

AFTER
1932 German pharmaceutical company Bayer introduces Prontosil (sulfonamide), the first drug broadly effective against bacteria.

1943 Penicillin, the first naturally occurring antibiotic to be developed as a drug, is prescribed to treat syphilis and becomes the standard therapy for this disease.

1970s Tamoxifen, a targeted cancer therapy, is launched.

At the dawn of the 20th century, German scientist Paul Ehrlich devised an entirely new way of treating disease using chemical drugs. He described his compounds as "magic bullets," because they were formulated to hit disease-causing microbes (pathogens) hard while leaving the body unharmed.

The idea occurred to Ehrlich while he was investigating the synthetic dyes discovered in 1856 by teenage British chemistry student William Henry Perkin. Ehrlich was fascinated by the way that some dyes, particularly methylene blue, stained animal tissues dramatically, while others didn't, allowing cells to be differentiated in the laboratory. It was clear to Ehrlich that there was some connection between the chemical structure of the dyes and living cells. He became convinced that the chemical structure of drugs needed to match the organisms that they were targeting in order to be effective.

In 1890, German physiologist Emil von Behring and Japanese physician Shibasaburo Kitasato discovered that antitoxins made by the body in response to a pathogen could be used to prevent disease. Ehrlich theorized that the antitoxins involved in this immune response were chemical receptors or "side-chains" attached to cells, just like the structures he had observed on dyes. He believed that these side-chains (antibodies) exactly fitted the side-chains on pathogens like a lock and key. If he could find a dye with exactly the right side-chain, he would have his magic bullet.

Targeting syphilis
In 1905, German scientists Erich Hoffmann and Fritz Schaudinn, working together in Berlin, found *Treponema pallidum*, the bacterium responsible for syphilis, a disease

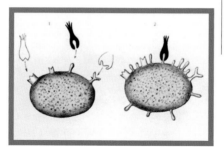

Ehrlich's illustration of side-chain theory, from his Croonian Lecture, 1900, proposed that body cells form receptors specific to a particular substance or pathogen, which lock together.

See also: Pharmacy 54–59 ▪ Cancer therapy 168–175 ▪ Bacteriophages and phage therapy 204–205 ▪ Antibiotics 216–223 ▪ Monoclonal antibodies 282–283

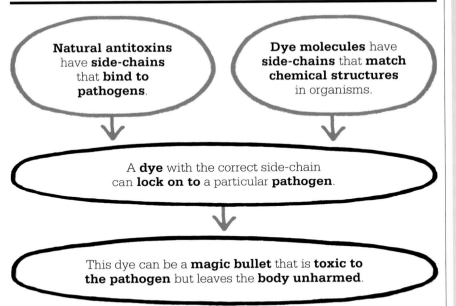

> **Natural antitoxins** have **side-chains** that **bind to pathogens**.

> **Dye molecules** have **side-chains** that **match chemical structures** in organisms.

> A **dye** with the correct side-chain can **lock on to** a particular **pathogen**.

> This dye can be a **magic bullet** that is **toxic to the pathogen** but leaves the **body unharmed**.

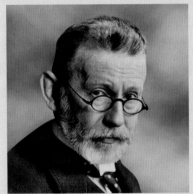

Paul Ehrlich

Born in 1854 in Strehlen, Germany, Paul Ehrlich studied medicine before concentrating his research on how dyes stain animal tissues. His work on dye classification and tissue staining laid the foundations for the science of hematology.

In 1890, Ehrlich joined Robert Koch at the Institute for Infectious Diseases and began to focus on immunology. Over the next 20 years, Ehrlich proved that the body makes antibodies that can target specific germs using chemical structures that hook together. For this groundbreaking discovery, he was awarded the Nobel Prize in Physiology or Medicine in 1908, along with Élie Metchnikoff for his discovery of macrophages. Ehrlich's magic bullet drug Salvarsan was launched in 1910, but controversies surrounding the drug took a toll on his health, and he died from a heart attack in 1915.

Key works

1900 Croonian Lecture: "On immunity with special reference to cell life"
1906 "The Tasks of Chemotherapy"

that had ruined lives for centuries. Ehrlich decided to make this bacterium his first target.

Working in the laboratories of the Hoechst chemical company, Ehrlich and his team started with a dye synthesized from an arsenic compound, atoxyl. They tried hundreds of variations to find an exact match. In 1907, they found one: the arsenic-based arsphenamine, which they called "compound 606." The team tried this formulation on patients in the terminal stages of syphilis and found that several made a complete recovery. Clinical trials soon showed that 606, given the trade name Salvarsan, was most effective if administered in the early stages of the disease. Salvarsan was launched in 1910, and by the end of the year, nearly 14,000 ampoules a day were being produced.

While Salvarsan was the first effective treatment for syphilis, it was difficult to administer safely and could have devastating side effects if not stored correctly. In 1912, Ehrlich's laboratory developed a less toxic version, Neosalvarsan.

While Ehrlich's dream of finding a chemical magic bullet to treat every disease has not been realized, his immunological breakthrough established the concept of chemotherapy, launched a global pharmaceutical industry, and fueled the invention of countless other drugs. ▪

> 66
>
> Success in research needs … luck, patience, skill, and money.
> **Paul Ehrlich**
>
> 99

UNKNOWN SUBSTANCES ESSENTIAL FOR LIFE

VITAMINS AND DIET

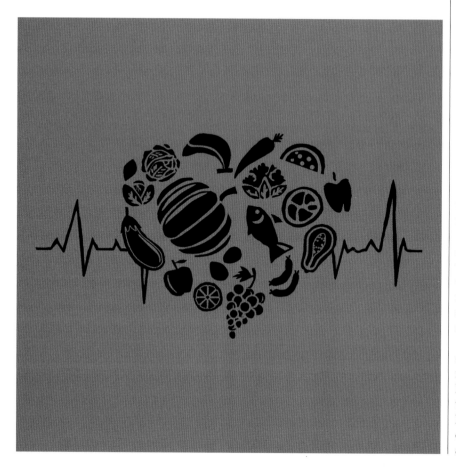

IN CONTEXT

BEFORE
c. 1500 BCE The ancient
Egyptians recognize that
night blindness can be
treated with specific foods.

1747 James Lind shows that
citrus fruit is an effective
treatment for scurvy.

1881 Russian biochemist
Nikolai Lunin proposes that
some foods contain "unknown
substances essential for life."

AFTER
1929 Christiaan Eijkman
and Frederick Hopkins are
awarded the Nobel Prize in
Physiology or Medicine
for their work on vitamins.

1931 Albert Szent-Györgyi
suspects that hexuronic acid
(since renamed ascorbic
acid) is vitamin C, and its
effectiveness in curing scurvy
is later confirmed.

Vitamins are essential
nutrients that every animal
needs in small amounts to
remain healthy. The human body
needs 13 different vitamins. Nearly
all must be obtained through diet,
as they cannot be produced by
the body. Vitamins work with
other nutrients to ensure that cells
function well. When any are absent,
ailments or diseases develop, and
some can prove fatal.

Despite their importance, the
discovery of vitamins is relatively
recent. In 1912, Casimir Funk, a
Polish-born biochemist, coined the
term "vitamine" when he published
his hypothesis that deficiency
diseases, such as rickets, pellagra,
and beriberi, are caused by a lack

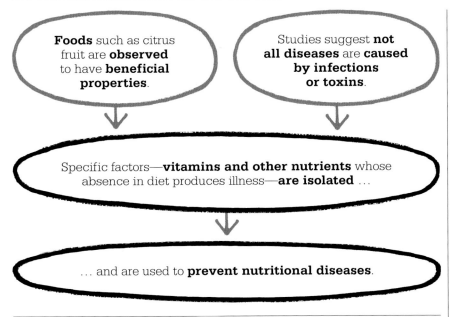

Foods such as citrus fruit are **observed** to have **beneficial properties**.

Studies suggest **not all diseases** are **caused by infections or toxins**.

Specific factors—**vitamins and other nutrients** whose absence in diet produces illness—**are isolated** …

… and are used to **prevent nutritional diseases**.

of vital substances in the diet. Funk initially believed that all these substances were amines (a compound crucial for the creation, growth, and metabolism of human cells), but the "e" was later dropped when it was discovered that most vitamins are not amines. Funk's work transformed understanding of diet and initiated a new era of nutritional science.

Misunderstood causes

Until Funk's research in the early years of the 20th century, the existence of vitamins had not been proven. Diseases related to nutrition that appeared to have no effective treatment, such as rickets, were common. Ironically, the revolution in medical thinking sparked by French chemist Louis Pasteur's discovery of microbes in the 1860s may have held back cures for these diseases, because it was assumed that most were caused by infections, and poor diet was mostly overlooked

as a cause. An exception was scurvy, which was known to be treated effectively by including citrus fruit in the diet, although the vitamin C responsible for preventing this disease was only isolated by Hungarian physiologist Albert Szent-Györgyi in 1931.

Searching for a cure

Funk's attempts to isolate the substances in food that affect health were inspired by the work of earlier researchers, especially that of Christiaan Eijkman. In the 1890s, Eijkman, a Dutch physician working in Indonesia, was tasked with finding a cure for beriberi, which was commonplace in Southeast Asia. Causing immense suffering, symptoms include dramatic weight loss, swelling and paralysis of the limbs, and brain damage, often resulting in death.

Eijkman stumbled across the link between diet and beriberi by accident in 1897. He noticed that

chickens fed with polished rice developed beriberi, but they soon recovered when their diet reverted to kitchen scraps. He concluded that white rice lacked an essential ingredient, which he called the "anti-beriberi factor."

Later, his colleague Adolphe Vorderman conducted controlled experiments with prison inmates, some eating polished rice and some eating unpolished rice, showing that the "anti-beriberi factor" was present in rice husks and kernels.

Isolating vitamins

The "anti-beriberi factor" was finally identified by Japanese researcher Umetaro Suzuki. In 1911, Suzuki described a nutrient (he called it aberic acid), which he had extracted from rice bran and given to patients as a cure for beriberi. The article was not widely read, but his discovery was later found to be thiamine, or vitamin B_1.

The following year, British biochemist Frederick Gowland Hopkins proposed that some foods contain "accessory factors," which the human body needs in addition »

> Protein supply
> and energy supply
> do not alone secure
> normal nutrition.
> **Frederick Gowland Hopkins**
> *Journal of Physiology*, 1912

Table of vitamins

	Chemical compound	Main food sources	Deficiency-related disease
A	Retinol	Oily fish, fish liver oils, liver, dairy products	Night blindness
*B₁	Thiamine	Whole grains, meat	Beriberi
*B₂	Riboflavin	Dairy products, meat, green vegetables	Inflammation of tongue
*B₃	Niacin	Meat, fish, whole grains	Pellagra
*B₅	Pantothenic acid	Meat, whole grains	Skin paresthesia
*B₆	Pyridoxine	Meat, vegetables	Anemia
*B₇	Biotin	Meat, eggs, nuts, seeds	Dermatitis
*B₉	Folic acid	Leafy vegetables, legumes	Anemia, birth defects
*B₁₂	Cobalamin	Meat, fish, dairy products	Anemia
*C	Ascorbic acid	Citrus fruit	Scurvy
D	Calciferol	Fish oils, dairy products	Rickets
E	Tocopherol	Unrefined vegetable oils, nuts, seeds	Mild anemia
K	Phylloquinone	Leafy vegetables	Excessive bleeding

*water-soluble vitamins

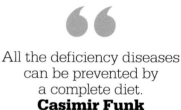

All the deficiency diseases
can be prevented by
a complete diet.
Casimir Funk
Journal of State Medicine, **1912**

British biochemist Edward Mellenby experimented with dogs' diets between 1918 and 1921. Inspired by the work of Funk and McCollum, Mellenby found that when fed on oatmeal alone, puppies developed rickets, but when given a diet rich in cod-liver oil or suet, they recovered. He had demonstrated beyond doubt that the disease is the product of a dietary deficiency.

Mellenby explained that in the absence of "accessory food factors" (which we now know are vitamins), the phytic acid present in the oats suppressed the absorption of calcium and phosphorus (needed for healthy bone growth). However, the vitamin D in fish (and in milk, eggs, and suet) helps that absorption. His work changed attitudes toward the prevention of rickets so dramatically that by the early 1930s, London was thought to be free from the disease.

Pellagra—whose symptoms include dermatitis, diarrhea, mouth sores, and dementia—affected 3 million Americans between 1906 and 1940, causing 100,000 deaths in areas where corn was the dominant food crop. In the early 20th century, scientists assumed that corn either carried the disease or contained a toxic substance. However, pellagra

to proteins, carbohydrates, fats, and minerals. Also in 1912, Funk presented the results of studies he had performed after reading about Eijkman's earlier work on beriberi.

Funk had fed pigeons polished rice and found that they became unwell, but if they were given the extract from rice hulls, they soon recovered. He realized that some chemical in these extracts was required, albeit in tiny quantities, to maintain health. While it took until 1936 for the chemical structure of this "anti-beriberi factor" (later named thiamine, or vitamin B₁) to be described, Funk had identified the existence of vitamins.

Shortly afterward, in 1913, Elmer Verner McCollum, an American biochemist, identified a substance he called "fat-soluble factor A" while researching the nutritional needs of animals. He found that without this factor (later named vitamin A), his laboratory rats died.

Tackling dietary disorders
By establishing nutrition as an experimental science, Funk's work paved the way for research into cures for disorders such as rickets, which ravaged populations in the 19th and early 20th centuries, contributing to high child mortality, especially in newly industrialized cities.

Rickets is a skeletal disease that produces weak, soft bones; stunted growth; and skeletal deformities in young children. Finding a cure had long challenged physicians, and diet had not been considered until

wasn't prevalent in Mesoamerica, where corn had been a dietary staple for centuries.

In 1914, the US government tasked physician Joseph Goldberger with finding a cure. Observing a higher incidence of pellagra among people with a poor diet, he tested a range of supplements. Goldberger concluded that a diet that included meat, milk, eggs, and legumes—or small amounts of brewer's yeast— prevented pellagra. The vitamin link was finally confirmed in 1937, when American biochemist Conrad Elvehjem demonstrated that niacin (vitamin B_3) cured the disease.

Filling the gaps

Between 1920 and 1948, vitamins E and K and seven more B-complex vitamins were identified, bringing the total to 13. These are all essential for body function; vitamins given the letters F to J and L to Z are substances that are nonessential, have been renamed or reclassified as they are not true vitamins (vitamin F, for example, is a fatty acid), or are not recognized scientifically.

Of the 13 essential vitamins, the eight B-complex vitamins and vitamin C are water-soluble, which

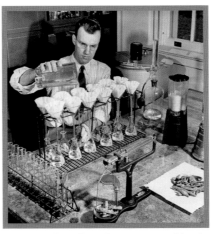

Testing the vitamin content of foods during the 1940s allowed nutritionists to understand the components of a balanced diet—one that would protect against deficiency diseases.

means they are readily excreted from the body, so a regular dietary supply is needed. Vitamins A, D, E, and K are fat-soluble and can be stored in the body.

Vitamins work in many different ways, and research continues to investigate all their functions and actions in the body, many of which remain unclear. Scientists know, for example, that the eye needs a form of vitamin A for its rods and

cones to detect light. Its absence leads to deteriorating eyesight and, ultimately, blindness, but research has yet to establish whether vitamin A can protect against particular eye disorders, such as the development of cataracts and age-related macular degeneration.

Synthesizing vitamins

The growth of nutritional science during the 1920s spurred attempts to synthesize vitamins. In 1933, British chemist Norman Haworth was the first to manufacture a vitamin—vitamin C—and by the 1940s, a new vitamin industry had developed. From an original focus on the use of vitamins for treating nutritional disorders, mass production allowed their use as a popular dietary supplement. It is now possible to reproduce every vitamin from either plant or animal materials or to make vitamins synthetically. Vitamin C, for example, can be taken from citrus fruits but is synthesized more cheaply from keto acid. With new research into how vitamins are taken up by the body, additives are also often included in vitamin pills to aid their absorption. ■

Casimir Funk

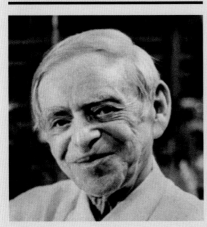

Born in Warsaw, Poland, in 1884, Casimir (originally Kasimierz) Funk studied chemistry at the University of Berne before working at the Pasteur Institute in Paris, and then at the Lister Institute in London. It was at the latter that he conducted his pioneering work on vitamins, researching beriberi, scurvy, pellagra, and rickets.

Funk moved to New York in 1915. Sponsored by the Rockefeller Foundation, he returned to Warsaw in 1923 before founding the Casa Biochemica research institution in Paris four years later. As he was a Jew, the outbreak of

World War II meant it was not safe for him to remain in France, so he returned to New York and set up the Funk Foundation for Medical Research. Apart from his work on vitamins, Funk also carried out research into animal hormones and the biochemistry of cancer, diabetes, and ulcers. He died in New York in 1967.

Key works

1912 "The Etiology of the Deficiency Diseases"
1913 "Studies on Pellagra"
1914 *Vitamins*

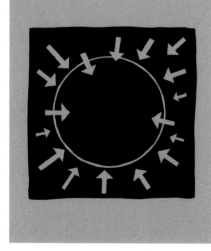

AN INVISIBLE, ANTAGONISTIC MICROBE

BACTERIOPHAGES AND PHAGE THERAPY

Bacteriophages are viruses that infect bacteria. There are an estimated 10 million trillion trillion of them in the world—around twice as many as there are bacteria. Félix d'Hérelle, a French-Canadian microbiologist, described them in 1917 and realized they could have potential for treating bacterial diseases—called phage therapy.

Dead patches

British microbiologist Frederick William Twort was the first to encounter bacteriophages in 1915. He was trying to culture the vaccinia bacteria used to create the smallpox vaccine but kept finding transparent patches of dead bacteria. Twort speculated that a virus could be killing the bacteria, but his research was curtailed by World War I.

That same year, d'Hérelle was working in Tunisia for the Paris-based Pasteur Institute and made a similar discovery to Twort while he cultured a bacillus to use against locusts. Back in Paris, in 1917, he found patches much the same in a culture of dysentery bacillus. It was clear that something was actively attacking bacteria, which d'Hérelle believed was a virus and called it a bacteriophage (bacteria-eater).

Miracle cure?

No one knew for certain what a bacteriophage was for some time. D'Hérelle believed it was a microbe, while others believed it was a chemical. But he immediately saw phages' medical possibilities. If they could kill bacteria, surely they could treat bacterial diseases? In 1919, after testing it on himself, d'Hérelle successfully treated several dysentery patients in Paris. Soon he repeated his success with treatments of a cholera epidemic in India and plague in Indochina. For

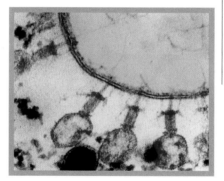

Enterobacteria T2 phages attack *E. coli* bacteria cells, shown here in an electron micrograph. Their tail fibers inject genetic material, which may replicate in the cells or remain dormant.

See also: Epidemiology 124–127 ▪ Germ theory 138–145 ▪ The immune system 154–161 ▪ Virology 177 ▪ Antibiotics 216–223 ▪ Monoclonal antibodies 282–283

Advantages and disadvantages of phage therapy

Advantages	Disadvantages
Phages destroy harmful bacteria; bacteria can become resistant to antibiotics.	Some bacteria may evolve resistance to phage attack.
Phages are effective against treatable and antibiotic-resistant bacteria.	While taking over a bacterial cell, a phage may acquire DNA harmful to humans.
Unlike antibiotics, phages have few adverse effects on good bacteria and are also less harmful to the environment.	Finding the exact phage or cocktail of phages to treat an illness effectively is difficult and time-consuming.
Phages multiply naturally during treatment, so only one dose may be necessary.	More research is required to determine which phages to use and in what dosages they are safe and effective.

a while, there was a boom in plans for phage therapy. Phage therapy, d'Hérelle believed, depends on a "cocktail" of phages to bombard the bacteria, just in case they develop resistance to one.

Other scientists, however, found that they were unable to replicate d'Hérelle's success, and doubts began to spread about the usefulness of phage therapy. By the time antibiotics came along in the 1940s, enthusiasm for it had faded. In the Soviet Union (USSR), however, it had been pioneered in the 1930s by microbiologist Georgi Eliava. D'Hérelle went there to work with him, but was forced to flee in 1937 when Eliava was suddenly executed as an enemy of the people. Nevertheless, with no access to the West's antibiotics, the USSR was soon using phage therapy as a key weapon against bacterial infections, and it continues to be popular in Russia today.

Phages rediscovered
By the late 1930s, though, the huge biological, if not medical, importance of phages was beginning to be widely understood. Steered by the famous Phage Group of scientists set up in Cold Spring Harbor in the US in 1940, phages became central to the discovery of DNA's structure. Alfred Hershey and Martha Chase used them to prove in 1952 that DNA is the genetic material of life.

Researchers have now discovered two ways in which phages take over bacterial cells. In both cases, the phage's tail fibers attach to the cell wall, then puncture it to inject their double-stranded DNA genome into the cell. In the "lytic" cycle, the phage uses the cell's resources to replicate multiple times until the cell ruptures. But in the "lysogenic" cycle, the DNA lies dormant within the cell, replicating as the host cell divides but leaving its host relatively unharmed.

As bacteria become resistant to antibiotics, enthusiasm for phage therapy has revived; many trials are now underway. Key benefits include the phages' swift replication rate and their ability to target specific bacteria. Phages could also be used to test for pathogens and to create antibodies that can work against illnesses such as rheumatism and gastrointestinal disorders. ▪

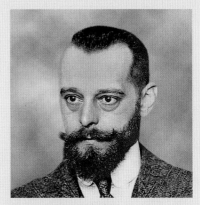

Félix d'Hérelle

Born in 1873 in Paris, France, Félix d'Hérelle was schooled in Paris, traveled widely, and moved to Canada at the age of 24, where his interest in microbiology began. Largely self-taught, he worked first in Guatemala, then in Mexico, where he found a bacteria that infects locusts. He began working on this in Tunis for the Pasteur Institute and observed something killing the bacteria.

At the Institute in Paris, d'Hérelle pursued his work on the bacteria killer and identified bacteriophages for the first time. From there, he moved to Leiden, Holland, and then to Alexandria, Egypt. He taught at Yale University and worked in the USSR before returning to Paris in 1938 to develop phage therapy.

Despite many nominations for the Nobel Prize, d'Hérelle never received it, but continued his work until his death in 1949.

Key works

1917 "An invisible, antagonistic microbe of the dysentery bacillus"
1921 *The Bacteriophage: Its Role in Immunity*
1924 *The Bacteriophage and its Behaviour*

A WEAKENED FORM OF THE GERM

ATTENUATED VACCINES

IN CONTEXT

BEFORE
1796 Edward Jenner tests the first vaccine on smallpox.

1881 Louis Pasteur immunizes farm animals against anthrax.

1885 Pasteur introduces the first rabies vaccine.

AFTER
1937 Based in the US, South African–born virologist Max Thieller creates the 17D vaccine against yellow fever.

1953 American virologist Jonas Salk announces he has found a vaccine against polio.

1954 Thomas C. Peebles, an American physician, identifies and isolates the measles virus. A vaccine is made in 1963 by John F. Enders and improved in 1968 by Maurice Hilleman.

1981 A plasma-based vaccine against hepatitis B is approved for use in the US.

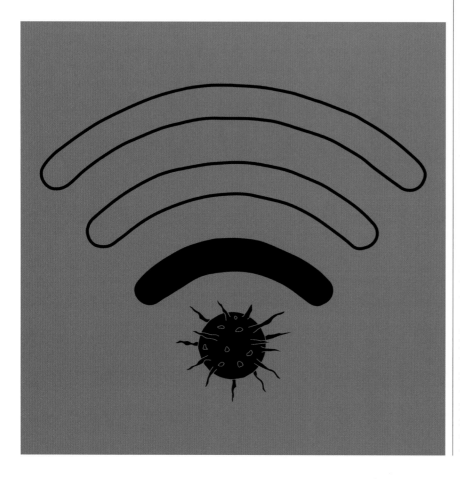

Following Louis Pasteur's success in the 1880s with finding vaccines for anthrax in livestock and for human rabies, interest in vaccination grew rapidly. Countless scientists began to hunt for new vaccines, believing that vaccination might one day rid the world of disease.

The quest proved more difficult and dangerous than anyone could have imagined and involved both terrible losses and huge heroism from the scientists and also many ordinary people willing to be used for trials. New methods had to be found for creating vaccines and enhancing their effectiveness, yet vaccines were gradually found for

See also: Vaccination 94–101 ▪ Germ theory 138–145 ▪ The immune system 154–161 ▪ Global eradication of disease 286–287 ▪ Genetics and medicine 288–293 ▪ HIV and autoimmune diseases 294–297 ▪ Pandemics 306–313

> Where youth grows pale,
> and spectre-thin,
> and dies …
> **John Keats**
> **British poet, who died from TB**
> **at the age of 25, in his poem**
> ***Ode to a Nightingale*, 1819**

many deadly diseases, including cholera, diphtheria, tetanus, whooping cough, and bubonic plague. Most famously, French scientists Albert Calmette and Camille Guérin created the BCG vaccine in 1921, saving millions of lives from tuberculosis.

New methods

Today, many vaccine researchers look for genetic material to find new vaccines, but in the 1880s, they tried to make vaccines from the pathogens themselves or from the toxic chemicals they secreted. Edward Jenner had used a less dangerous cousin, cowpox, to make his smallpox vaccine; Pasteur attenuated (weakened) the pathogen to make his anthrax vaccine. The difficulty with these "live" vaccines lay in robbing the pathogen of its power to make the patient ill while keeping it potent enough to activate the immune system.

In 1888, French bacteriologist Émile Roux and his Swiss-born assistant Alexandre Yersin found that diphtheria bacteria do their damage partly by secreting a toxin. In 1890, in Germany, Emil von Behring and his Japanese colleague Shibasaburo Kitasato showed in experiments on animals that the body gains immunity to diphtheria by developing antitoxins. Having captured some of these antitoxins from blood serum, they went on to develop an antiserum that could be used to cure diphtheria victims. "Serotherapy" provided the first effective treatment of diphtheria and prevented tens of thousands of deaths before a vaccine was developed in the 1920s.

Killed vaccines

The hunt for a cholera vaccine was led by Ukrainian bacteriologist Waldemar Haffkine. Haffkine came up with a method that began with a "passage": passing the pathogen on through a series of animals such as pigeons to give it the right form. With some vaccines, the idea was to weaken the germ. But Haffkine's aim was to boost its virulence to ensure it would provoke the human immune system. He then "killed" the pathogen by boiling it in a broth to prevent it from causing the disease. In 1892, Haffkine bravely tested the vaccine on himself.

Initially, Haffkine's vaccine was met with skepticism, despite a courageous demonstration later in 1892 by *New York Herald* reporter Aubrey Stanhope. Having been injected with the newly developed vaccine, Stanhope went right into the midst of a cholera epidemic in Hamburg, Germany. He slept among cholera sufferers and even drank the same water but survived unharmed. The next year, Haffkine went to India, where there was a desperate need for an answer to cholera. As with serotherapy, there were setbacks, but Haffkine's cholera vaccine saved hundreds of thousands of Indian lives. »

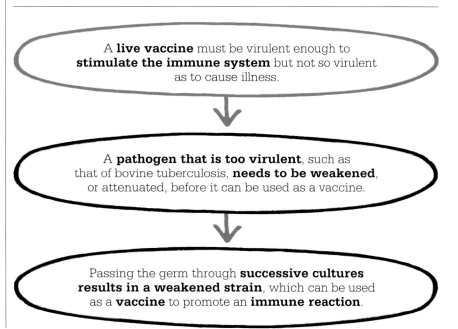

A **live vaccine** must be virulent enough to **stimulate the immune system** but not so virulent as to cause illness.

A **pathogen that is too virulent**, such as that of bovine tuberculosis, **needs to be weakened**, or attenuated, before it can be used as a vaccine.

Passing the germ through **successive cultures results in a weakened strain**, which can be used as a **vaccine** to promote an **immune reaction**.

Other scientists, including British bacteriologist Almroth Wright, followed suit, and a typhoid vaccine was produced in 1896 using a killed pathogen. Like Haffkine, Wright tested the vaccine on himself. Despite nasty side effects at first, it worked, and the entire British army was immunized against typhoid at the start of World War I.

Creating BCG

Perhaps the most significant breakthrough in the search for new vaccines was the tuberculosis (TB) vaccine created by Calmette and Guérin, known as BCG (Bacillus Calmette-Guérin) in their honor.

In the 1890s, scientists had looked to cattle for a TB vaccine, as Jenner had done with smallpox. But bovine tuberculosis proved too virulent for humans, and a trial in Italy ended disastrously. On the other hand, TB bacteria killed by boiling or chemical treatment had no effect on the human immune system. Calmette and Guérin knew they had to use a live germ but weaken it enough to make it safe.

Using a strain of *Mycobacterium bovis* (bovine TB) taken from the milk of an infected cow, in 1908,

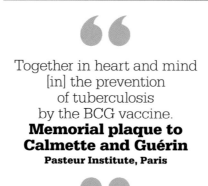

Together in heart and mind [in] the prevention of tuberculosis by the BCG vaccine.
Memorial plaque to Calmette and Guérin
Pasteur Institute, Paris

Calmette and Guérin began to culture the bacteria in their lab in glycerine and potatoes, with ox bile added to stop the germs from clumping. Every three weeks, they removed the bacteria and started another culture. The bacteria became less virulent with each successive culture. It was a slow process, and only after five years were the pair ready to test their vaccine on cows.

The trials were interrupted by the outbreak of World War I, but the culturing went on through the war. After 11 years and 239 subcultures,

Calmette and Guérin had created BCG—an attenuated form of bovine tuberculosis bacteria. BCG did not cause TB when injected in animals but provoked an immune response. In 1921, Calmette decided to test BCG on the baby of a woman who had died of TB after giving birth. Following vaccination, the baby became immune to the disease.

Ever-safer vaccines

By 1930, thousands of infants in France had been successfully vaccinated with BCG. Yet scientists still feared that the bacteria might revert to their more virulent form and give those who had been vaccinated the disease. That year, the fear seemed confirmed. When 250 babies were vaccinated with BCG at Lübeck hospital in Germany, 73 died of tuberculosis and 135 fell ill but recovered.

The investigation that ensued concluded that BCG was not to blame; the vaccine had been contaminated with virulent TB in the Lübeck laboratories, and two doctors were sent to prison. It took decades for confidence in BCG to return, but it is now recognized as one of the safest of all vaccines.

Albert Calmette

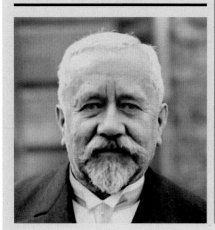

Born in Nice, southern France, in 1863, Albert Calmette went on to train as a doctor in Paris. As a student, he spent some time in Hong Kong learning about tropical medicine, and after graduating, he worked in the French Congo and Newfoundland, Canada. When the Pasteur Institute set up a branch in Indo-China (now Vietnam), Calmette became its head and organized vaccination campaigns against smallpox and rabies. After illness forced him to return home, he continued his studies of snake venom and made one of the first successful antivenoms.

In 1895, Calmette was made head of the new Pasteur Institute in Lille, and it was here he was joined by Camille Guérin, with whom he created BCG. The Lübeck disaster took its toll on Calmette, even though the BCG vaccine turned out not to be the culprit. He died shortly afterward, in 1933.

Key work

1920 *The Infection by Tuberculosis Bacilli in the bodies of humans and animals*

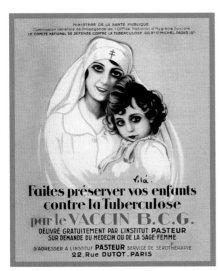

This French Ministry of Health poster from 1917 urges parents to take part in free BCG vaccinations to protect their children against tuberculosis.

Meanwhile, other scientists at the Pasteur Institute where Calmette and Guérin worked were devising a new way of creating a vaccine, this time for diphtheria. Serotherapy was a lifesaver for those who fell ill with the disease, but a vaccine would stop many more from falling ill in the first place. In 1923, French veterinarian Gaston Ramon found that formalin neutralizes the toxin secreted by diphtheria. In the UK, immunologists Alexander Glenny and Barbara Hopkins discovered that formaldehyde did the same.

Back in 1913, Behring had made a diphtheria vaccine by combining the toxin that provokes the immune reaction with an antitoxin to stop it from causing damage. But this toxin-antitoxin (TA) mixture often went wrong—as in Dallas, Texas, in 1919, when 10 vaccinated children died. Ramon and Glenny's neutralized toxin, or "toxoid," could still provoke the body's immune reaction, but it was much safer.

Adjuvants

Ramon and Glenny also discovered that certain substances called adjuvants enhance the potency of vaccines, although it was unclear why this was the case. Ramon's adjuvant was tapioca; Glenny's was alum, an aluminum salt, the most widely used adjuvant today. The combined diphtheria vaccine (toxoid with adjuvant) was so effective that within five years, it was being used across the world. In New York City in 1922, 22 people in 100,000 were dying of diphtheria each year. By 1938, the rate had dropped to just one person. The immunity provided by the vaccine does not always last a lifetime, but with occasional boosters, it is very effective, and this deadly disease is now rare.

The search goes on

By 1930, medics had three main ways to create vaccines: using a live, attenuated form of the germ (as in the smallpox vaccine and BCG); using killed organisms (as in the typhoid, cholera, plague, and whooping cough vaccines); and using neutralized toxins, or toxoids (as in the diphtheria and tetanus vaccines). Vaccination was never foolproof, but hundreds of millions of lives were saved and, in developed countries, the experience of major diseases began to fade into memory.

Since the mid-1980s, genetic engineering has led to subunit and conjugate vaccines against diseases such as human papillomavirus (HPV) and hepatitis. Scientists are now developing DNA vaccines, in which a short DNA length containing a germ's antigen sequence triggers an immune response. As shown by the COVID-19 pandemic, the quest for new vaccines is as critical today as ever. ∎

Types of vaccine

Living viruses or bacteria are weakened to make live vaccines.

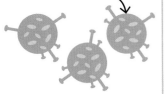

Live attenuated vaccines such as BCG contain living germs. In healthy people, they create a strong and lasting immune response.

Killing germs using chemicals or heat makes them safe to use in a vaccine.

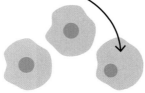

Inactivated "whole killed" vaccines such as polio use bacteria or viruses that have been killed. Boosters may be needed to maintain immunity.

Toxins are removed from bacteria or viruses and neutralized.

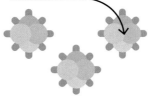

Toxoid vaccines such as tetanus use inactivated toxins (toxoids). They target the part of the germ that causes illness (its toxins), not the whole germ.

Specific parts of a germ, such as sugars or proteins, are used.

Subunit and conjugate vaccines such as HPV are made from parts of an organism that stimulate an immune response (such as its antigens).

TO IMITATE THE ACTION OF THE PANCREAS

DIABETES AND ITS TREATMENT

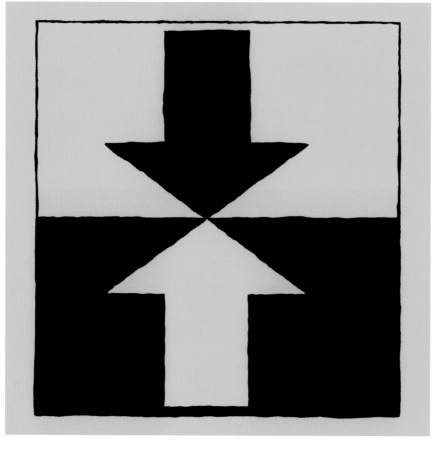

IN CONTEXT

BEFORE
1776 Matthew Dobson confirms an excess of sugar in the blood and urine of diabetics.

1869 Paul Langerhans discovers distinctive cell clusters—the islets of Langerhans—in the pancreas.

1889 A link between the pancreas and diabetes is confirmed by Joseph von Mering and Oskar Minkowski.

AFTER
1955 British biochemist Frederick Sanger determines the molecular structure of insulin.

1963 Insulin becomes the first human protein to be synthesized in the laboratory.

1985 The insulin pen is launched in Denmark, making the delivery of insulin easier for diabetics.

W hen Frederick Banting discovered the cause of diabetes in 1920, he cracked a medical mystery that had perplexed physicians for centuries. The earliest recorded mention of what is thought to be diabetes—a reference to frequent urination—is contained in ancient Egypt's Ebers papyrus, dating from around 1550 BCE.

More detailed accounts of the disorder appeared during the Golden Age of Islamic medicine in the 9–11th centuries CE. Ibn Sina and others describe the sweet urine, abnormal appetite, gangrene, and sexual dysfunction associated

See also: Ancient Egyptian medicine 20–21 ▪ Hormones and endocrinology 184–187
▪ Genetics and medicine 288–293 ▪ HIV and autoimmune diseases 294–297

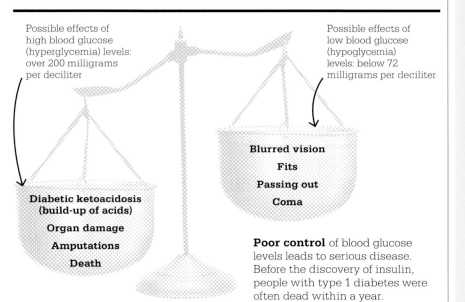

Possible effects of
high blood glucose
(hyperglycemia) levels:
over 200 milligrams
per deciliter

Possible effects of
low blood glucose
(hypoglycemia)
levels: below 72
milligrams per deciliter

Blurred vision

Fits

Passing out

Coma

**Diabetic ketoacidosis
(build-up of acids)**

Organ damage

Amputations

Death

Poor control of blood glucose
levels leads to serious disease.
Before the discovery of insulin,
people with type 1 diabetes were
often dead within a year.

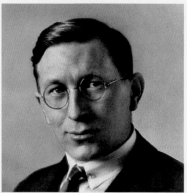

Frederick Banting

Born in 1891 in the Canadian
town of Alliston, Ontario,
Banting was the youngest
son of farmers. On finishing
his medical degree at the
University of Toronto in 1916,
he served as a battalion
medical officer in Europe
during World War I.

Banting returned home to
Canada in 1919 and opened
a surgical practice in London,
Ontario, while also lecturing
and teaching. It was while he
was preparing a lecture on the
function of the pancreas that
he began to investigate the
organ's link with diabetes.

In 1923, Banting received
the Nobel Prize in Physiology
or Medicine for his work
on diabetes and was also
made head of the University
of Toronto's Banting and
Best Department of Medical
Research. On the outbreak of
World War II in 1939, Banting
rejoined the Royal Canadian
Army Medical Corps. He died
in 1941, following a plane
crash in Newfoundland.

Key work

1922 "Pancreatic extracts
in the treatment of diabetes
mellitus"

with diabetes, and examination of
the color, odor, and taste of urine
was a common means of diagnosis.
In 1776, British physician Matthew
Dobson published a paper in which
he suggested that the sweet taste of
the urine was due to excess sugar
(glucose) in the urine and the blood.
He also observed that diabetes
was fatal in some instances but
not in others, which was the first
indication of there being two types
of diabetes: type 1 and type 2.

The role of the pancreas
In the mid-19th century, Apollinaire
Bouchardat, a French chemist and
physician, developed treatments
for diabetes. He recommended
reducing starchy foods and sugar
from the diet and emphasized the
importance of exercise. He was
among the first to suggest that
diabetes was linked to problems
with the pancreas. This idea was
supported by experiments on dogs.
In 1889, German physicians Joseph
von Mering and Oskar Minkowski

found that dogs developed the
symptoms of diabetes when their
pancreas was removed.

The exact nature of the link
between the pancreas and diabetes
was not yet known. Twenty years
earlier, German medical student
Paul Langerhans had discovered
clusters of cells in the pancreas
whose function was unknown to
him. In 1901, American pathologist
Eugene Opie linked damage to
these cells (now named the islets
of Langerhans) with the onset of
diabetes. In 1910, British physiologist
Edward Sharpey-Schafer proposed
that diabetes developed when a
substance produced by the beta
cells in the islets of Langerhans
was deficient. He called this
substance *insuline* (from *insula*,
the Latin for island); it was later
identified as a protein hormone.

In 1920, Frederick Banting, a
Canadian physician and scientist,
realized that pancreatic secretions
might hold the key to treating
the symptoms of diabetes. He »

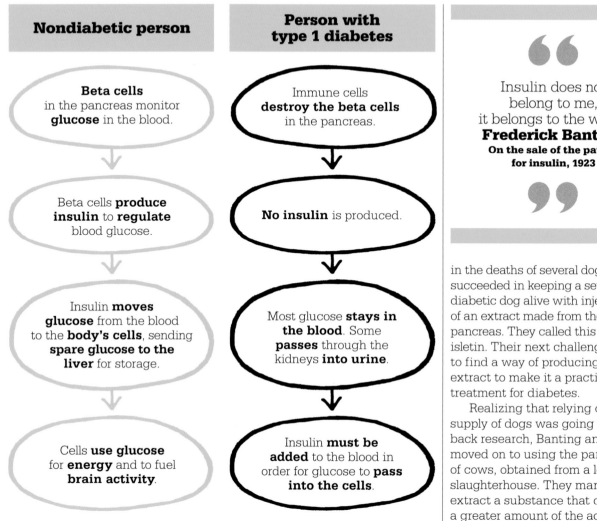

Nondiabetic person

Beta cells in the pancreas monitor **glucose** in the blood.

↓

Beta cells **produce insulin** to **regulate** blood glucose.

↓

Insulin **moves glucose** from the blood to the **body's cells**, sending **spare glucose to the liver** for storage.

↓

Cells **use glucose** for **energy** and to fuel **brain activity**.

Person with type 1 diabetes

Immune cells **destroy the beta cells** in the pancreas.

↓

No insulin is produced.

↓

Most glucose **stays in the blood**. Some **passes** through the kidneys **into urine**.

↓

Insulin **must be added** to the blood in order for glucose to **pass into the cells**.

Insulin does not belong to me, it belongs to the world.
Frederick Banting
On the sale of the patent for insulin, 1923

in the deaths of several dogs, they succeeded in keeping a severely diabetic dog alive with injections of an extract made from the tied-off pancreas. They called this extract isletin. Their next challenge was to find a way of producing enough extract to make it a practicable treatment for diabetes.

Realizing that relying on a supply of dogs was going to hold back research, Banting and Best moved on to using the pancreas of cows, obtained from a local slaughterhouse. They managed to extract a substance that contained a greater amount of the active ingredient and injected it into one of the laboratory dogs that had had its pancreas removed. The dog's blood sugar dropped significantly.

Human testing
At the end of 1921, Macleod invited James Collip, a skilled biochemist, to help purify Banting and Best's pancreatic extract for clinical testing in humans. On January 11, 1922, the extract was injected into 14-year-old Leonard Thompson, a diabetic patient who was close to death, at the Toronto General Hospital. The first test proved disappointing, but it was repeated

took his ideas to John Macleod, a Scottish expert in carbohydrate metabolism. Thinking Banting's theories were worth investigating further, Macleod made a laboratory available for him at the University of Toronto and provided an assistant, Charles Best.

The discovery of insulin
In May 1921, Banting and Best began to conduct experiments on dogs. They removed the pancreas of some dogs and tied off the pancreatic duct of others. The dogs whose pancreas had been removed

altogether developed diabetes, as expected, while the dogs whose ducts had been tied did not. While the pancreatic cells that produced digestive secretions degenerated in the dogs whose pancreatic duct had been tied, the islets of Langerhans remained undamaged. Clearly, the islets of Langerhans produced the secretions that prevented diabetes from occurring.

Banting and Best wanted to extract and isolate these secretions, but it was difficult to keep the dogs alive long enough to carry out tests. After numerous setbacks, resulting

with a purer version of the extract around two weeks later, this time with much better results. Thompson's blood sugar returned to normal levels and his other symptoms abated.

In May 1922, Macleod delivered a paper, "The Effects Produced on Diabetes by Extracts of Pancreas," on behalf of the team at the annual conference of the Association of American Physicians. He received a standing ovation. The paper used the word "insulin" for the first time.

The triumph of an effective treatment for diabetes was marred by rivalries. In Banting's opinion, it was his idea and his and Best's experiments that had led to the breakthrough. Others thought they would not have succeeded without the help of Macleod and Collip. The Nobel committee awarded the 1923 Prize in Physiology or Medicine to Banting and Macleod jointly. Banting shared his prize money with Best; Macleod shared his with Collip.

Manufacturing insulin

Insulin was not a cure for diabetes, but it was an extremely effective treatment with the potential to save millions of lives. Banting, Best, and Collip held the patent rights for insulin but sold them to the

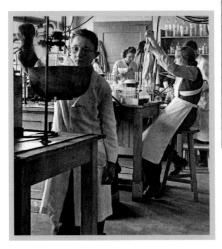

Workers at a factory in postwar Germany make insulin from pancreatic tissue derived from animals. Before the manufacture of insulin, diabetics had to control the condition by diet alone.

Types of diabetes

There are two forms of diabetes. Type 1 is caused by the body's inability to make insulin as a result of the immune system mistakenly attacking the cells involved in insulin production in the pancreas. It can be treated, but not cured, by administering artificial doses of insulin. People with type 2 diabetes produce insulin, but they may not produce enough or are unable to use it effectively. Type 2 diabetes is by far the most common. It is usually diagnosed in later life, generally in people over 30, although it is becoming common among younger age groups, too.

Research is ongoing into why people develop type 2 diabetes, but lifestyle seems to play a role. Obesity, for example, is a known risk factor. If exercise and a healthy diet fail to make a difference, doctors may prescribe insulin. As this can reduce blood glucose levels too much, type 1 and type 2 diabetics who use insulin must measure their glucose levels by testing their blood several times a day.

University of Toronto for just $1. However, producing sufficient quantities of insulin commercially was no easy undertaking, and the university allowed American pharmaceutical company Eli Lilly and Company to take on the task.

The scientists at Eli Lilly began work on insulin in June 1922, but they found it difficult to increase the yield from the pig pancreases they used or to achieve full-strength insulin consistently. Lilly started shipments to the newly opened diabetes clinic at Toronto General Hospital, but the potency varied so much that doctors were constantly on the lookout for the symptoms of hypoglycemia (low blood sugar) caused by too much insulin. These included sweating, dizziness, tiredness, and even passing out.

Toward the end of that year, Lilly's chief chemist, George Walden, made an important breakthrough. The isoelectric precipitation method

of extraction that he pioneered produced a much purer and more effective form of insulin than anything obtained previously. Now that the production problem had been solved, the company was able to build up large reserves of insulin.

Further breakthroughs

Over the next few decades, researchers continued to make improvements in the way insulin was produced and delivered. Scientists had succeeded in decoding the chemical structure of insulin in the 1950s and then identified the exact location of the insulin gene in human DNA.

In 1977, a rat insulin gene was successfully spliced into the DNA of a bacterium, which then produced rat insulin. By 1978, the first human insulin was being produced using genetically engineered *E. coli* bacteria. Marketed under the name Humulin by Eli Lilly in 1982, this was the first genetically engineered human medication. Today, the vast majority of people with diabetes rely on insulin produced in this way. ∎

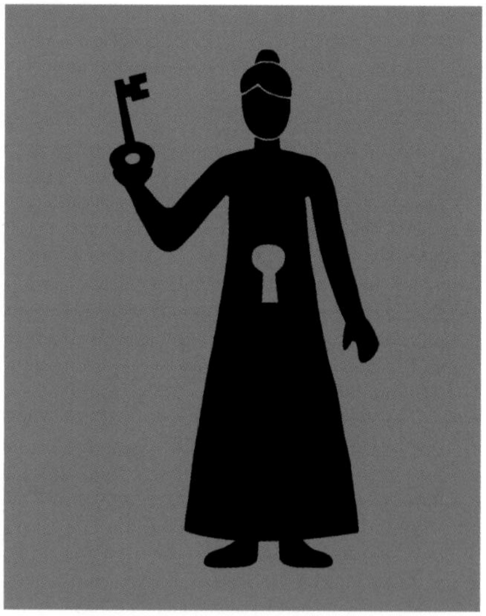

NO WOMAN IS FREE WHO DOES NOT OWN HER BODY

BIRTH CONTROL

IN CONTEXT

BEFORE

1484 Pope Innocent VIII approves the killing of "witches" who provide contraceptive advice to women.

1855 American chemist and engineer Charles Goodyear manufactures condoms from vulcanized rubber.

1873 In the US, the Comstock Act prohibits the distribution of birth control.

AFTER

1942 The Planned Parenthood Federation of America is formed.

1960 The US government approves the first oral contraceptive, later known as "the Pill."

1973 In the US, the Supreme Court rules that women have the right to seek an abortion.

2012 The UN declares access to birth control to be an essential human right.

Unwanted pregnancies can subject women to **ill health**, **botched abortions**, and even **death**.

→

Removing legal barriers to birth control allows women to take charge of their **health and their lives**.

↓

With safe, accessible birth control, a woman can call herself free and own her body.

American nurse and feminist Margaret Sanger viewed birth control as a fundamental women's right. Working in the slums of New York's Lower East Side, she was familiar with the devastation caused by unwanted pregnancies among the suburb's poverty-stricken immigrants. Sanger was often called to the homes of women who had undergone dangerous backstreet abortions, usually performed by an untrained person with unsterilized instruments. She discovered that many of these women did not have even a basic understanding of their own reproductive systems and sometimes asked her to share "the secret" to limiting their family's size.

Legal obstacles

America's Comstock Act of 1873 had deemed all contraceptives and literature about them "obscene" and outlawed their distribution. Sanger made it her mission to defy this Act and provide contraceptives to as many women as possible. She believed it was every woman's right to control when she became pregnant, and that contraception was an essential first step in ending the cycle of female poverty. With no

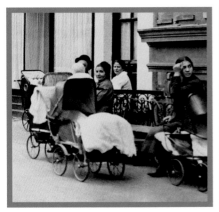

Women wait outside America's first birth control clinic, set up by Margaret Sanger in Brooklyn, New York, in 1916. The clinic was closed down by the government after just 10 days.

control over the size of her family, a woman would always struggle to make ends meet and have no means to educate herself. The number of dangerous, illegal abortions would also continue to rise.

In 1914, Sanger launched *The Woman Rebel*, a feminist publication in which she insisted that all women should have access to contraception and coined the term "birth control." After being charged with breaking the law, Sanger fled to the UK, but she returned a year later. The charges were dropped in the face of public sympathy following the death of Sanger's 5-year-old daughter.

In 1916, Sanger was sent to jail for 30 days after opening a birth control clinic in Brooklyn, New York. During her appeal, the court ruled that physicians could prescribe contraceptives for medical reasons. To exploit this legal loophole, in 1923, Sanger opened the Birth Control Clinical Research Bureau, staffed solely by female doctors. The organization would later become

part of the Planned Parenthood Federation of America, the vehicle used by Sanger over the next 30 years to bring birth control to the American masses.

Hard-won reform

Sanger lobbied for changes in the law and achieved many victories. In 1936, for example, New York, Connecticut, and Vermont were the first states to make it legal for family doctors to prescribe contraceptives; later, in 1971, reference to contraception was removed from the Comstock Act.

By then, the oral contraceptive known as the Pill was widely available. Sanger, who had always been frustrated by the small number of contraceptives available to women, had spearheaded the Pill's development. She had enlisted the financial help of heiress Katharine McCormick and the expertise of biologist Gregory Pincus. When the US government approved the Pill's manufacture in 1960, Sanger had finally won the fight for American women to control their own fertility. ▪

Our laws force women into celibacy … or abortion … Both conditions are declared by eminent medical authorities to be injurious to health.
Margaret Sanger

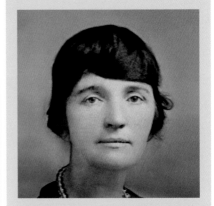

Margaret Sanger

Born Margaret Higgins in Corning, New York, in 1879, Sanger was one of 11 children in a working-class Irish family. Her father was progressive-thinking and supported women's suffrage. In 1902, after training to be a nurse, Margaret married William Sanger, an architect. The couple campaigned for various causes, and Sanger joined the Women's Committee of the New York Socialist Party and the Industrial Workers of the World.

Sanger fought against US contraception laws all her adult life. This included being an enthusiastic supporter of eugenics, which sought to reduce "undesirable" populations through enforced birth control and sterilization. She did not support eugenics on the base of race or class, but her views tarnished her reputation. She died in 1966.

Key works

1914 "Family Limitations"
1916 *What Every Girl Should Know*
1931 *My Fight for Birth Control*

MARVELOUS MOLD

THAT SAVES LIVES

ANTIBIOTICS

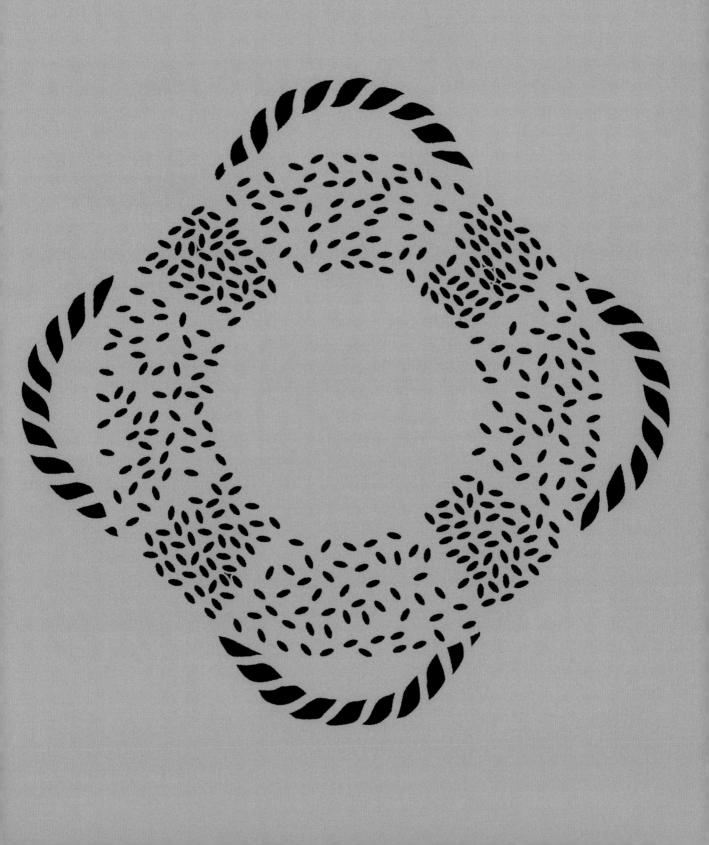

IN CONTEXT

BEFORE

1640 English pharmacist John Parkington advises the use of molds to treat wounds.

1907 Paul Ehrlich discovers arsphenamine, which is later released as Salvarsan, the first synthetic antimicrobial.

AFTER

1941 Howard Florey, Ernst Chain, and Norman Heatley treat a septicemia patient with penicillin, and mass production of the drug begins.

1948 Benjamin Duggar discovers the first tetracycline antibiotic, which has its origin in a soil sample.

1960 In Britain, Beecham, a pharmaceutical company, launches the new antibiotic methicillin to tackle pathogens that are resistant to penicillin.

2017 The WHO publishes a list of pathogens to be prioritized in antibiotic research.

Before the 20th century, there were no effective treatments for bacterial infections, including pneumonia, tuberculosis, diarrhea, rheumatic fever, urinary tract infections, and sexually transmitted diseases such as syphilis and gonorrhea. In 1928, this all changed with the work of Scottish bacteriologist Alexander Fleming, who was working at St. Mary's Hospital, London. Fleming was experimenting on the bacteria *Staphylococcus*—which cause illnesses such as septicemia (blood poisoning) and food poisoning—when an error occurred that proved to be a major medical breakthrough.

The first antibiotic

Returning from a vacation, Fleming found that a mold had contaminated the culture growing in one of his Petri dishes. On closer examination, he noticed the mold had cleared a ring of bacteria from around it. This mold was the fungus *Penicillium notatum*, which is now called *P. chrysogenum*. By chance, Fleming had discovered the first naturally occurring antibiotic drug that would be produced for therapeutic use—it would change the world of medicine.

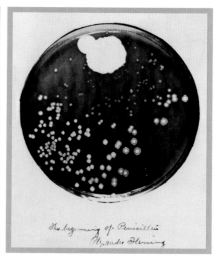

Alexander Fleming's original culture of *Penicillium notatum* (shown here) resulted in the groundbreaking discovery of antibiotics and marked a turning point in the history of medicine.

Initially, he called the substance "mold juice," but he then used the name "penicillin" in 1929.

Fleming demonstrated that penicillin could kill some kinds of bacteria but not others. Scientists divide bacteria into two categories: Gram-positive and Gram-negative. In 1884, Danish bacteriologist Hans Christian Gram had devised a new

Alexander Fleming

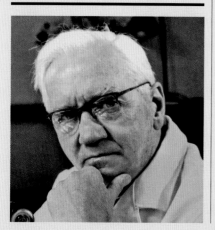

Born in Ayrshire, Scotland, in 1881, Alexander Fleming followed his brother into medicine. In 1906, Fleming graduated from St. Mary's Hospital Medical School in London, where he assisted Almroth Wright, a pioneer of immunology as well as vaccine therapy, in the hospital research department.

In World War I, Fleming served in the Royal Army Medical Corps, witnessing the effects of sepsis on injured soldiers. Returning to St. Mary's Hospital, he discovered the first lysozyme, an enzyme in tears and saliva that inhibits bacteria. Fleming was modest about his

role in the development of penicillin, but he was knighted for his work in 1944, and in 1945, he accepted the Nobel Prize in Physiology or Medicine, jointly with Florey and Chain. He also received the US Medal for Merit in 1947. Fleming died in 1955.

Key works

1922 "On a remarkable bacteriolytic element found in tissues and secretions"
1929 "On the antibacterial action of cultures of a penicillin"

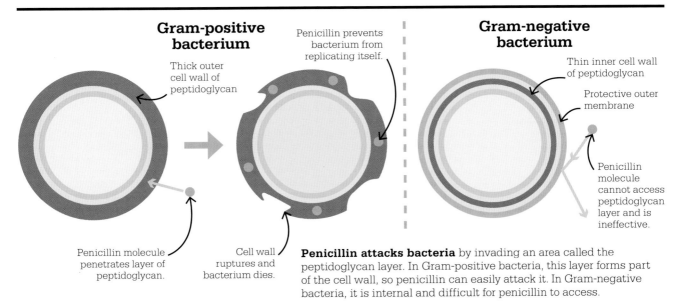

Gram-positive bacterium

Thick outer cell wall of peptidoglycan

Penicillin prevents bacterium from replicating itself.

Gram-negative bacterium

Thin inner cell wall of peptidoglycan

Protective outer membrane

Penicillin molecule cannot access peptidoglycan layer and is ineffective.

Penicillin molecule penetrates layer of peptidoglycan.

Cell wall ruptures and bacterium dies.

Penicillin attacks bacteria by invading an area called the peptidoglycan layer. In Gram-positive bacteria, this layer forms part of the cell wall, so penicillin can easily attack it. In Gram-negative bacteria, it is internal and difficult for penicillin to access.

method of staining that separated bacteria with an outer membrane around the cell wall from those without. This technique is still widely used by microbiologists: bacteria with no membrane (Gram-positive) retain the purple staining, visible under a microscope; those with a membrane (Gram-negative) do not retain the color.

Fleming showed that penicillin affected Gram-positive bacteria, including those responsible for pneumonia, meningitis, and diphtheria. It also killed the Gram-negative gonorrhea bacteria but not those responsible for typhoid or paratyphoid. Fleming published his findings in 1929, but they aroused little interest at the time.

Mass production

The idea of developing penicillin as an antibiotic lay dormant until 1938, when Australian pathologist Howard Florey assembled a team of biochemists at Oxford University's Dunn School of Pathology to realize

penicillin's potential. Florey's team included Ernst Chain, a Jewish refugee from Germany, and Norman Heatley and Edward Abraham, who were both British. The team faced formidable obstacles: the mold contained just one part in 2 million of penicillin, which was unstable and difficult to work with. Producing the penicillin was very slow, but Heatley devised a way to separate it from its impurities and then return it to water for easier processing.

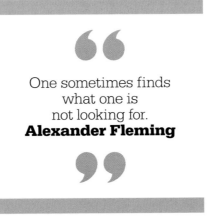

One sometimes finds
what one is
not looking for.
Alexander Fleming

Early in 1941, the team carried out the first clinical trials on Albert Alexander, a patient suffering from acute septicemia on his face. No one knew how much penicillin to administer, nor the necessary length of treatment, so they worked by trial and error. Alexander was given an intravenous infusion of the antibiotic. Within 24 hours, his temperature had fallen and the infection had subsided. However, Florey's team only had access to a small supply of penicillin, which ran out after five days, and the patient relapsed and died.

Florey realized that far larger quantities of *Penicillium* mold were needed. His team began to grow the cultures inside different vessels, including laboratory flasks, bedpans, and ceramic pots—yet the production remained slow.

With World War II raging, the need for penicillin was great, but the British pharmaceutical industry was working at full capacity on other drugs. Florey and Heatley »

The structure of penicillin

In 1945, British biochemist Dorothy Hodgkin used X-ray crystallography to discover the molecular structure of penicillin fungi. She saw that a penicillin molecule has a beta-lactam ring at its core, made up of one nitrogen atom and three carbon atoms. This was a vital discovery, as the beta-lactam ring is the reason for penicillin's effectiveness.

The outer wall of a Gram-positive bacteria cell consists of layers of peptidoglycan held together by cross-links of proteins. If the penicillin is present while bacterial cells are dividing, the beta-lactam rings bind to the cross-links while they are still under construction, preventing the completion of cell division. The bacteria cell wall is left weakened, osmotic pressure bursts it, and the cell dies.

In 1964, Hodgkin received the Nobel Prize in Chemistry for her work on the structure of biochemical substances.

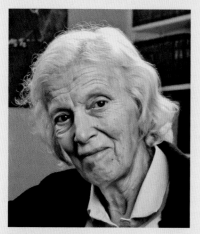

To recognize her work on the structure of penicillin, Dorothy Hodgkin was elected as a member of the Royal Society in 1947.

flew to the US for assistance, and by late 1941, the US Department of Agriculture had organized mass production of the antibiotic. A year later, a woman with streptococcal septicemia was successfully treated with penicillin in the US. Production increased exponentially, with 21 billion units produced in 1943 and 6.8 trillion units in 1945, saving thousands of lives. Also in 1945, British biochemist Dorothy Hodgkin discovered the molecular structure of penicillin, enabling the drug to be chemically synthesized. This meant that scientists could alter penicillin's structure to create new, derivative antibiotics able to treat a wider range of infections.

From natural to synthetic

For centuries, people knew that certain substances cured ailments. In ancient Egypt, moldy bread was applied to infected wounds, and mold treatments were prescribed in many other cultures, including in ancient Greece, Rome, and China, and in medieval Europe. While not understood at the time, these were antibiotic treatments in all but name. Experiments with the antibacterial properties of mold gathered speed

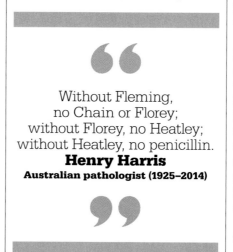

Without Fleming, no Chain or Florey; without Florey, no Heatley; without Heatley, no penicillin.
Henry Harris
Australian pathologist (1925–2014)

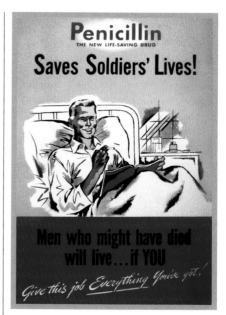

A poster issued during World War II shows an American penicillin ad targeting doctors. The US government ordered 20 companies to mass produce the drug, and it was heavily promoted.

in the 19th century. In 1871, British physiologist John Sanderson noted that bacterial growth was impeded by spores of *Penicillium*. The same year, British surgeon Joseph Lister observed the antibacterial effects of a mold on human tissue. Then in 1897, French physician Ernst Duchesne used *Penicillium notatum* to cure typhoid in guinea pigs.

In 1900, German scientist Paul Ehrlich embarked on a quest to find a "magic bullet" that would be able to seek and destroy all pathogens but leave healthy body cells alone. He noted that certain dyes would color some bacterial cells but not others. Methylene blue was one example, staining the single-celled parasite *Plasmodium*, which was known to be responsible for causing malaria.

Ehrlich aimed to find a cure for the sexually transmitted disease syphilis. His Japanese assistant

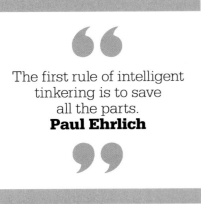

Sahachiro Hata trialed a series of synthetic arsenic compounds and found that one—arsphenamine—was able to select and destroy *Treponema pallidum*, the bacterium responsible for the disease. Ehrlich marketed it as the drug Salvarsan in 1910. However, it had nasty side effects, and the Russian Orthodox Church denounced the treatment, claiming that syphilis was a divine punishment for immorality. In 1912, Ehrlich introduced the improved version, Neosalvarsan, which then became the standard treatment for syphilis. As such, arsphenamine was the first synthetic antimicrobial. Yet as an arsenic-based compound, Neosalvarsan still carried bad side effects, and was also hard to store. In the 1940s, penicillin became the new treatment for syphilis, as it was considered a safer alternative.

Finding new antibiotics

Bacteriologists now understand that penicillin is a bactericide—it works by directly killing bacteria. Yet as Fleming discovered, penicillin

Leafcutter ants grow a fungus on harvested leaves. This fungus produces the bacteria *Pseudonocardia* (seen as a white powder). Some scientists believe this bacteria could be used to develop a new class of human antibiotic.

is not effective against every kind of bacterium. Over time, new varieties of antibiotics were developed that operate differently.

The 1950s and 1960s became known as a "golden era" of antibiotic discovery. Many pharmaceutical companies conducted wide-ranging searches for microorganisms that could be used to produce these new drugs. By 1968, 12 new groups of antibiotic had been discovered, and to date more than 20 groups exist.

There are three primary ways that antibiotics can attack bacteria. The first (as shown by penicillin) is to disrupt the pathogen's cell wall synthesis (see diagram on p.219). Vancomycin is another antibiotic that works this way. It was produced from the bacterium *Streptomyces orientalis* and became available in 1958. Vancomycin was effective against most of the Gram-positive pathogens, including penicillin-resistant bacteria. It was eclipsed by drugs that produced fewer adverse effects but regained popularity after the appearance of more antibiotic-resistant bacteria in the 1980s.

The second way that antibiotics attack bacteria is by inhibiting production of essential proteins, which stops the cells from multiplying. The first antibiotic to do this was streptomycin. It was discovered after soil samples taken in 1943 by American microbiology student Albert Schatz revealed the bacteria *Streptomyces griseus*, from which streptomycin was produced; it was effective against bacterial infections, including tuberculosis.

The tetracyclines are another family of antibiotics that work as protein inhibitors. In 1948, plant biologist Benjamin Duggar identified the bacterium called *Streptomyces aureofaciens* from a soil sample in Missouri. Chlortetracycline was isolated from the bacteria, the first of the large family of tetracycline antibiotics. Marketed as the drug Aureomycin, it was subsequently used to treat infections in animals, as well as humans.

Microbiologists developed other tetracyclines during the 1950s, and many have since been used to treat a range of conditions, including »

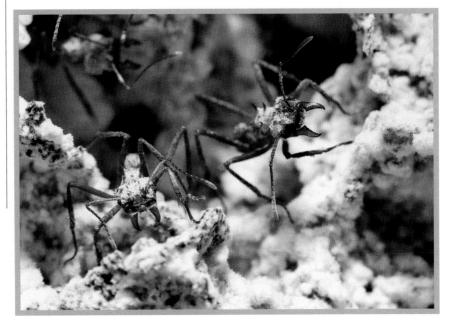

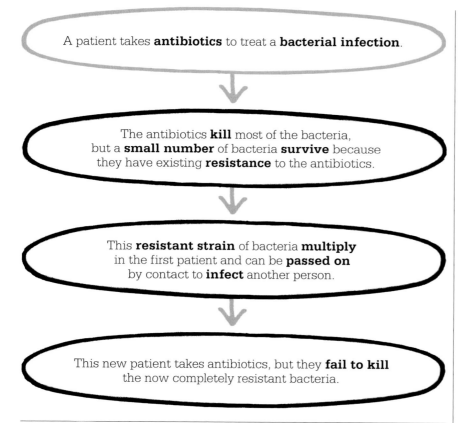

A patient takes **antibiotics** to treat a **bacterial infection**.

↓

The antibiotics **kill** most of the bacteria, but a **small number** of bacteria **survive** because they have existing **resistance** to the antibiotics.

↓

This **resistant strain** of bacteria **multiply** in the first patient and can be **passed on** by contact to **infect** another person.

↓

This new patient takes antibiotics, but they **fail to kill** the now completely resistant bacteria.

acne, respiratory tract infections, stomach ulcers, chlamydia, and Lyme disease. They are also used to tackle the *Plasmodium* protozoan parasites that cause malaria. Unlike some antibiotics, tetracyclines can work against both Gram-negative and Gram-positive bacteria.

Tetracyclines inhibit protein synthesis by entering the pathogen cell and preventing key molecules from binding to its ribosomes (tiny cellular structures, or "organelles"). The proteins that build and run the cell are made by these ribosomes, and when this process is stopped, the cell cannot multiply.

Almost half of all tetracyclines are used in animal husbandry. The drugs are given to pigs, cattle, and other intensively reared animals to prevent gastrointestinal infections and to increase meat and dairy

production by stimulating growth. Their overuse in agriculture is likely to have caused the increased resistance among many pathogens: now, tetracyclines are no longer as effective for animals or humans.

Quinolones, another class of antibiotics, use the third method of attack: preventing the bacteria from reproducing their genetic material so they cannot multiply. Quinolones include ciprofloxacins, which were introduced in the late 1980s. They work by damaging the DNA of targeted pathogen cells. These antibiotics are used to treat

The bacteria in this image were taken from the back of a cell phone, which provides an optimal breeding ground due to its warmth. Bacteria identified on phone handsets include *E. coli* and the superbug MRSA.

bone and joint infections, typhoid fever, diarrhea, and respiratory and urinary infections.

Rise of the superbugs
Staphylococcus aureus (SA) was discovered by German scientist Friedrich Rosenbach in 1884. It is the bacterium responsible for infections including septicemia, respiratory illnesses, and food poisoning. Scientists estimate that of those infected with SA before 1941, 82 percent died. However, since the introduction of antibiotics, an "arms race" has begun between the bacteriologists inventing new drugs and pathogens developing resistance to them.

Bacteria reproduce very rapidly; therefore, mutation and evolution also take place quickly. Chain and Abraham, two members of Florey's research team, had first noticed penicillin resistance in the bacteria *Escherichia coli* (*E. coli*) in 1940, before the drug had even gone into production. *E. coli* can be harmless, but certain strains (genetic variants) are linked to food poisoning, as well as gastrointestinal infections. Resistance to penicillin became more common in the late 1940s. Scientists developed alternative antibiotics, vancomycin and methicillin, to try and defeat the resistant strains in the 1950s and

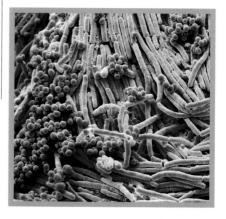

early 1960s—but methicillin-resistant SA (MRSA) appeared in the same decade and is now classed as one of the "superbugs."

These superbugs are resistant to antibiotics and are more virulent than their ancestors. An example is *Pseudomonas aeroginos*, which is a bacterium once found in burn-wound infections. In the early 21st century, it developed resistance to certain antibiotics and became a more virulent and common infection in hospitals. In the first decade of the 21st century, new categories of extremely drug-resistant (XDR) and totally drug-resistant (TDR) strains of pathogen were described.

Global health problem

Superbugs pose a major threat to humanity. Tuberculosis treatments have been compromised because the *Mycobacterium tuberculosis* bacterium responsible has evolved resistance to both isoniazid and rifampin, previously the two most powerful antibiotics used against it. Cholera (caused by the *Vibrio cholerae* bacterium) is also harder to treat, having developed resistance in Asia and South America.

> The world is headed for a postantibiotic era, in which common infections and minor injuries which have been treatable for decades can once again kill.
> **Keiji Fukada**
> **Assistant director general of the World Health Organization, 2010–2016**

Resistance to common antibiotics

The increasing misuse of antibiotics has led to bacterial resistance against drugs that were previously effective. In the US alone, prescriptions in 2018 reached 258.9 million. The global antibiotics market was valued at $45 billion in 2018, and is predicted to reach $62 billion by 2026.

Antibiotic	Release	First resistance identified
Penicillin	1941	1942
Vancomycin	1958	1988
Methicillin	1960	1960
Azithromycin	1980	2011
Ciprofloxacin	1987	2007
Daptomycin	2003	2004
Ceftazidime-avibactam	2015	2015

The World Health Organization (WHO) has identified antibiotic resistance as one of the biggest risks to global health and food security, one that threatens to roll back many achievements of modern medicine. Physicians find it harder to treat pneumonia, tuberculosis, food poisoning, and gonorrhea because the appropriate antibiotics are less effective. Even standard procedures, such as Cesarean sections and organ transplants, are more dangerous due to the reduced effectiveness of antibiotics used for postoperative infections. Each year in the US, 2.8 million people are infected with antibiotic-resistant bacteria or fungi, and more than 35,000 die as a result.

Misuse of antibiotics

While antibiotic resistance occurs naturally, misuse of the drugs has accelerated the process. Misuse falls into two main categories. First, antibiotics are overprescribed for humans, often being used to treat viral infections for which they are entirely ineffective. Added to this, patients frequently fail to complete their course of antibiotics, which enables bacteria to survive and gain immunity. The second form of misuse is the inappropriate administration of these drugs to animals. In 1950, food scientists in the US discovered that adding antibiotics to livestock feed accelerated the animals' growth, probably by affecting their gut flora. Because these drugs were cheaper than traditional supplements, many farmers embraced the practice.

By 2001, the Union of Concerned Scientists estimated that around 90 percent of antibiotic use in the US was for nontherapeutic purposes in agriculture. The WHO now campaigns for antibiotics not to be given to healthy animals, whether the intention is to prevent disease or to promote growth.

The need for antibiotics can be minimized by maintaining the basic rules of hygiene, including handwashing, as such practices will reduce the spread of bacteria. Antibiotics have saved millions of lives, but microbiologists now face the challenge of finding new and effective models to beat infection. ■

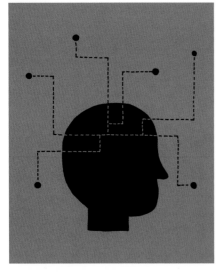

NEW WINDOWS INTO THE BRAIN
ELECTROENCEPHALOGRAPHY

In 1935, British neurophysiologist William Grey Walter diagnosed a patient with a brain tumor using an electroencephalogram (EEG). This technique, measuring electrical activity ("brain waves") in the human brain, had already been used by German neuropsychiatrist Hans Berger in the 1920s; Walter improved the technology to detect a range of brain waves, enabling EEG to be used as a diagnostic tool.

The brain contains billions of neurons (nerve cells) that form a vast, complex network. Neurons communicate with one another at junctions within the network called synapses—any activity at a synapse creates an electrical impulse. The voltage at any one synapse is too small for an electrode to detect, but when thousands of neurons fire simultaneously—which is what happens all the time in a human

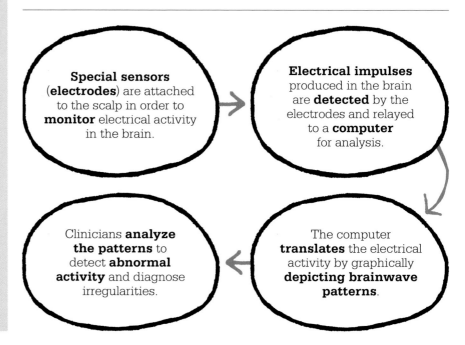

Special sensors (**electrodes**) are attached to the scalp in order to **monitor** electrical activity in the brain.

Electrical impulses produced in the brain are **detected** by the electrodes and relayed to a **computer** for analysis.

The computer **translates** the electrical activity by graphically **depicting brainwave patterns**.

Clinicians **analyze the patterns** to detect **abnormal activity** and diagnose irregularities.

See also: X-rays 176 ▪ The nervous system 190–195 ▪ Alzheimer's disease 196–197 ▪ Ultrasound 244 ▪ MRI and medical scanning 278–281

William Grey Walter

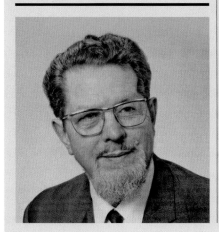

Born in Kansas City, MO, in 1910, William Grey Walter moved to the UK aged 5. He graduated with a degree in natural sciences from Cambridge University. Fascinated by Hans Berger's work with EEG, Walter then worked with British neurologist Frederick Golla at the Maudsley Hospital, London, using self-built EEG equipment.

In 1939, Walter moved to the Burden Neurology Institute in Bristol, where he conducted his most famous work as a pioneer of cybernetics, building electronic robots. Walter referred to these as his "tortoises" because of their shape and slow movement, and used them to show how a small number of instructions can give rise to complex behaviors—something he believed was applicable to the human brain.

In 1970, Walter crashed his motorcycle while trying to avoid a runaway horse. He spent three weeks in a coma and lost sight in one eye. Walter died in 1977.

Key works

1950 "An imitation of life"
1951 "A machine that learns"
1953 *The Living Brain*

brain—they generate an electric field that is strong enough to be measured by electrodes.

Walter performed experiments during which he placed detecting devices (electrodes) around each patient's head to map electrical activity of the brain beneath. His EEG machines differentiated a range of brain signals reflecting various states of consciousness, from high-frequency waves to low-frequency (delta) waves. Walter's great breakthrough was to discover a correlation between disrupted delta waves and the presence of brain tumors and epilepsy.

Different wave bands

While much is still not understood about electrical impulses in the brain, neurophysiologists now recognize five main frequency bands. Very low-frequency delta waves dominate when someone is in deep sleep. Theta waves occur if the brain is awake but relaxed—on autopilot or daydreaming. Higher-frequency alpha waves occur during periods of targeted rest in the day, such as in meditation or reflection. Beta waves are typical of an alert or strongly engaged mind. Finally, gamma waves, which have the highest frequency, are linked to periods of peak concentration.

EEG techniques have increased in sophistication since Walter first developed his model, but the basic principles remain unchanged. Electrodes placed around the scalp detect electrical signals when the neurons in the brain send messages to one another. These are recorded and a neurologist then analyzes the results. EEG is used primarily to diagnose and monitor epilepsy, as well as disorders of the brain such as tumors, encephalitis (brain inflammation), stroke, dementia, and sleep disorders. EEG is noninvasive and entirely safe.

Scanning alternatives

There are now other tools used for analyzing the human brain's health, although these do not measure electrical activity directly. Positron emission tomography (PET) measures the brain's metabolic activity, while functional magnetic resonance imaging (fMRI) records changes in blood flow. However, EEG is the only technique that can measure the extremely rapid changes in the brain's electrical activity, detecting these to the level of 1 millisecond or less. EEG's disadvantage is that the electrodes located on the scalp are not always able to precisely identify the exact sources of electrical activity that occurs at depth in the brain. ▪

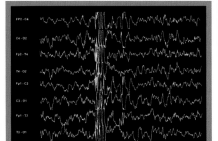

This EEG shows the chaotic brain waves of a patient during an epileptic episode (or seizure). Seizures are often recurrent and are caused by sudden surges in the brain's electrical activity.

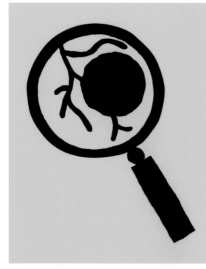

SILENT DISEASE CAN BE FOUND EARLY

CANCER SCREENING

IN CONTEXT

BEFORE

1908 Austrian gynecologist Walther Schauenstein notes observable differences between a healthy cervix and one that will become, or is, cancerous.

1927 Aurel Babeș suggests that cervical cells can be used to detect cancer.

1930 Austrian pathologist Walter Schiller charts the progression of cancer from cells to lesions and promotes the idea of routine testing.

AFTER

1963 A trial in New York City finds that mammography reduces mortality from breast cancer by 30 percent.

1988 The world's first mass breast cancer screening program begins in the UK for women aged 50–70 years.

2020 The World Health Organization (WHO) proposes a global strategy to eliminate cervical cancer by 2030.

Early diagnosis of cancer is crucial to **improve treatment outcomes**.

→

Screening the apparently healthy population can identify those with the **potential to develop cancer** but who have **no symptoms**.

↓

If **abnormal cells** are detected, they can be **removed before they develop** into cancerous cells.

←

Screening can reveal early signs of **certain cancers**, including **precancerous cells**.

---

lobally, cancer is estimated to cause almost 10 million deaths per year. That figure would be much higher if scientists had not found ways to identify certain cancers before they develop. The most effective way to do this is by screening—testing apparently healthy individuals to identify those who have the disease but are not showing symptoms.

Using a smear test introduced in 1943, the first mass screening program was established in the US during the 1950s and aimed to identify cases of cervical cancer, the

fourth most common cancer among women. Prevention depends on the early detection of cell abnormalities (precancerous lesions) that can develop into full-blown cancer.

In the 1920s, Greek American physician George Papanicolaou and Romanian gynecologist Aurel Babeș devised tests that used swab samples of cells from a woman's cervix. Working independently, they discerned that differences could be observed between healthy and cancerous cells. Crucially, Babeș established that malignant cells were often preceded by a detectable

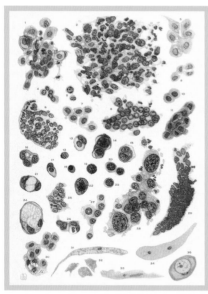

George Papanicolaou's *Atlas of Exfoliative Cytology* aimed to train other clinicians in his screening method and used drawings to help them identify changes in cervical cells.

precancerous stage. Papanicolaou's "Pap smear" test became a standard screening procedure for cervical cancer after 1943, and has since reduced mortality significantly.

Successful screening

The Pap smear proved that early cancer detection was key to saving lives, and its success fueled interest in developing tests for other cancers. By the late 1960s, tests had been devised for two of the most prevalent forms: breast and colorectal cancers.

Mammograms became standard procedure for breast screening. These X-ray tests detect tumors too small to see or feel. New technology has improved the test since 2000, with 3D digital imaging allowing analysis of breast tissue layer by layer. Colorectal cancer is one of the most treatable cancers if it is

identified early. Exploratory procedures such as colonoscopy, sigmoidoscopy (examining the lower colon), and fecal occult (hidden) blood testing (FOBT) have proven effective in detecting the disease. It is estimated that 60 percent of deaths from colorectal cancer can be avoided through screening.

Mixed results

Screening has not always proved successful. Prostate cancer is the second most common cancer in men. Since the 1990s, physicians have been able to test for it using a prostate-specific antigen (PSA) test. Above-average blood levels of this antigen may indicate the presence of cancer but may also be produced by other factors. There is no clear evidence that mortality rates have fallen since PSA testing was introduced and several countries have now abandoned it.

Balancing the gains of screening programs against the costs and risks (such as falsely positive results) therefore remains key in establishing successful cancer tests. Research continues to develop new tests and to establish which existing policies are most effective. ■

❝
A mammogram is nothing to be afraid of. It's not an enemy, but a friend.
Kate Jackson
American actor (1948–)
❞

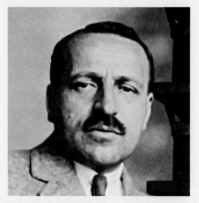

George Papanicolaou

Born on the Greek island of Euboea in 1883, George Papanicolaou studied medicine at Athens University. In 1913, he and his wife Mary emigrated to the US. He obtained posts at New York University's Pathology Department and at Cornell University Medical College's Anatomy Department, where his wife was also employed as his technician.

From 1920, Papanicolaou began studying changes in the structure of cervical cells, performing the first "Pap test" on his wife. A larger study followed, which revealed the first instances of cancer cells obtained using a smear test. Papanicolaou's initial findings had gained little interest, but the publication of these results in 1943 was well received and the Pap test became widely adopted. Papanicolaou moved to Florida to head the Miami Cancer Institute in 1961, but died just three months later from a heart attack in 1962.

Key works

1943 *Diagnosis of Uterine Cancer by the Vaginal Smear*
1954 *Atlas of Exfoliative Cytology*

GLOBAL
1945–1970

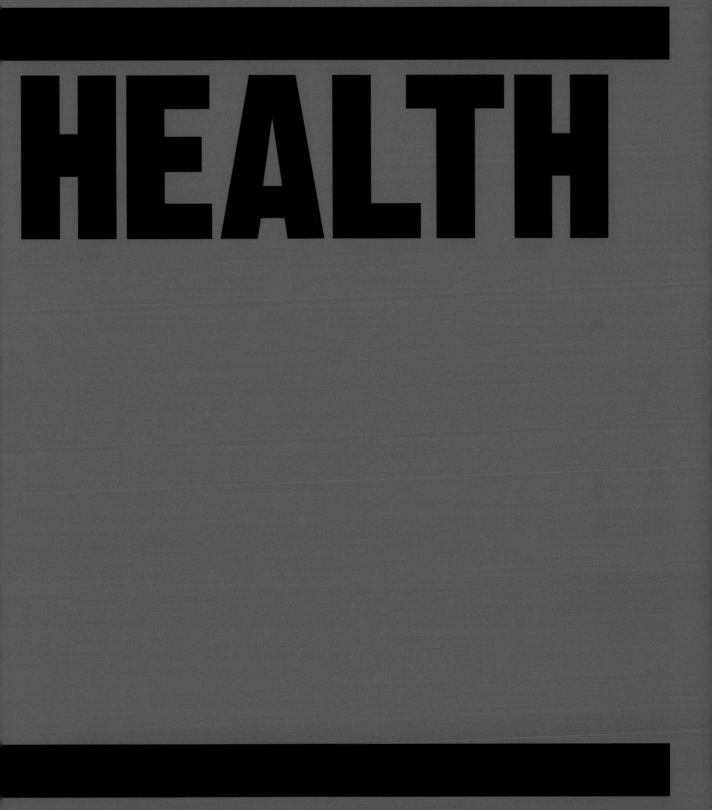

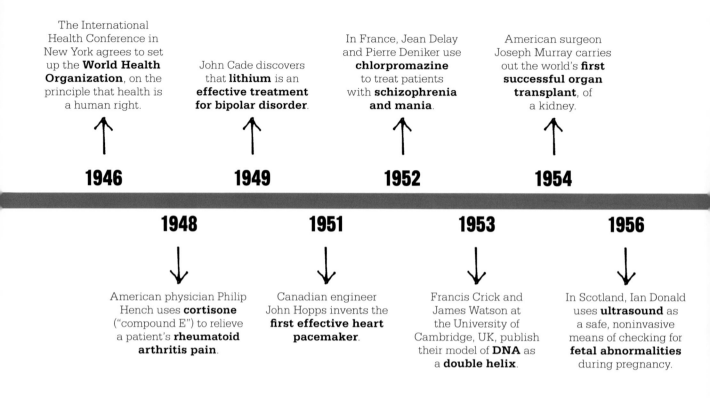

The International Health Conference in New York agrees to set up the **World Health Organization**, on the principle that health is a human right.

1946

John Cade discovers that **lithium** is an **effective treatment for bipolar disorder**.

1949

In France, Jean Delay and Pierre Deniker use **chlorpromazine** to treat patients with **schizophrenia and mania**.

1952

American surgeon Joseph Murray carries out the world's **first successful organ transplant**, of a kidney.

1954

1948

American physician Philip Hench uses **cortisone** ("compound E") to relieve a patient's **rheumatoid arthritis pain**.

1951

Canadian engineer John Hopps invents the **first effective heart pacemaker**.

1953

Francis Crick and James Watson at the University of Cambridge, UK, publish their model of **DNA** as a **double helix**.

1956

In Scotland, Ian Donald uses **ultrasound** as a safe, noninvasive means of checking for **fetal abnormalities** during pregnancy.

I n the wake of World War II, the bloodiest conflict in history, the World Health Organization (WHO) was officially established on April 7, 1948. Its vision of universal health included the notion that the highest possible standards of care should be available to all. Over the following decades, millions of lives were improved or saved thanks to the development of new drugs; advances in genetics, immunology, and orthopedics; a revolution in organ transplant techniques; and new ways of treating mental illness.

Healing the mind

War had left millions of combatants and civilians alike suffering from disease, injury, and psychiatric conditions such as depression. American psychologist B. F. Skinner believed that humans could be conditioned to relearn previously learned behaviors and emotional responses, enabling them to act more appropriately. From the 1940s, he honed his behavioral therapy techniques, which were influential in the development of cognitive behavioral therapy in the 1960s.

Other psychiatric treatments involved the use of drugs. In 1949, Australian psychiatrist John Cade found that lithium—previously used to treat gout—was effective as a treatment for bipolar disorder. Likewise, chlorpromazine initially had another use, as an anesthetic, but in 1952, it was used successfully to treat schizophrenia and mania.

Changing lives

Life for those with long-term physical conditions also improved in the postwar era. Kidney failure was an untreatable and life-threatening disorder until 1945, when Dutch physician Willem Kolff's dialysis machine was used successfully to filter toxic material and excess fluid from a patient's blood. Although dialysis techniques improved over the next few years, patients still had to be connected to a machine for long periods.

In 1952, French surgeon Jean Hamburger transplanted a healthy kidney from a mother to her son, who had renal failure. But donor and recipient were not closely related enough—the boy's body rejected the organ and he died soon after. The first successful organ transplant (of a kidney) took place in the US between identical twins in 1954.

The main issue with transplant surgery was in finding suitable donors. South African heart surgeon

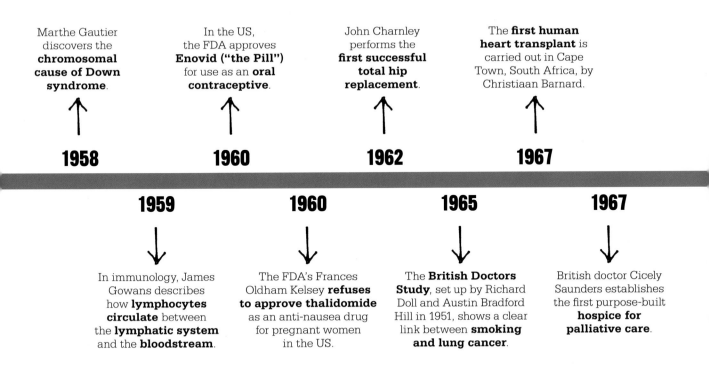

Marthe Gautier discovers the **chromosomal cause of Down syndrome**.

1958

In the US, the FDA approves **Enovid ("the Pill")** for use as an **oral contraceptive**.

1960

John Charnley performs the **first successful total hip replacement**.

1962

The **first human heart transplant** is carried out in Cape Town, South Africa, by Christiaan Barnard.

1967

1959

In immunology, James Gowans describes how **lymphocytes circulate** between the **lymphatic system** and the **bloodstream**.

1960

The FDA's Frances Oldham Kelsey **refuses to approve thalidomide** as an anti-nausea drug for pregnant women in the US.

1965

The **British Doctors Study**, set up by Richard Doll and Austin Bradford Hill in 1951, shows a clear link between **smoking and lung cancer**.

1967

British doctor Cicely Saunders establishes the first purpose-built **hospice for palliative care**.

Christiaan Barnard performed the first successful heart transplant in 1967, but it was not until the 1980s that an effective immunosuppressant drug to reduce the risk of rejection—cyclosporine—was licensed for use.

Understanding the body
As the 1950s progressed, more of the mysteries of the human body were explained. In genetics, the structure of DNA was discovered in 1953, and in 1956, scientists at the University of Lund, Sweden, established that humans have 46 chromosomes, arranged in 23 pairs. In 1958, French researcher Marthe Gautier found that Down syndrome was caused by having three copies of chromosome 21 instead of two.

British physician James Gowans made a huge contribution to the understanding of the immune system in 1959, when he showed that lymphocytes (a type of white blood cell) do not vanish but travel in the lymph system, and that they produce antibodies—a central part of the body's immune response.

Medical advances were not confined to the cellular level. In orthopedics, British surgeon John Charnley performed a total hip replacement in 1962, and in 1968, Canadian surgeon Frank Gunston carried out the world's first total knee replacement. In obstetrics, ultrasound—a new, noninvasive method for looking inside the body without using X-rays—became the technique of choice to examine pregnant women.

For those who wished to avoid pregnancy, the oral contraceptive, or "Pill," transformed the lives of millions of women after it was

approved for use in 1960. Not only a medical advance, this added pace to the female liberation movement and contributed to the counterculture campaigns gaining prominence in Western culture from the mid-1960s.

The need for caution
Although new treatments and drugs usually improve lives, there is always an element of risk—and it is crucial that they are thoroughly trialed. In 1961, it emerged that thalidomide—a drug introduced in some countries to relieve nausea in pregnant women—had caused birth defects in at least 10,000 children worldwide. A year earlier, pharmacologist Frances Oldham Kelsey at the Food and Drug Administration (FDA) had refused to authorize its use in the US, not satisfied it was risk-free. Her action saved many lives. ∎

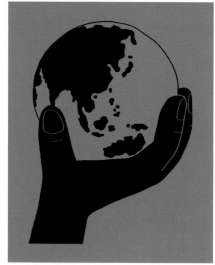

WE DEFEND EVERYONE'S RIGHT TO HEALTH

THE WORLD HEALTH ORGANIZATION

IN CONTEXT

BEFORE

1902 The Pan American Health Organization is founded; it becomes the first international health agency.

1923 The Health Organization at the League of Nations is established.

AFTER

1974 The WHO launches its immunization program against six diseases: measles, tetanus, pertussis, diphtheria, poliomyelitis, and tuberculosis.

1980 Smallpox is the first human disease to be eradicated worldwide.

1988 The WHO launches its Global Polio Eradication Initiative; by 2020, cases of polio worldwide have decreased by 99 percent.

2018 The first WHO global conference on air pollution, climate change, and health is held.

The concept of a specialty body responsible for international public health was first raised by Chinese doctor Szeming Sze in 1945. Sze had been stationed in the US as an aide to the Chinese foreign minister T. V. Soong, and it was only by chance that Soong asked Sze to attend the United Nations Conference on International Organization on April 25, 1945, in San Francisco. The US and UK delegates had explicitly stated that health would not be on the agenda, but Sze, with support from Brazilian Dr. Geraldo de Paula Souza and Norwegian Dr. Karl Evang, put forward a declaration

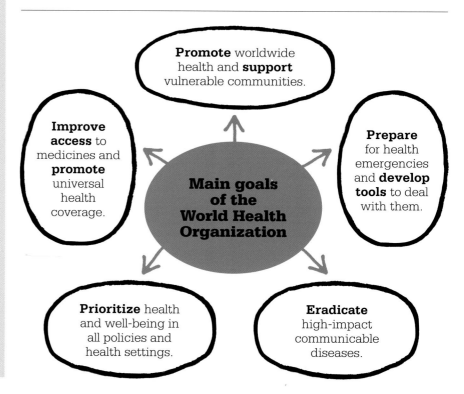

Promote worldwide health and **support** vulnerable communities.

Improve access to medicines and **promote** universal health coverage.

Main goals of the World Health Organization

Prepare for health emergencies and **develop tools** to deal with them.

Prioritize health and well-being in all policies and health settings.

Eradicate high-impact communicable diseases.

that a conference be called to discuss the establishment of an international health organization. Sze's declaration received overwhelming support, and one year later, an International Health Conference in New York approved the constitution of the World Health Organization (WHO).

Earlier organizations

For Sze, the WHO represented a new age in which international health would engender a postwar era of global cooperation. Previous attempts at health cooperation between countries had taken place in Europe during the 19th century. In 1851, an International Sanitary Convention was held in France to try and form a collective response to cholera outbreaks (which killed thousands), but political differences prevailed until the Convention reconvened in 1892 and agreed joint policies to tackle the disease.

From the early 20th century, new international health agencies sprang up on both sides of the Atlantic, such as the Pan American Health Organization in 1902, the European L'Office International d'Hygiène Publique in 1907, and the Health Organization at the League of Nations in 1923. These organizations mainly worked in disease control and eradication (for smallpox and typhus), with quarantining measures where needed.

The WHO formally began work on April 7, 1948. It inherited the tasks and resources of the earlier organizations and was given a broad mandate to promote "the highest possible level of health" for all peoples. With a budget of $5 million, funded by its 55 member states, it began by addressing

outbreaks of malaria, tuberculosis, and venereal diseases; developing strategies against leprosy and trachoma; and exploring ways to improve children's health.

The WHO today

By 2020, the WHO had grown to 194 member states and a budget of $4.2 billion. Among its key functions are the issuing of global public health guidelines; providing sanitary regulations, health education, and mass vaccination campaigns; and collecting global data on health problems. Its most celebrated achievement to date is the eradication of smallpox.

In response to the COVID-19 pandemic that erupted in 2020, the WHO acted as a worldwide information center on the deadly respiratory illness, issuing practical advice for governments, updates on scientific research, and news on the virus's spread—including global mortality figures.

The establishment of the WHO is celebrated each year on April 7 as World Health Day, which aims to promote global health awareness. ▪

> Health is a state of complete physical, mental, and social well-being and not merely the absence of disease or infirmity.
> **WHO Constitution**

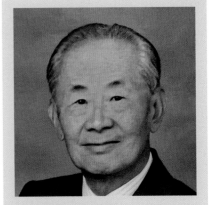

Szeming Sze

Born in Tientsin, China, in 1908, Szeming Sze was the son of the Chinese ambassador in the UK and later the US. Sze was educated at Winchester College and then Cambridge University, where he studied chemistry and medicine.

Sze worked as an intern at St. Thomas's Hospital in London, but returned to China in 1934 in order to devote his life to public service. During World War II, Sze worked in the US as part of its Lend-Lease program, supplying the Chinese government with defense aid. Instrumental in helping establish the WHO in 1945, Sze then joined the newly formed United Nations in 1948. He became the UN's medical director in 1954, a role that he held until his retirement in 1968. Sze died in 1998.

Key works

1982 *The Origins of the World Health Organization: a personal memoir, 1945–1948*
1986 *Working for the United Nations: a personal memoir, 1948–1968*

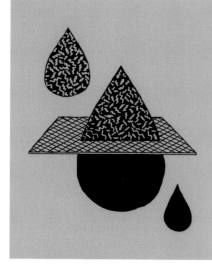

THE ARTIFICIAL KIDNEY CAN SAVE A LIFE

DIALYSIS

IN CONTEXT

BEFORE

1861 Scottish chemist Thomas Graham coins the term "dialysis" and uses the process to extract urea from urine.

1913 In the US, doctors John Abel, B. B. Turner, and Leonard Rowntree test their kidney dialysis machine on animals.

1923 German physician Georg Ganter pioneers peritoneal dialysis, which uses the lining of the abdomen (peritoneum) as the dialyzing membrane.

AFTER

1950 Ruth Tucker of Illinois is the first to receive a successful kidney transplant.

1960 American physician Belding Scribner develops a shunt that allows permanent access to veins for repeated dialyses.

1962 In the US, a team led by physician Fred Boen develops the first automated home peritoneal dialysis device.

Acute and chronic kidney (renal) failure are serious, potentially life-threatening disorders. The function of kidneys is to eliminate excess salts, fluids, and waste materials from the body, which accumulate in the blood if kidneys fail. Until the late 19th and early 20th centuries, there was little understanding of kidney problems and no effective treatment until the 1940s, when Dutch physician Willem Kolff's kidney dialysis machine successfully filtered out the toxic materials and excess fluid from a patient's blood.

German physician Georg Haas had attempted the first kidney dialysis on human patients in the 1920s, using varying machines of his own design. His original choice of anticoagulant (to stop the blood forming clots, impeding its flow) was hirudin from the saliva of leeches, which caused allergic reactions. Haas later used heparin, an anticoagulant that occurs naturally in humans and is still used today. However, the dialysis procedures were too short to have a therapeutic effect, and none of Haas's patients survived.

Kolff's machine

The breakthrough came in 1945, when Kolff performed a week-long dialysis on a 67-year-old patient with acute kidney failure using a rotating drum dialyzer, the forerunner of the modern kidney dialysis machine. He built it with materials he could easily access,

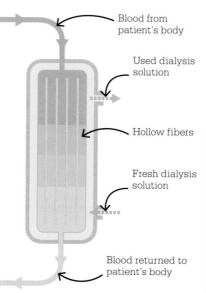

During dialysis, blood from the body passes through thin, hollow fibers, which filter out excess salt and waste products into a dialysis solution flowing in the opposite direction. The filtered blood then flows back into the body.

Blood from patient's body

Used dialysis solution

Hollow fibers

Fresh dialysis solution

Blood returned to patient's body

See also: Blood circulation 68–73 ▪ Scientific surgery 88–89 ▪ Blood transfusion and blood groups 108–111
▪ Physiology 152–153 ▪ Transplant surgery 246–253

including wooden bed slats for the drum, semipermeable cellophane sausage casing for the tubes, and an electric motor.

During treatment, blood from the patient's body, with the added heparin anticoagulant, passed through the cellophane tubes. These were wrapped around the wooden drum, which rotated through an electrolyte solution (dialyzate) in a tank. As the drum turned, the blood was filtered by diffusion: small molecules of toxins passed through the semipermeable tubes from the more concentrated fluid (blood) to the less concentrated dialyzate until an equilibrium was reached. The filtered blood, retaining its larger molecules of proteins and blood cells, then flowed back into the body.

Further refinements

Kolff's machine was adapted and improved at the Peter Bent Brigham Hospital in Boston, MA. The new Kolff-Brigham dialyzer was shipped to 22 hospitals around the world and used in the Korean War (1950–1953) to treat soldiers who were suffering

> I don't hesitate
> to try something that
> most other people will not try
> if I see a possibility.
> **Willem Kolff**
> **Interview after receiving the Russ
> Prize for bioengineering, 2003**

from posttraumatic kidney failure. Later machines used ultrafiltration, first proposed by Swedish doctor Nils Alwall in 1947, which removes more excess fluid from the blood as a result of differing pressures in the blood and dialyzate.

A further refinement in 1964 was the development of the first hollow-fiber dialyzer, which is still the most common type today. It uses around 10,000 capillary-sized

hollow membranes to create a larger surface area, which allows more efficient filtration of the blood.

Modern dialysis

Hemodialysis, filtering the blood through a dialyzer, is still the most common form of kidney dialysis, but for an estimated 300,000 kidney patients worldwide, peritoneal dialysis is a viable alternative. In this home procedure, dialysis solution flows via a catheter into the abdomen, and the abdominal lining (peritoneum) filters out waste products from the blood, which are then drained out of the body. The patient repeats the procedure four to six times a day, or a machine can operate the dialysis during sleep.

The challenge today is no longer the technology that Kolff pioneered, but the sheer number of patients with kidney failure. More than 2 million people worldwide undergo dialysis (of whom around 90,000 receive a kidney transplant), but this is thought to represent a mere tenth of those in need who cannot access or afford treatment. ■

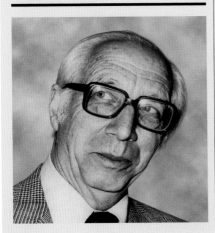

Willem Kolff

Born in Leiden in the Netherlands in 1911, Willem "Pim" Kolff studied medicine in his home city and, as a postgraduate at the University of Groningen, became interested in the possibilities of artificial kidney function. After Nazi Germany's invasion of the Netherlands in 1940, Kolff founded Europe's first blood bank in The Hague, then moved to a small hospital in Kampen. There, he developed his first kidney dialysis machine in 1943. Two years later, he used it for the first time to save the life of a woman imprisoned for collaborating with the Nazis.

Kolff moved to the US in 1950 and next turned his skills to cardiovascular problems and the development of an artificial heart. He was inducted into the Inventors Hall of Fame in 1985 and continued to work until he retired in 1997. Kolff died of heart failure in 2009.

Key works

1943 "The artificial kidney: a dialyzer with a large surface area"
1965 "First clinical experience with the artificial kidney"

NATURE'S DRAMATIC ANTIDOTE

STEROIDS AND CORTISONE

IN CONTEXT

BEFORE
1563–1564 In Italy, anatomist Bartolomeo Eustachi first describes the adrenal glands, located just above the kidneys.

1855 British physician Thomas Addison describes a disorder, later called Addison's disease, which occurs when the adrenal glands produce too little of the hormone cortisol.

1930s Researchers in the US and Switzerland begin to isolate adrenal hormones.

AFTER
1955 The Schering Corporation in the US first synthesizes prednisone, a new safer corticosteroid for treating inflammatory diseases.

2020 The WHO welcomes the positive UK clinical trial results for the use of the corticosteroid dexamethasone to treat severe COVID-19 symptoms.

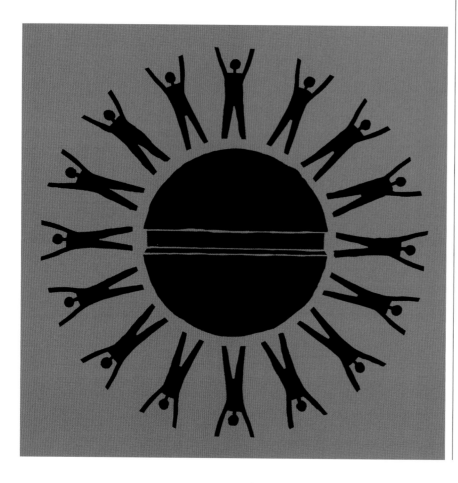

Rheumatoid arthritis is an autoimmune condition that occurs when the body's immune system misfires and attacks healthy cells that line the joints, causing inflammation and swelling. First described in 1800 and named in 1859, it was poorly understood, and there was little to relieve the pain when American physician Philip Hench began to study the disorder in the 1930s.

The 1948 discovery that cortisol, a hormone naturally produced in the adrenal cortex (the outer part of the adrenal gland above each kidney), could alleviate the condition led to the first effective treatments and paved the way for the

See also: Cellular pathology 134–135 ▪ The immune system 154–161 ▪ Hormones and endocrinology 184–187
▪ Transplant surgery 246–253 ▪ Monoclonal antibodies 282–283 ▪ Genetics and medicine 288–293

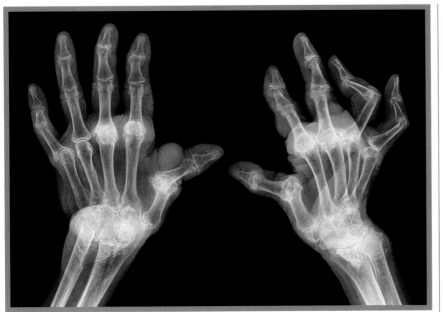

Rheumatoid arthritis can produce severe, crippling deformities of the hands, as shown in this X-ray. It mainly affects the capsule (synovium) around the joints, causing painful swelling.

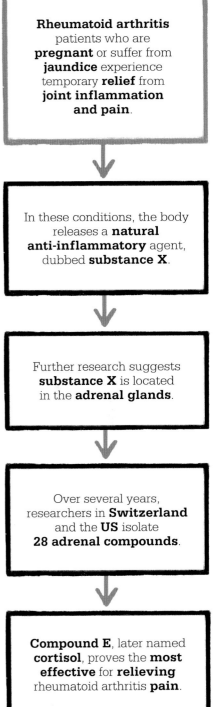

Rheumatoid arthritis patients who are **pregnant** or suffer from **jaundice** experience temporary **relief** from **joint inflammation and pain**.

In these conditions, the body releases a **natural anti-inflammatory** agent, dubbed **substance X**.

Further research suggests **substance X** is located in the **adrenal glands**.

Over several years, researchers in **Switzerland** and the **US** isolate **28 adrenal compounds**.

Compound E, later named **cortisol**, proves the **most effective** for **relieving** rheumatoid arthritis **pain**.

development of a new class of anti-inflammatory drugs called corticosteroids, or steroids. Hench, his colleague Edward Kendall, and Swiss researcher Tadeus Reichstein were awarded the Nobel Prize in Physiology or Medicine in 1950 for their work.

Jaundice brings a clue

In the mid-19th century, British physician Alfred Garrod laid the groundwork for rheumatoid arthritis research by distinguishing the disorder from gout, which involves an excess of uric acid in the blood; Garrod noted that this was not evident in any form of arthritis.

By the 1920s, most cases of rheumatoid arthritis were thought to be the result of infection. Hench, however, was not convinced. In 1929, while head of the Mayo Clinic's department of rheumatic diseases in Minnesota, he noticed that a patient's rheumatoid arthritis became less severe the day after he developed jaundice. For several months after his recovery from jaundice, the patient continued to experience less arthritic pain. Hench observed similar effects when other arthritic patients developed jaundice.

By 1938, Hench had detailed studies of more than 30 cases in which jaundice temporarily relieved his patients' arthritic symptoms. He observed that other conditions, especially pregnancy, induced the same relief. Knowing that the concentration of steroid hormones in the blood is higher than normal under these conditions, Hench reasoned that a natural steroid hormone might be responsible for the effect. Allergic conditions, such as asthma, hay fever, and food sensitivity, also improved when a »

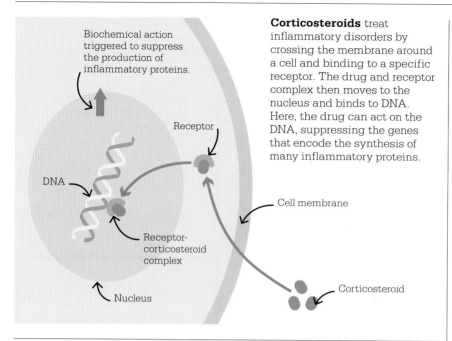

Biochemical action triggered to suppress the production of inflammatory proteins.

Receptor

DNA

Receptor-corticosteroid complex

Nucleus

Cell membrane

Corticosteroid

Corticosteroids treat inflammatory disorders by crossing the membrane around a cell and binding to a specific receptor. The drug and receptor complex then moves to the nucleus and binds to DNA. Here, the drug can act on the DNA, suppressing the genes that encode the synthesis of many inflammatory proteins.

patient developed jaundice or became pregnant, suggesting that in these conditions, too, the same hormone was responsible.

The search for substance X

In collaboration with Kendall, a professor of physiological chemistry at the Mayo Clinic, Hench began to investigate the possibility that the adrenal glands were the source of the hormone he called substance X. Kendall was one of several American researchers who, throughout the 1930s, had been studying cortin, an extract of the adrenal cortex that contains a mixture of hormones that have important biological actions. By 1940, the Mayo Clinic, other American laboratories, and the Basel laboratory where Reichstein worked had isolated 28 compounds. By 1941, Hench and Kendall were convinced that one of these—which they had named compound E—was what they had been searching for.

World War II brought all their research to a temporary halt. Hench was appointed chief of the Medical Service and director of the US Army's Rheumatism Center at the Army and Navy General Hospital. Unfounded reports that German Luftwaffe pilots could fly at high altitudes thanks to injections of adrenal extract persuaded the US government to increase funding for adrenal hormone research. After the war, Kendall collaborated with Lewis Sackett of pharmaceutical company Merck to produce larger amounts of compound E, and Hench obtained enough of it to use in rheumatoid arthritis studies.

Immediate success

For his first subject, Hench chose 29-year-old Mrs. Gardner. For five years, she had suffered from such severe rheumatoid arthritis that she was confined to a wheelchair and had been an inpatient at the Mayo Clinic for almost two months. Hench began giving her daily injections of compound E in 1948. The effect was spectacular. Within two days, Mrs. Gardner noticed significantly reduced joint pain. Within three

days, she was walking with a slight limp and, four days after starting treatment, she was spending three hours shopping. Over the following months, 13 more patients, all with symptoms as severe as those of Mrs. Gardner, received compound E and found the same level of relief. When Hench described his results to a meeting of fellow doctors in April 1949, he received a standing ovation. The Nobel Prize awarded a year later to Hench, Kendall, and Reichstein had never been offered at such speed.

Potential side effects

News of compound E, which Hench renamed cortisone (the naturally occurring compound was later named cortisol), spread quickly. *The New York Times*, among other newspapers, touted it as a "miracle cure," and patients with rheumatoid arthritis began bombarding their doctors to prescribe it. Yet Hench himself never claimed it was a perfect solution. He soon became aware that cortisone was not a cure; when the treatment was withdrawn, the patient always suffered a relapse. In a 1950 paper, he wrote that its use should be considered only as an "investigative procedure." The adverse side effects he had started to observe also troubled him.

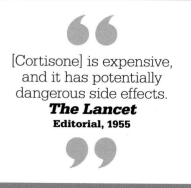

[Cortisone] is expensive, and it has potentially dangerous side effects.
The Lancet
Editorial, 1955

Corticosteroids, such as cortisone, mimic the effects of hormones produced naturally in the adrenal glands. In the body, naturally occurring cortisol is involved in the conversion of proteins to carbohydrates and also in the regulation of salt levels. When used as the anti-inflammatory drug cortisone, however, the dose prescribed is much larger than the amount normally present in the body. This leads to imbalances that can result in dangerous side effects, such as edema (swelling), high blood pressure, osteoporosis, and psychiatric disorders. These were apparent in Mrs. Gardner and other patients with prolonged use of high-dose cortisone. Hench subsequently refused to prescribe cortisone to patients he considered especially susceptible to these side effects.

The rise of corticosteroids

The use of cortisone as a treatment for rheumatoid arthritis declined from the late 1950s, as medicines with fewer side effects, such as new nonsteroidal anti-inflammatory drugs (NSAIDs), came on the scene. However, by this time, researchers had identified the potential of

Current uses of corticosteroids	
Corticosteroid	**Treats**
Betamethasone	Severe dermatitis (skin conditions)
Budesonide	Asthma, allergic rhinitis, autoimmune hepatitis
Dexamethasone	Croup, macular edema, joint and soft tissue inflammation
Hydrocortisone	Diaper rash, eczema, and other mild inflammatory skin disorders; severe acute asthma; Addison's disease; severe inflammatory bowel disease
Methylprednisolone	Joint inflammation, inflammatory and allergic disorders, organ transplants, relapse in multiple sclerosis
Prednisolone	Chronic obstructive pulmonary disease, severe croup, mild to moderate acute asthma, ulcerative colitis, Crohn's disease, systemic lupus, acute leukemia
Triamcinolone acetonide	Allergic rhinitis, inflammation of joints and soft tissues

cortisone and other corticosteroids for treating other disorders. In 1950, four separate studies had described the beneficial effects of cortisone for conditions including asthma, eye diseases such as conjunctivitis, and connective tissue disorders such as lupus. When treating these conditions, the side effects of the drugs are less of a consideration because the doses required are far lower than those used to treat rheumatoid arthritis.

Since the 1950s, the powerful effects of synthetic corticosteroids have transformed many branches of medicine—from rheumatology to dermatology, gastroenterology, ophthalmology, and respiratory medicine—and proved effective in treating conditions from hepatitis to psoriasis. They are also helpful during organ transplantation as, by suppressing the immune response, they reduce the risk of the body rejecting the transplant. ∎

Philip Hench

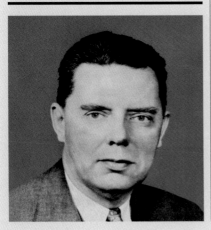

Born in 1896, Philip Showalter Hench grew up in Pittsburgh, Pennsylvania. He enlisted in the US Army Medical Corps in 1917, and in 1920 received a doctorate in medicine from the University of Pittsburgh. In 1923, he joined the Mayo Clinic, and became head of its department of rheumatic diseases in 1926. He married in 1927 and had four children.

Hench was a founding member of the American Rheumatism Association and its president in 1940 and 1941. He served in senior medical posts during World War II, then returned to the Mayo Clinic, where he became professor of medicine in 1947. Hench retired in 1957 and died of pneumonia while on vacation in Jamaica in 1965.

Key works

1938 "Effect of spontaneous jaundice on rheumatoid arthritis"
1950 "Effects of cortisone acetate and pituitary ACTH on rheumatoid arthritis, rheumatic fever and certain other conditions" (with Edward Kendall, Charles H. Slocumb, et al.)

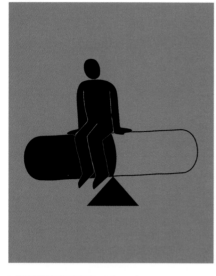

THE QUIETENING EFFECT
LITHIUM AND BIPOLAR DISORDER

IN CONTEXT

BEFORE
1871 In the US, neurologist William Hammond uses lithium "salts" to treat mania.

1894 Danish psychiatrist Frederik Lange proposes using lithium to treat "melancholic depression."

AFTER
1963 During trials at Hellingly Hospital in Sussex, UK, doctor Ronald Maggs finds lithium has "value during the acute manic illness."

1970 Mogens Schou publishes an article showing that lithium has a preventative effect in bipolar mood disorders.

1970 The US Food and Drug Administration approves the use of lithium to treat acute mania, becoming the 50th country to do so.

1995 The advent of "mood stabilizers" provides an alternative to lithium.

Australian psychiatrist John Cade made a breakthrough with the drug lithium to treat bipolar disorder in 1949. He had noticed that autopsies on the brains of bipolar patients often revealed physical symptoms, such as blood clots, and thought there could be an organic cause for bipolar illness. Cade hypothesized that a manic bipolar patient was in a state of intoxication due to an excess of a certain chemical in the body; when the patient was melancholic, it was caused by a deficit of that chemical.

Guinea pig theory

Cade injected urine from bipolar patients into guinea pigs and found the urine from manic patients was more lethal for the animals than urine from nonbipolar patients. He added lithium (formerly used to treat gout) to the urine and realized that it made the urine less toxic and that large doses of lithium made the guinea pigs passive. Reasoning it could also pacify bipolar patients, Cade gave 10 patients lithium and noted dramatic improvements. His

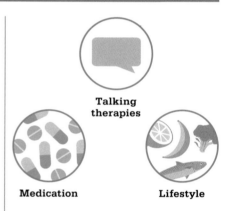

Bipolar patients may be treated with medication, talking therapies such as cognitive behavioral therapy, and lifestyle management techniques such as better diet and regular exercise.

findings, published in 1949, gained little acclaim, yet work with lithium continued, and it was adopted as a medication for mania in various European countries from the 1960s.

Danish psychiatrist Mogens Schou published research in 1970 showing lithium was effective for bipolar disorder. Accepted by the US in 1970, lithium is the main bipolar medicine used today. ■

See also: Pharmacy 54–59 ▪ Humane mental health care 92–93 ▪ The nervous system 190–195 ▪ Chlorpromazine and antipsychotics 241

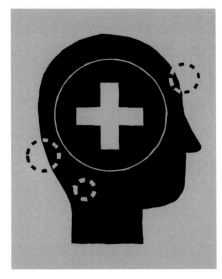

A PSYCHIC PENICILLIN
CHLORPROMAZINE AND ANTIPSYCHOTICS

In the 1940s, French surgeon Henri Laborit suggested the drug company Rhône-Poulenc should develop an antihistamine that would have an effect on the central nervous system, claiming that the sedative effect would be a useful anesthetic for patients before surgery. The drug produced in 1950 was chlorpromazine.

Two French psychiatrists at St. Anne's Hospital, Paris, Jean Delay and Pierre Deniker, began using chlorpromazine in 1952 to treat inpatients experiencing mania and schizophrenia. The drug proved effective in controlling patients' agitation or overexcitement. It was labeled as a "major tranquilizer," later known as an "antipsychotic."

World's first antipsychotic
After small but highly successful trials by Canadian psychiatrist Heinz Lehmann, chlorpromazine was used in the US from 1954. By the 1960s, it was widely prescribed in Europe and North America for patients with schizophrenia and bipolar disorder. The drug worked by blocking dopamine receptors in the brain, which lessened the transmission of messages between brain cells. This relieved psychotic symptoms, such as delusions and hallucinations. Chlorpromazine also reduced reliance on treatments such as electroshock therapy.

Despite new antipsychotics being developed from the 1960s, none has proved as successful as chlorpromazine, now recognized as the world's first antipsychotic. ∎

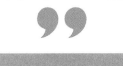

I couldn't believe that psychotic symptoms … could be affected by a simple pill.
Heinz Lehmann
Recollections of the History of Neuropsychopharmacology, 1994

See also: Pharmacy 54–59 ▪ Aspirin 86–87 ▪ Lithium and bipolar disorder 240 ▪ Behavioral and cognitive therapy 242–243

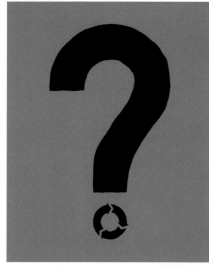

CHANGING THE WAY YOU THINK

BEHAVIORAL AND COGNITIVE THERAPY

IN CONTEXT

BEFORE
1897 Ivan Pavlov describes the principles of a classic conditioned response.

1913 John Watson outlines a new philosophy of psychology, which he calls "behaviorism."

1924 American psychologist Mary Cover Jones is dubbed "the mother of behavior therapy" after her study of desensitization involving a boy named Peter.

AFTER
1955 American psychologist Albert Ellis launches cognitive therapy based on confronting irrational beliefs.

1962 Australian physician Claire Weekes publishes *Self Help For Your Nerves*, a bestseller on treating anxiety with CBT.

1967 Aaron Beck publishes his cognitive model to explain depression.

In the 1940s, the need for effective, short-term therapies to treat anxiety and depression among troops returning from World War II combined with advances in behavioral research to produce a new approach to psychological disorders: "behavioral" therapy. Supporters of behaviorism rejected Sigmund Freud's introspective and more subjective psychoanalytical approach, which focused on the role of the unconscious mind. Instead, they maintained that measurable external factors, such as events and environment, were more important influencers of behavior and emotion. Pioneering this theory, American psychologist B. F. Skinner formulated a science of behavior by 1953 that now underpins much of modern psychotherapeutic practice and which led to the development of cognitive behavioral therapy.

Conditioning behavior

Skinner's theories were based on the research of earlier behaviorists Russian physiologist Ivan Pavlov and American psychologist John Watson. Pavlov's experiments with dogs in the 1890s showed that responses

---

Behavioral theory
shows that repeated positive or negative **responses** to behaviors **condition our future actions** and emotions.

Cognitive theory
suggests that the way we **perceive**, **interpret**, and **attribute meaning** to events influences our behavior and emotions.

⬇ ⬇

By **modifying** our **behaviors and changing our thought patterns** using **cognitive behavioral therapy**, we can **regulate our emotions** and solve psychological problems.

See also: Humane mental health care 92–93 ▪ Psychoanalysis 178–183 ▪ The nervous system 190–195 ▪ Lithium and bipolar disorder 240 ▪ Chlorpromazine and antipsychotics 241

can be learned through "classical conditioning": repeatedly ringing a bell (an unrelated stimulus) just before presenting food taught the dogs to salivate at the sound of the bell alone. Watson later suggested that conditioning could explain all human psychology.

In 1938, Skinner first theorized that if all behaviors and emotional responses are learned (conditioned), we have the capacity to relearn how to behave more appropriately. This relearning process, which he called "operant conditioning," involved positive or negative reinforcement— shaping behavior by rewarding small movements toward a desired behavior and disincentivizing undesired behavior.

Cognitive revolution

In the 1960s, interest in how thinking (the process of cognition) affects emotions and behavior led to a reevaluation of Skinner's work and a second wave of psychological therapies. Cognitive therapists, such as American psychiatrist Aaron Beck, maintained that the

conditioned responses demonstrated by Skinner could not explain or control all behaviors, and that unhelpful or inaccurate thinking must also play a role. Identifying and evaluating these negative perceptions or automatic thoughts— and then correcting them, so that they reflect reality rather than a distorted or dysfunctional view of reality—formed the basis of Beck's cognitive approach.

Therapists began to combine behavioral and cognitive theories, developing a practice termed "cognitive behavioral therapy" (CBT). Studying and amending visible behaviors, as well as assessing and reprogramming conscious thoughts, gained support as studies repeatedly showed the efficacy of this combined approach.

A third wave

Since the 1990s, a third wave of therapies has emerged, broadening the field of CBT. With a focus on changing people's relationship with their thoughts and emotions rather than changing the content of their

Permanent recovery lies in the patient's ability to know how to accept the panic until he no longer fears it.
Claire Weekes, 1977

thoughts, these methods include mindfulness, visualization, and acceptance-based therapies.

Although CBT continues to evolve, it is still rooted in scientific experiments and clinical case studies to obtain measurable results and quantifiable data, as were Skinner's efforts to develop psychotherapy and psychology as a science. His emphasis on the value of reinforcement as a means of effecting behavioral change has also had a long-lasting impact. ▪

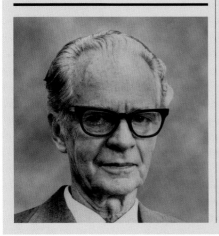

B. F. Skinner

Born in 1904 in Pennsylvania, Burrhus Frederick Skinner initially planned to become a writer, but he became interested in the scientific study of human behavior after reading about the research of Ivan Pavlov and John Watson. Inspired by their work, he set out to prove that behavior is controlled by the surrounding environment, not by subjective mental processes or free will.

Between 1948 and 1974, while professor of psychology at Harvard University, Skinner conducted behavioral experiments using inventions such as his "Skinner box." This featured levers for rats to pull or pigeons to peck in order to receive food or water, proving that behavior can be modified and reinforced by the process Skinner termed "operant conditioning." This pioneering research influenced approaches to psychology and education. He died in 1990 from leukemia.

Key works

1938 *The Behavior of Organisms*
1953 *Science and Human Behavior*
1957 *Verbal Behavior*

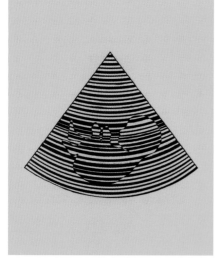

A NEW DIAGNOSTIC DIMENSION
ULTRASOUND

The first person to apply ultrasound technology to the field of obstetrics was British physician Ian Donald at the University of Glasgow, Scotland. In 1956, Donald, helped by engineer Tom Brown and obstetrician John McVicar, built the first successful ultrasound diagnostic scanner.

Ultrasound—high-frequency sound waves above the range of human hearing—enables doctors to obtain key information on the fetus. Also called medical sonography, it is noninvasive and safer than X-rays, which expose the fetus to radiation. A device called a transducer sends the ultrasound into the body and detects the returning echoes. A computer then converts the echoes into images.

Diagnostic firsts
Ian Donald was not the first medic to experiment with ultrasound as a diagnostic tool. In 1942, Austrian neurologist Karl Dussik and his brother, Friedrich, attempted to locate brain tumors by measuring the transmission of an ultrasound beam through the skull. Other pioneers include American George Ludwig, who used ultrasound to detect gallstones in animals in the late 1940s, and British physician John Wild, who developed the first handheld contact scanner with the help of electrical engineer John Reid in 1951. In 1953, Swedish cardiologist Inge Edler and German physicist Hellmuth Hertz performed the first successful echocardiogram, using ultrasound to study the workings of the heart. ■

> Any new technique becomes more attractive if its clinical usefulness can be demonstrated without harm ...
> **Ian Donald**

See also: Midwifery 76–77 ▪ X-rays 176 ▪ Electrocardiography 188–189 ▪ Electroencephalography 224–225 ▪ MRI and medical scanning 278–281

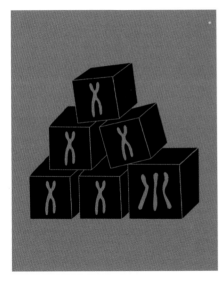

ALL THE CELLS HAD 47 CHROMOSOMES
CHROMOSOMES AND DOWN SYNDROME

IN CONTEXT

BEFORE

1866 British physician John Langdon Down describes the features of the syndrome now named after him.

1879 German biologist Walther Flemming discovers vertebrate chromosomes.

1956 Sweden's Albert Levan and Joe Hin Tjio from the US discover that humans have 46 chromosomes.

AFTER

1999 The Human Genome Project to map all the genes in the human body reveals the first full genetic code of a chromosome (chromosome 22).

2000 Chromosome 21, the one that is associated with Down syndrome, is sequenced.

2013 Researchers in the US find that the characteristics of Down syndrome may be linked to low levels of a particular protein in brain cells.

I n 1958, Marthe Gautier, a French researcher in pediatrics in Paris, discovered the cause of Down syndrome. Examining slides in a hospital laboratory, she found that Down syndrome children had three copies of chromosome 21 instead of two.

Two years before Gautier made her discovery, geneticists at Lund University, Sweden, had discovered that most people have 23 pairs of chromosomes (46 altogether) in almost all of their body cells—one in each pair inherited from their mother, and the other from their father. Sperm and egg cells, however, each have a single set of 23 unpaired chromosomes. When an egg is fertilized by a sperm, it becomes a cell with 23 pairs of chromosomes.

Trisomy

Geneticists now know that the presence of a third copy or extra bit of a chromosome—a condition called trisomy—can arise during meiosis, the production of sperm and egg cells in the reproductive organs. Trisomy can occur in any

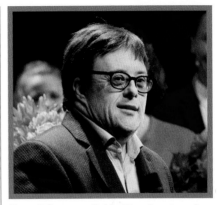

Spanish actor Pablo Pineda, star of the film *Yo, también* (*Me Too*), is the first person with Down syndrome in Europe to obtain a university degree.

chromosome, but trisomy 21, which causes Down syndrome, is the most common, affecting about one birth in every 1,000. It results in distinctive physical characteristics, such as a flatter facial profile and poor muscle tone, and learning disabilities that range from mild to moderate. Edwards syndrome, causing heart defects, arises from trisomy 18 and affects about one in 6,000 babies. ■

See also: Inheritance and hereditary conditions 146–147 ▪ Genetics and medicine 288–293 ▪ The Human Genome Project 299 ▪ Gene therapy 300

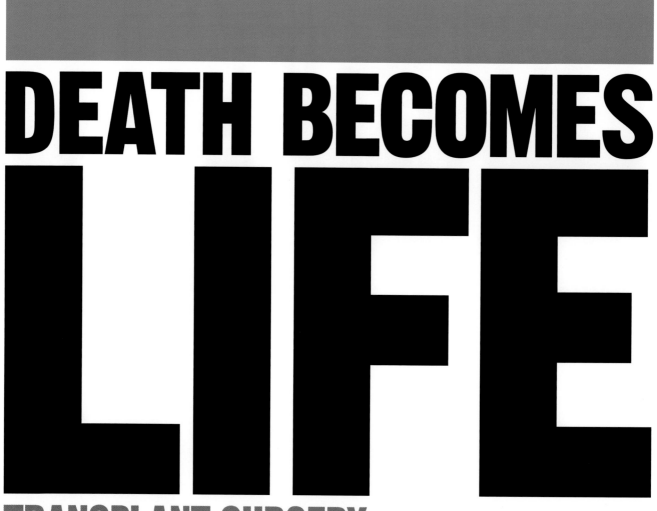

DEATH BECOMES LIFE

TRANSPLANT SURGERY

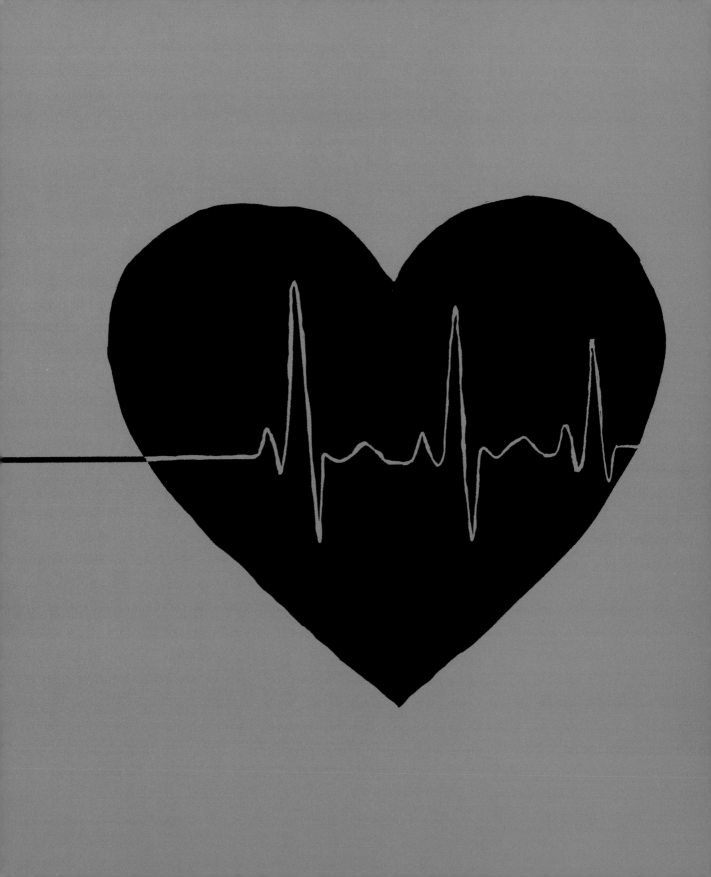

IN CONTEXT

BEFORE

1668 The first successful bone graft is performed by Job van Meekeren in the Netherlands.

1838 In the US, Richard Kissam transplants the cornea of a pig into a young man, who temporarily regains his sight.

AFTER

1979 Spain passes legislation establishing presumed consent for organ donation after death; it is the first country to have an "opt-out" system.

1998 French surgeon Jean-Michel Dubernard performs the first hand transplant.

2002 In the US, cloned pigs are specially bred for research into animal-to-human organ transplants. The pigs are genetically engineered to reduce the chances of rejection.

2008 French surgeon Laurent Lantieri claims to have carried out the first full face transplant.

Transplant surgery—the replacement of damaged or failing body parts with healthy ones—is one of modern medicine's most astonishing feats. A successful kidney transplant in 1954 led the way, and just 13 years later the world's first human heart transplant was hailed as the pinnacle of transplant surgery. Since then, hundreds of thousands of lives have been saved by heart, kidney, lung, and liver transplants. While transplants are still major medical procedures for the patients, many surgeons now consider such operations routine.

Early experiments

Surgeons did not entertain the possibility of organ transplantation until the discovery of general anesthesia in the mid-19th century. This allowed surgeons to operate inside the body without causing the patient unbearable pain or sending their muscles into spasm.

At the beginning of the 20th century, surgeons began to practice transplant surgery on animals. In 1902, Hungarian surgeon Emerich Ullmann performed the world's first kidney transplant on a dog when he moved a kidney from the dog's abdomen up to its neck and reconnected it using brass tubes. Young French surgeon Alexis Carrel performed similar operations and even transplanted the heart of a dog to its neck.

Carrel's experiments also led him to invent the micro-sewing techniques that were later used to reattach severed blood vessels in human transplant operations. In 1894, Carrel had witnessed the stabbing of French president Sadi Carnot and was appalled that surgeons were unable to save the president simply because they had no way to repair a damaged vein. Determined to avoid such tragedies in the future, Carrel spent months learning how to sew with tiny needles from Madame Leroidier, the finest embroiderer in Lyons. "Carrel's suture" is still used in transplant operations today.

Success and failure

In 1905, Austrian eye surgeon Eduard Zirm performed a successful corneal transplant on Czech farmworker Alois Glogar, who had been blinded in an accident while working with lime.

Carrel's suture is a simple but ingenious way of joining the blood vessels of a new organ to those of its host. In 1912, Carrel was awarded the Nobel Prize in Physiology or Medicine for his method of suturing blood vessels.

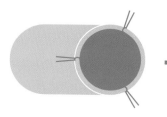

The ends of the blood vessels are brought into contact. They are united by three stitches at equidistant points around the circumference of the vessels.

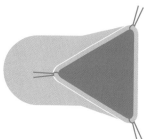

By gently pulling the stitches outward, the circumference of the blood vessel is transformed into a triangle.

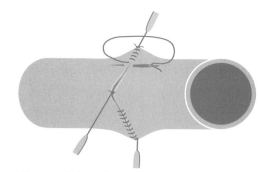

The straight edges are then easily stitched together without the need for forceps to hold the tissue in place, thus avoiding the risk of tearing or bruising.

See also: Blood transfusion and blood groups 108–111 ▪ Anesthesia 112–117 ▪ Skin grafts 137 ▪ The immune system 154–161 ▪ Electrocardiography 188–189 ▪ Dialysis 234–235 ▪ Regenerative medicine 314 ▪ Face transplants 315

> It's the gift
> of life itself.
> **Dick Cheney**
> **46th US vice president (2001–2009),**
> **on his heart transplant**

Zirm used corneas from an 11-year-old boy. The effects of the operation lasted. Glogar was back at work within three months of the surgery and retained his sight for the rest of his life.

Carrel and other surgeons began to believe that a human organ transplant was just a matter of time. Yet whenever attempts were made to transplant organs between dogs, the dog receiving the organ died within weeks, even if the operation had initially seemed successful. By the 1940s, many surgeons had the surgical skills to perform organ transplants on humans, but any attempt always ended in the death of the patient.

New insight

Research into skin transplants during World War II helped throw light on the problem. During the war, many bomber pilots suffered horrific burns, but skin grafts from donors were never successful. To find out why, British biologist Peter Medawar conducted experiments on rabbits. He found that bodies actively reject a "foreign" piece of skin. Just as the body develops

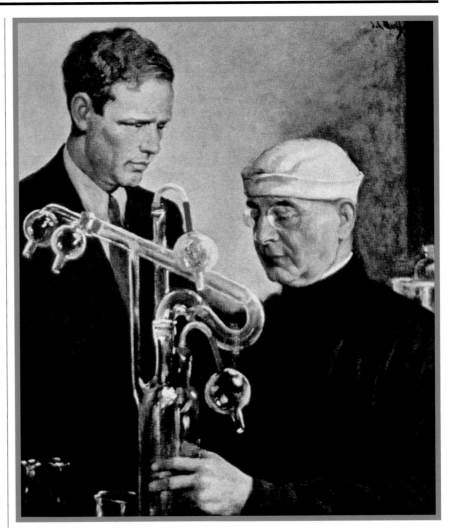

In 1935, Alexis Carrel (right) joined forces with American aviator Charles Lindbergh (left) to design a perfusion pump—a precursor to the heart–lung machine used in open-heart surgery.

antibodies against infection, so it produces antibodies against transplants. The body appears to accept the transplant at first, but it slowly builds antibodies against the invader, and within a few weeks, the body's immune system begins to attack it.

Medawar then found that skin grafts between identical twins were not rejected. Nor were grafts between cows, which are closely interbred and have the same immunological tolerance as twins.

Organ transplants had little chance of success, while rejection was a major problem. Yet surgeons were desperate to save lives and clung to the hope that if closely related donors could be found, the same immunological tolerance would help the patient survive. **»**

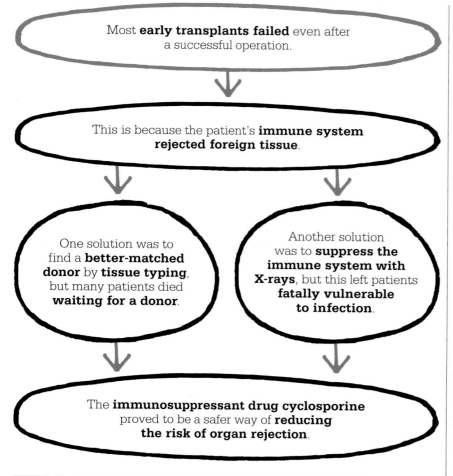

Most **early transplants failed** even after a successful operation.

This is because the patient's **immune system rejected foreign tissue**.

One solution was to find a **better-matched donor** by **tissue typing**, but many patients died **waiting for a donor**.

Another solution was to **suppress the immune system with X-rays**, but this left patients **fatally vulnerable to infection**.

The **immunosuppressant drug cyclosporine** proved to be a safer way of **reducing the risk of organ rejection**.

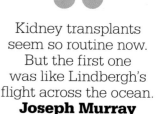

> Kidney transplants seem so routine now. But the first one was like Lindbergh's flight across the ocean.
> **Joseph Murray**
> *The New York Times*, 1990

kidney was rejected. Only the transplants between identical twins were successful. Doctors were desperate to find a solution.

Overcoming rejection

To reduce the chances of organ rejection, transplant surgeons tried bombarding the patient with X-rays to suppress the body's immune system. However, this weakened the body's defenses so much that even the mildest infection made the patient very ill. American blood specialist William Dameshek proposed using the anti-cancer drug 6-mp, which stops cancer cells from multiplying by interfering with their chemistry. He hoped that the drug would slow the proliferation of the immune system's white blood cells, which recognize foreign tissue, and therefore reduce the chances of organ rejection.

In the early 1960s, British doctor Roy Calne tried the idea out on dogs. After performing kidney transplants on the animals, he gave them azathioprine, a similar drug to 6-mp. Azathioprine worked so well with a dog called Lollipop that Calne made the decision to

Meanwhile, in 1945, Dutch inventor and physician Willem Kolff pioneered the dialysis machine, a mechanical filter that took over from damaged kidneys for a short period of time, giving the kidneys the chance to recover. Physicians began to wonder if dialysis could help a patient survive during a kidney transplant.

In 1952, at a hospital in Paris, French surgeon Jean Hamburger transplanted a mother's kidney to her son, whose single kidney had been damaged in a fall, and used a dialysis machine to keep the boy alive during the operation. The donor could not have been more closely related to the recipient (aside from identical twins), and the operation initially seemed to be successful. In less than two weeks, however, the kidney was rejected and the boy died.

Two years later, at a hospital in Boston, Joseph Murray made the world's first successful organ transplant when he took a kidney from Ronald Herrick and gave it to his identical twin brother Richard. Richard survived for eight years, during which he married and had children. He died from heart failure, with the donated kidney still working.

Inspired by Murray's success, other surgeons tried their hand at kidney transplants. Yet nearly every patient died, as the new

prescribe the drug to human transplant patients. Nonetheless, only a few of his patients survived.

A breakthrough came in 1963, when American surgeon Thomas Starzl gave his transplant patients azathioprine immediately after the operation. If it looked as though their body was going to reject the donor heart, he also gave them a huge dose of steroid drugs, which suppress the immune system. The combination of azathioprine and steroids significantly boosted patients' chances of survival.

Around this time, biochemists at the Swiss drug company Sandox were investigating soil samples for fungi that might be a source of antibiotics. Examining a soil sample from Norway, they found the fungus *Tolypocladium inflatum*, from which they extracted a substance called cyclosporine, an immunosuppressant with few toxic side effects. Licensed for use in the early 1980s, the drug revolutionized transplant surgery, reducing the chance of organ rejection and stopping patients from succumbing to infections.

Researchers were also finding better ways to identify suitable donors by using marker proteins

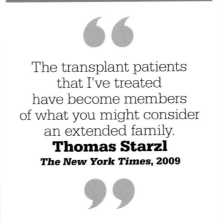

> The transplant patients that I've treated have become members of what you might consider an extended family.
> **Thomas Starzl**
> *The New York Times*, 2009

called human leukocyte antigens (HLAs) on the outside of cells. These are like chemical passports. From the pattern of HLAs on a cell, the body's immune system can instantly recognize whether cells are its own or foreign and therefore to be rejected. No two people have the same HLAs (apart from some identical twins), but some are more similar than others. Blood relatives are more likely to have similar HLAs than people who are unrelated. Blood tests on potential donors can show how closely their HLAs

match those of the patient. The closer the match, the less likely it is that an organ will be rejected. This is called tissue typing.

Liver transplants

As kidney transplants became more common in the 1960s, surgeons began to explore the possibility of liver and heart transplants. Livers were much bigger and more complex than kidneys, and there was no machine to stand in for the liver during an operation. In addition, whole livers can only come from dead donors and are sensitive to a lack of blood supply. They must be taken out of the body and chilled within 15 minutes of the donor's death.

In 1963, Thomas Starzl in the US and Roy Calne in the UK both attempted the first liver transplants on patients who would certainly die otherwise. The patients survived the operations, but the livers were then rejected and both patients died. This remained the pattern for the next 20 years, with three out of four liver transplant recipients dying within a year. But when cyclosporine became available in the early 1980s, the situation was transformed. Today, nine out of »

Christiaan Barnard

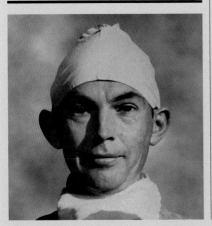

Born the son of an impoverished preacher in Western Cape, South Africa, in 1922, Christiaan Barnard decided to become a heart surgeon when one of his brothers died from heart disease at the age of 5. He became world famous in 1967, when he carried out the first human heart transplant in Cape Town, South Africa.

Barnard went on to perform "auxiliary transplants," which involved placing a healthy heart alongside the patient's ill heart. He also pioneered the use of monkey hearts to keep patients alive while waiting for a suitable

donor. He retired from heart surgery at the age of 61 after developing rheumatoid arthritis in his hands. During his remaining years, he wrote a novel and two autobiographies, and established the Christiaan Barnard Foundation to aid underprivileged children. Barnard died in 2001, aged 78.

Key works

1970 *One Life*
1993 *The Second Heart*
1996 *The Donor*

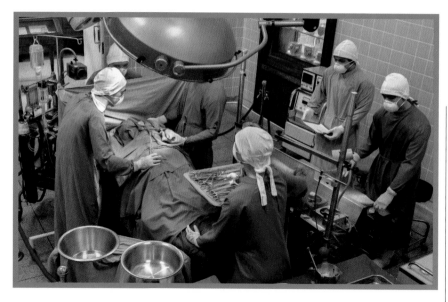

The operation was successful. Washkansky's new heart started to beat, and everything looked fine for a few days. However, his immune system was badly weakened by the drugs he had taken to stop rejection of the new heart. Washkansky died from pneumonia 18 days after the operation. Nevertheless, the era of heart transplants had begun. With the arrival of cyclosporine in the early 1980s, the success rate soared.

Donor shortages

Heart transplants are limited by a shortage of donors. Almost half the kidneys for transplants come from living donors. They are carefully selected to be a good match, with many willingly donated by relatives. Hearts, however, have to come from donors who have died. A patient can die waiting for a donor. Donor hearts may become available in a location

10 liver transplant patients survive for at least a year, and many regain full health.

Heart transplants

The ultimate challenge in transplant surgery was a heart transplant. In the early 1950s, Russian scientist Vladimir Demikhov carried out heart transplants on dogs, but his success rate was patchy. It was difficult to take the old heart out and insert the new heart without the dogs dying. In the late 1950s, surgeon Norman Shumway of Stanford University discovered he could stop a patient's heart beating and the blood flowing while it was taken out simply by chilling it with ice-cold water. He also invented an improved artificial heart machine to pump the blood until the new heart was working. Together with pioneering cardiac surgeon Richard Lower, Shumway practiced taking hearts out of dead bodies and putting them in again.

After practicing on dog hearts for several years, Shumway decided it was time to try a human heart transplant, even though there was still a major risk of rejection. While

Shumway waited for a suitable patient and donor, South African surgeon Christiaan Barnard beat him to it. Making headlines around the world, Barnard used Shumway and Lower's techniques to carry out the world's first human heart transplant on December 3, 1967, at Groote Schuur hospital in Cape Town. Barnard's patient was Louis Washkansky, a 54-year-old grocer. The donor heart came from a young woman who had been killed by a car while crossing the road.

Heart–lung transplants

Many heart transplant patients have damaged lungs as well. As heart transplants began to seem feasible, surgeons also started to think about combined heart–lung transplants.

In 1968, just a year after the first heart transplant, American surgeon Denton Cooley carried out the world's first heart–lung transplant on a 2-month-old baby. The baby survived just 14 hours. The idea was then abandoned until 1981, when surgeon Bruce Reitz of Stanford

University decided to try again because the newly licensed drug cyclosporine gave a better chance of success. The patient was 45-year-old Mary Gohlke. The operation worked, and Mary survived for five years.

Nowadays, almost half of heart–lung transplant patients survive for at least five years. However, a shortage of donors and the rapid deterioration of lung tissue after the donor's death limit the number of heart–lung operations.

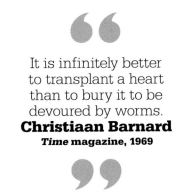

> It is infinitely better to transplant a heart than to bury it to be devoured by worms.
>
> **Christiaan Barnard**
> *Time* magazine, 1969

far away from the patient, or at the wrong time. Procuring and transporting the heart and setting up the operation is a race against the clock. Starved of oxygen, the heart tissue starts to deteriorate within four to six hours of being harvested from the donor.

Electric hearts

Powered by an electric battery, "total artificial hearts" (TAHs) could be the answer to donor heart shortages. In the 1960s, Domingo Liotta, an Argentinian cardiac specialist working in the US, and American surgeon O. H. "Bud" Frazier tried using TAH technology at the Texas Heart Institute in Houston. These early artificial hearts were called bridges because they were meant to keep a patient alive only until a donor could be found. They included an external air pump kept by the side of the patient.

In 1969, American heart surgeon Denton Cooley, who had already carried out 29 transplants, was confronted with a patient called Haskell Karp who would die within days because no donor heart was available. Cooley implanted a TAH. A donor heart was found two and a half days later, but Karp died from an

The list of organs and tissues that can be transplanted is growing. Hands and faces have recently been added to the organ transplant list. So far, only a few hundred hand or face transplants have taken place around the world.

Face transplants are particularly complex, because multiple types of tissue are involved.

Corneal donors don't have to match recipients like organ donors do.

50 percent of patients who have received lung transplants are alive five years later.

72 percent of heart transplant patients survive for at least five years. Some live for more than 30 years.

Living donors can donate a portion of their liver, pancreas, or intestine.

Hand transplants can restore function in ways that artificial limbs cannot.

Kidneys can be donated by living as well as deceased donors.

Tissues can also be transplanted. Skin is used by burn victims.

infection a short while after the natural heart was implanted. Some surgeons condemned Cooley for implanting a device that they did not consider ready to be tried on humans. Nonetheless, as more patients rejected their new heart and died, some surgeons wondered whether electric hearts could be the answer, and not just as bridges.

An electric heart called the Jarvik-7 was given to a number of dying cardiac patients in the US in the early 1980s, one of whom survived for two years. Interest in electric hearts began to wane when the immunosuppressant cyclosporine boosted the survival rate of donor heart transplants, but

it revived when the shortage of donors became more acute in the 21st century, partly because TAH technology allowed patients with end-stage heart failure to wait longer for a transplant.

Electric hearts have not become long-term replacements for diseased hearts as first hoped. Most cardiac surgeons believe it will be hearts grown in a laboratory from stem cells and other cloned organs that will revolutionize transplant surgery, though their use is still some way off. Meanwhile, kidney, liver, and heart transplants continue to save tens of thousands of lives each year and are among the medical world's most remarkable achievements. ∎

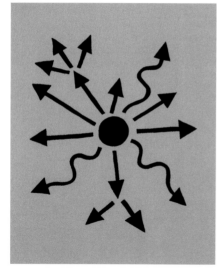

A PROMISING BUT UNRULY MOLECULE

INTERFERON

IN CONTEXT

BEFORE

1796 Edward Jenner performs the first effective inoculations against the smallpox virus.

1882 Élie Metchnikoff discovers phagocytes—cells, including macrophages (large white blood cells), that attack, engulf, and destroy germs.

1931 German physicist Ernst Ruska invents the electron microscope, which enables the first detailed studies of viruses and their effects on the body.

AFTER

1959 Jacques Miller discovers T-cells, which are essential for the immune response to viruses; T-cells are later found to produce the gamma form of interferon.

2016 In the US, Matthew Halpert and Vanaja Konduri pin down the role of dendritic cells which, together with macrophages, produce the alpha form of interferon.

Interferon—named for its ability to interfere with infections—is any of several proteins in the large class of cytokines and is part of the body's natural defense against viruses. Alick Isaacs and Jean Lindenmann, virologists at the UK's National Institute for Medical Research, first described it in 1957.

Viruses spread within the body by hijacking cells. Cells infected by viruses release interferons to slow down cell replication, curtailing the progress of the virus, and to block future infections. Interferons also spread to healthy cells, alerting them to the danger and limiting their replication. There are three main types of interferon—alpha, beta, and gamma—with slightly varying roles.

Initially, there was considerable excitement about the potential of interferon to make antiviral drugs and, because it interferes with cell growth, to treat cancer. In the 1960s, Finnish scientist Kari Cantell found that infecting white blood cells with the Sendai virus triggered them to produce alpha interferon. In 1980, genetic engineering of the

In science, as in show business, there really is no such thing as an overnight sensation.
Mike Edelhart and Jean Lindenmann
Interferon, 1981

alpha interferon gene at a Swiss laboratory led to the mass production of alpha and other interferons.

In animal research, interferon's ability to suppress cancer had appeared highly promising, but patients experienced serious side effects, including flulike symptoms, nausea, and severe depression. In low doses, however, interferon is still used to treat various cancers, hepatitis, and multiple sclerosis. ∎

See also: Vaccination 94–101 ▪ The immune system 154–161 ▪ Virology 177 ▪ Antibiotics 216–223 ▪ HIV and autoimmune diseases 294–297

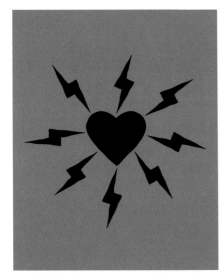

A SENSATION FOR THE PATIENT

PACEMAKERS

IN CONTEXT

BEFORE
1887 Augustus D. Waller measures the electrical activity that precedes every heartbeat.

1903 Willem Einthoven's electrocardiograph measures cardiac activity and displays a reading—known as an electrocardiogram (ECG).

1928 Australian doctors Mark Lidwill and Edgar Booth use a needle attached to an electrical power source to revive the heart of a stillborn baby.

AFTER
1990s Microprocessor-driven pacemakers modify pacing automatically according to the patient's needs.

2012 Heart surgeons at Homolka Hospital in Prague, Czech Republic, implant a wireless pill-sized pacemaker.

2019 American and Chinese scientists invent a battery-free pacemaker that harvests its energy from the beating heart.

The human heart beats more than 2 billion times in the average lifetime—usually with great regularity. However, the hearts of around 3 million people across the world rely on the stimulus provided by an artificial pacemaker to keep their heartbeat on track.

From bulky to minute

In 1951, Canadian engineer John Hopps developed the first effective pacemaker—an external, bulky, electricity-powered machine, which the patient wheeled around on a cart. Seven years later, aided by the invention of small batteries and tiny transistors to control the signal, Swedish engineer Rune Elmqvist and cardiac surgeon Åke Senning created a pacemaker that could be implanted in the chest.

Else-Marie Larsson persuaded the pair to try out the device on her dying husband, Arne. Short on time,

An X-ray shows a pacemaker implanted just below the collarbone. Its wire, guided into the right ventricle, carries an electrical pulse to the heart.

Elmqvist molded the components from resin in a plastic cup, and Senning implanted it on October 8, 1958. Although it had to be replaced the next morning, a second model worked perfectly. Larsson went on to receive 25 more pacemakers over the next 43 years and died aged 86.

Patient-controlled, variable-rate pacemakers arrived in 1960, and lithium batteries, introduced in 1972, extended battery life from around two to 10 years. Recent innovations include pill-sized pacemakers and sensors that enable the devices to change the heart pace automatically according to body activity. ∎

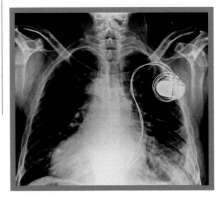

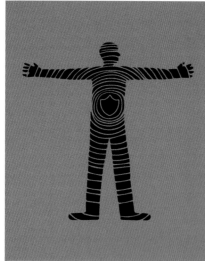

THE CENTER OF OUR IMMUNE RESPONSE
LYMPHOCYTES AND LYMPHATICS

IN CONTEXT

BEFORE

1651 French scientist Jean Pecquet highlights the role of the thoracic duct (the main lymphatic vessel).

1652 Thomas Bartholin shows the lymphatic vessels extend throughout the body and coins the term "lymphatics."

1701 Dutch anatomist Frederik Ruysch describes lymphatic circulation.

1770 William Hewson identifies tiny round cells that are later called lymphocytes.

1784 Italian anatomist Paolo Mascagni describes how lymphatics must drain the spaces between body cells and end up in lymph nodes.

AFTER:

1959 French-born scientist Jacques Miller discovers T-lymphocytes, or T-cells.

1980 Researchers establish the way T- and B-lymphocytes give adaptive immunity.

The lymphatic system is the body's main circulating drainage system and a key defense against infection. Its many vessels, or lymphatics, wash toxins and other waste away in lymph fluid, while lymphocytes (a type of white blood cell) identify and fight germs that enter the system.

The discovery that lymphocytes circulate between the lymphatic system and the blood was made by British physician James Gowans in 1959. This was a crucial step in understanding the central role that lymphocytes and lymphatic circulation play in the body's immune system.

The lymphatic system includes key organs—such as the thymus, bone marrow, and spleen—in which lymphocytes are produced and matured. Activation of lymphocytes takes place in lymph nodes (small "glands"), where the lymphocytes detect antigens.

The thymus enables T-cells to mature.

Lymphocytes travel in the lymph and are activated on contact with an antigen.

The spleen filters blood and brings it into contact with lymphocytes.

Bone marrow produces precursors of T-cells and B-cells; B-cells remain and mature there.

Lymph vessels transport lymph and its infection-fighting lymphocytes around the body.

Lymph nodes filter lymph to remove damaged cells and germs and house lymphocytes that fight antigens. They cluster at the armpits, groin, and neck.

See also: Blood circulation 68–73 ▪ Vaccination 94–101 ▪ The immune system 154–161 ▪ Cancer therapy 168–75 ▪ Targeted drug delivery 198–199 ▪ Monoclonal antibodies 282–283

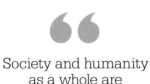

> Society and humanity
> as a whole are
> richer for [Gowans'] work.
> **Andrew Copson**
> CEO of Humanists UK (1980–)

Earlier knowledge

An early description of lymph nodes (small "glands" where lymphocytes cluster) was recorded by the Greek physician Hippocrates in the 5th century BCE, and Galen of Pergamum in the 2nd century CE wrote about lymphatic vessels. Only during the 1650s did Danish physician Thomas Bartholin and Swedish scientist Olaus Rudbeck independently discover that lymphatics extend throughout the whole body. Over the following centuries, scientists gradually pieced together how the system and its circulation worked.

A vital system

Once blood has delivered nutrients and oxygen to body cells, it carries away cell waste in blood plasma. Most of the plasma stays in the bloodstream, but some, along with other fluids, seeps into body tissues. From there, it drains into the lymphatic vessels as lymph.

Lymph is a clear fluid, like blood plasma. It slowly moves around the body, removing the cell waste, before returning to the bloodstream. Throughout the system are around 600 nodes filled with a meshlike tissue that filters the lymph to trap germs and toxins. Lymph also carries lymphocytes, tiny pale blood cells found in places such as the spleen and lymph nodes. They were first described in 1770 by British surgeon William Hewson, but their function was not understood. Lymphocytes had already been detected in inflammatory reactions and bacterial diseases, but until James Gowans' discovery, it was assumed that lymphocytes were short-lived cells because they seemed to vanish from the blood.

Gowans' breakthrough was to show these cells do not vanish, but are absorbed into the lymph system, then circulate through the tissues and lymph nodes before returning into the blood. Far from being short-lived, lymphocytes can live for up to 15 years, with the same cells continually recirculating. Gowans went on to suggest that lymphocytes are the cells that carry antibodies, and that by circulating through the tissues, they spread

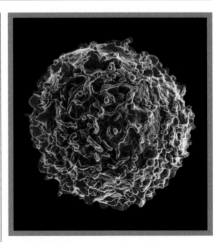

Lymphocytes are white blood cells, including B-cells and T-cells, which respond to and remember specific invaders. B-cells (shown here) release antibodies against a particular antigen.

the antibodies around the body. He showed that lymphocytes react with antigens (molecules on a pathogen's surface) to instigate an immune response. They are now recognized as the central cells of the body's targeted, adaptive immune system. ▪

James Gowans

Born in Sheffield, UK, in 1924, James Gowans got a degree in medicine at King's College, London. He graduated in 1947, after volunteering as a medical student at the newly liberated Bergen-Belsen concentration camp at the end of World War II. Gowans attended Oxford University, and in 1955–1960, was a medical research fellow at Exeter College, where he conducted his pioneering work on lymphocyte recirculation.

Gowans was elected to a fellowship of the Royal Society in 1963 for his work on the lymphatic system. He was the Society's research professor for 15 years, and head of the UK's Medical Research Council in 1977–1987. In 1989, he became the first secretary-general of the Human Science Frontier Program, based in Strasbourg, France. Gowans was knighted in 1982, and died in 2020.

Key works

1959 "The recirculation of lymphocytes from blood to lymph in the rat"
1995 *The mysterious lymphocyte*
2008 *The origin and function of lymphocytes*

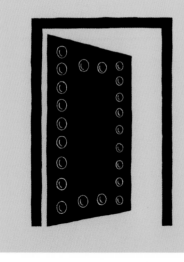

THE POWER TO DECIDE
HORMONAL CONTRACEPTION

IN CONTEXT

BEFORE

1920s American scientist George W. Corner pinpoints the role of progesterone and estrogen in the female reproductive cycle.

1930s Scientists in both Europe and the US isolate estrogen and progesterone.

AFTER

1965 Around 6.5 million American women are using the Pill, rising to 151 million women worldwide in 2019.

1968 Pope Paul VI issues an encyclical banning the use of contraceptives by Catholics.

1999 The FDA approves the morning-after pill, which prevents pregnancy if it is used up to 72 hours after sexual intercourse.

2014 In the US, *Bloomberg Businessweek* claims one-third of wage gains among women can be attributed to the Pill.

In the mid-20th century, the two main forms of contraception were condoms and diaphragms, yet the scientific basis of hormonal contraception had been understood since the 1920s. In the US in 1951, birth control crusader Margaret Sanger challenged Gregory Pincus, a biologist, to develop a hormonal contraceptive in pill form. Around the same time, chemist Carl Djerassi, working for the drug company Syntex in Mexico City, synthesized norethindrone, an artificial version of progesterone, the female sex hormone.

Pincus knew that high levels of progesterone inhibited ovulation in laboratory animals. By 1953, with gynecologist John Rocks, he had trialed a birth control pill for women, which became known as "the Pill." Anti-birth-control laws and opposition from the Catholic Church persuaded Pincus and Rocks to move their trials to Puerto Rico, a US territory, in 1955. Known as Enovid, their drug contained 10 times the estrogen and progesterone found in the modern Pill. The 200 volunteers were unaware of the Pill's possible side effects, such as dizziness, nausea, headaches, and blood clots.

In 1960, the US Food and Drug Administration approved Enovid as an oral contraceptive, despite the side effects of such high levels of hormones. (They were halved in 1961.) As it was based on the work of Pincus and Djerassi, both men are known as the "father of the Pill." ∎

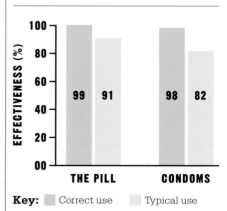

Key: Correct use | Typical use

There is only a 1 percent difference between the effectiveness of condoms and the Pill when they are consistently used correctly, but typical use results in a 9 percent difference.

See also: Women in medicine 120–121 ▪ Hormones and endocrinology 184–187 ▪ Birth control 214–215 ▪ The FDA and thalidomide 259

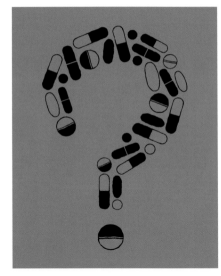

ASKING FOR PROOF OF SAFETY
THE FDA AND THALIDOMIDE

In 1937, more than 100 US citizens, many of them children, died in pain after taking a new drug called elixir sulfanilamide. The elixir had been tested for flavor and appearance, but there was no requirement to test it for toxicity. While sulfanilamide itself is safe and effective, diethylene glycol, in which it was dissolved, is a poison. Public outrage led to the 1938 Food, Drug, and Cosmetic Act, which set out the mechanism for the control of drugs in the US. The law required companies to demonstrate that new drugs were safe and allowed for government inspections of factories.

The team at the Food and Drug Administration (FDA) responsible for approving new drugs included pharmacologist Frances Oldham Kelsey, who was then studying for her doctorate. In 1960, the FDA appointed Kelsey to review a drug called thalidomide, which proved effective in reducing nausea in pregnant women. Although the drug had already been approved in 40 other countries, Kelsey turned

> [Kelsey's] exceptional judgment ... has prevented a major tragedy ... in the United States.
> **John F. Kennedy**
> **35th US president (1961–1963)**

it down, on the grounds that the risk assessment had not considered possible effects on the fetus.

In 1961, reports emerged in Germany and the UK that mothers who had taken thalidomide were having babies with severe birth defects. The drug was crossing the placenta and causing deformities in the fetus. At least 10,000 children worldwide were affected, half of whom died within months of being born, but only 17 were in the US. ∎

See also: Pharmacy 54–59 ▪ Women in medicine 120–121 ▪ Steroids and cortisone 236–239 ▪ Evidence-based medicine 276–277

A RETURN TO FUNCTION

ORTHOPEDIC SURGERY

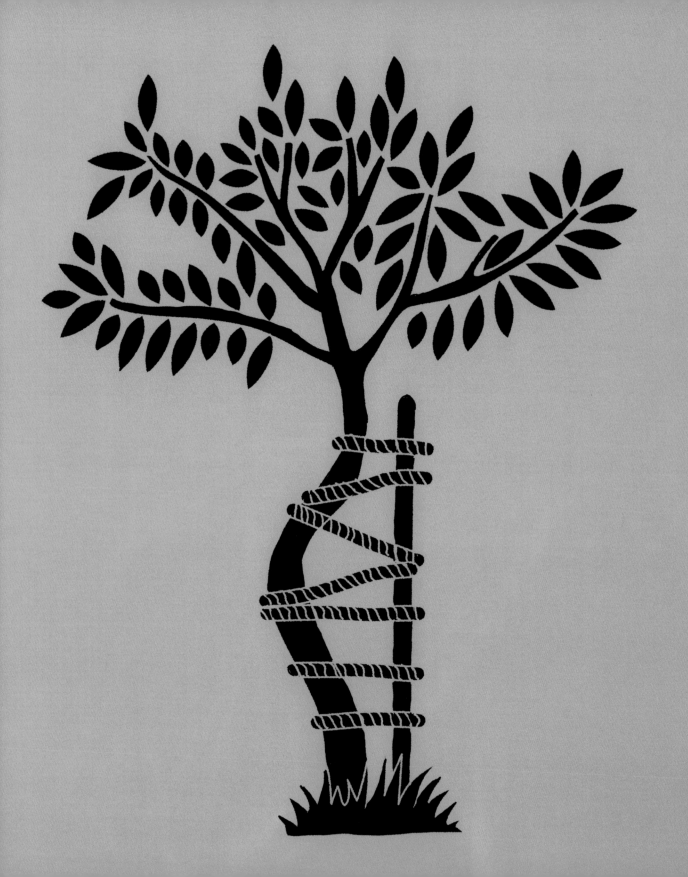

IN CONTEXT

BEFORE

1650 BCE Ancient Egyptians use splints to help mend fractured bones.

c. 1000 CE Al-Zahrawi compiles the medical encyclopedia *Kitab al-Tasrif*, which describes orthopedic practices in detail.

1896 X-rays are first used to evaluate skeletal damage, after being discovered by Wilhelm Röntgen the year before.

AFTER

1968 Frank Gunston carries out the first successful full knee replacement.

1986 Japanese biomedical engineer Kazunori Baba invents 3D ultrasound, which allows detailed bone imaging.

1990s Robot-assisted hip and knee replacement operations are introduced.

The total hip replacement performed at Wrightington Hospital, Wigan, UK, in 1962 was a landmark in 20th-century orthopedic surgery. The brainchild of British orthopedic surgeon John Charnley, it is now one of the most commonly performed major surgical procedures in the world.

Osteoarthritis of the hip joint disables an estimated 10 percent of people over the age of 60, with wear between the ball of the femur (thigh bone) and the hip socket becoming excruciatingly painful. Previous attempts to carry out the procedure had used a variety of materials, from steel to glass, but none had been completely successful.

After many years of research and several false starts, Charnley used a cobalt-chrome alloy ball-ended stem fitted into the femur and a socket made of a type of high-density polyethylene. This allowed the thigh bone to move in the socket with minimal friction—and therefore minimal wear. After five years of conducting joint replacements, Charnley declared the procedure safe, and other surgeons began to replicate it. By 2019, more than

> The cart has been put before the horse; the artificial joint has been made and used, and now we are trying to find out how and why it fails.
> **John Charnley**
> *The Journal of Bone and Joint Surgery, 1956*

300,000 total hip replacements were being conducted annually in the US alone. Charnley's work also initiated the development of replacement techniques for other joints.

Musculoskeletal repair

Orthopedic surgery is used to repair broken bones and their associated soft tissues (ligaments, tendons, and cartilage); correct skeletal deformities such as scoliosis (curvature of the spine); rebuild or replace damaged joints (a procedure known as arthroplasty); remove bone tumors; and treat a range of other bone conditions.

The word *orthopedic* comes from the Greek words *ortho*, which means straight, and *pais*, meaning child. It was coined by French physician Nicolas Andry in 1741, and describes one early focus of the discipline—attempts to straighten the crooked spines

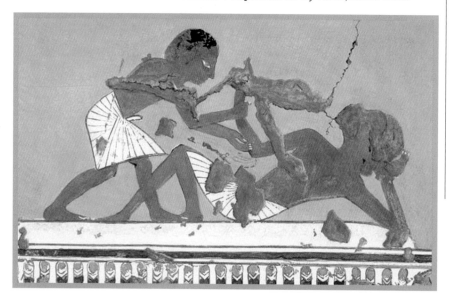

A painting from the tomb of Ipuy at Luxor in Egypt, dating to the reign of Ramesses II in the 13th century BCE, shows a physician fixing a dislocated shoulder with a method still used today.

> The **hip joint is worn or damaged by use** over time by high-impact **sports or by conditions** such as osteoarthritis or fractures.

> **Damage** to the hip joint **results in swelling**, stiffness, **pain, and reduced mobility**.

> The **difficulty of finding materials** that are not rejected by the body, that will last, and that will restore natural movement **hinder progress in finding a cure**.

> John Charnley pioneers a **total hip operation** in 1962, **which uses new materials to reduce friction** and **improve longevity**.

> Surgeons **attempt hip replacement operations** during the 1940s and '50s, but **none are completely successful**.

---

and limbs of children. Until the 1890s, the field of orthopedics was mainly concerned with correcting skeletal deformities in the young and mending broken bones.

Early practice

The origins of orthopedics are much older than its name, as many early civilizations developed ways to manage orthopedic injuries. Written in ancient Egypt, c. 17th century BCE, the Edwin Smith papyrus describes physicians placing padded boards of palm bark over broken limbs, held in place with linen bandages. In ancient Greece, Hippocrates (c. 460 BCE–c. 375 BCE) wrote of wrapping injured limbs in bandages soaked in wax and resin.

During the Islamic Golden Age, in Cordoba, Spain, renowned surgeon al-Zahrawi (936–1013 CE)

Hugh Owen Thomas's leg splint transformed outcomes for compound fractures when it was adopted during World War I. Prior to its use, amputation was the usual treatment offered.

operated on spinal injuries and skull fractures. In France, Guy de Chauliac, author of the surgical treatise *Chirurgia Magna* (1363), pioneered the concept of pulley traction to treat fractures.

While orthopedic surgery made little progress for several centuries, bonesetting—usually by self-taught practitioners without formal medical training—became established in many parts of the world. In China and Japan, the traditional art of bonesetting (known as *die-da* and *sekkotsu*, respectively) developed in association with martial arts schools, where practitioners refined techniques for treating injuries

sustained in training and combat. One of Britain's most famous bonesetters was "Crazy" Sally Mapp, who plied her trade near London in the early 18th century.

Modern pioneers

In 1876, Hugh Owen Thomas, son of a renowned Welsh bonesetter, described his revolutionary hip and knee splint in *Diseases of the Hip, Knee, and Ankle Joints*. The splint used a steel rod and leather straps to stabilize a fracture and help the bone heal. When his nephew Robert Jones, director of military orthopedics, advocated its use during World War I, the Thomas »

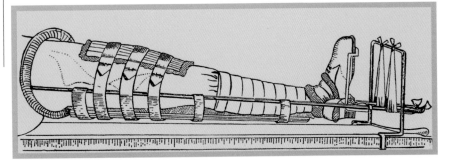

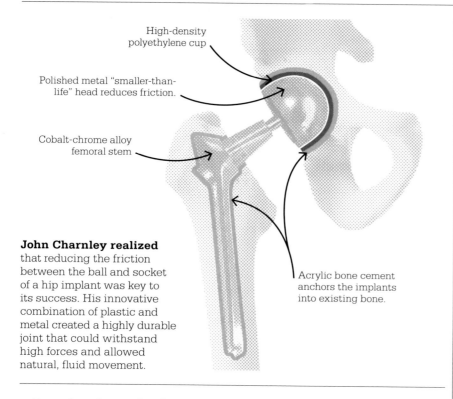

High-density polyethylene cup

Polished metal "smaller-than-life" head reduces friction.

Cobalt-chrome alloy femoral stem

Acrylic bone cement anchors the implants into existing bone.

John Charnley realized that reducing the friction between the ball and socket of a hip implant was key to its success. His innovative combination of plastic and metal created a highly durable joint that could withstand high forces and allowed natural, fluid movement.

splint reduced mortality from compound fractures of the femur from more than 80 percent to less than 20 percent. Thomas's other innovations included the Thomas collar (a brace for neck injuries), the Thomas test (for hip deformities), and the Thomas heel (a corrective children's shoe for flat feet).

Other important developments included the discovery, by Dutch military surgeon Anthonius Mathijsen in 1851, that bandages soaked in water and plaster of Paris (gypsum plaster) hardened in minutes and made excellent casts to support fractures. In 1896, newly invented X-rays were used to produce a radiograph showing the position of a bullet lodged in a boy's wrist bone. X-rays would play an ever-increasing role in orthopedics in the 20th century.

Early in World War II, in 1939, German surgeon Gerhard Küntscher introduced the intramedullary rod,

or nail, which was fitted into the central cavity of a fractured femur to give support while the bone healed. This enabled patients—not least German soldiers—to regain mobility quickly. Refined many times since, the technique is still used for fractures of the femur and tibia.

Another type of metal implant— a system of hooks attached to a steel rod—was developed by American surgeon Paul Harrington during the 1950s. Used to straighten curvature of the spine, the technique was replaced by the Cotrel-Dubousset double rod in the 1980s. From the 1950s, Russian surgeon Gavriil Ilizarov devised fixators (now known as Ilizarov apparatuses)—frames fixed to limb bones to correct angular deformities, rectify leg-length differences, and mend bones that failed to heal in a cast.

John Charnley's revolutionary advances in hip replacement surgery in the early 1960s soon

inspired Canadian surgeon Frank Gunston to tackle the challenge of making a knee joint. This was even more complex because the knee has three parts: the bottom of the femur, the top of the tibia, and the kneecap. German surgeon Thermistocles Gluck had made the first attempt with an ivory implant in 1860, but efforts to reproduce a knee that worked like a healthy joint had foundered until 1968, when Gunston used the same materials as Charnley's hip replacement.

Gunston attached a curved cobalt-chromium alloy component to the end of the femur, which rocked on a polyethylene platform attached to the tibia, replicating the natural bending and extension of the knee. Surgeons now carry out about 600,000 total knee replacements every year in the US. Although designs have evolved since Gunston performed the first procedure, the materials used are similar.

Orthopedics today

The scope of modern orthopedics is broad and continues to expand as lengthening lifespans, changing occupational demands, and evolving lifestyles present new challenges

Sir John was a perfectionist … he would not be satisfied until an instrument did exactly what he wanted it to in his mind.
Maureen Abraham
British scrub nurse

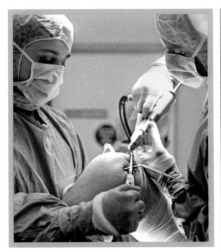

Recent technological advances have initiated a new era of minimally invasive orthopedic procedures, such as this keyhole surgery on a knee.

and drive innovation. Charnley's seminal work on replacement joints has retained its significance as factors such as an aging population and rising obesity levels worldwide continue to increase the incidence of musculoskeletal conditions such as osteoarthritis. According to a 2013 prediction by the World Health Organization, 130 million people globally will have osteoarthritis by 2050. The disease affects mostly knees, hips, and the spine when cartilage wears away, causing the bones to rub together. While walking frames and other devices can help mobility and palliative medicines can ease pain, joint replacement is often the only effective approach.

Bone fractures remain one of the largest areas of treatment, affecting more than 6 million people a year in the US. Wrist fractures are the most common breaks in those aged under 75, with hip fractures the most common in the over-75s. Fractured bones are still treated using methods similar to those that were practiced in ancient times: movement of the broken bone is restricted and a splint or cast is applied. However, new research and advances in medical technology continue to refine procedures and attempt to promote the faster healing of bone.

Continuing innovation

The invention of 3D ultrasound in 1986 enabled noninvasive mapping of bones and joints. Assisting the diagnosis and treatment of disorders, it has also facilitated better training in orthopedics. The more recent development of video-assisted keyhole surgery with computer-aided navigation means that many procedures can now be completed less invasively.

Keyhole surgery has especially advanced orthopedic oncology, a specialty dealing with cancerous tumors in bone and surrounding soft tissues. Previously, amputation was often the recommended early treatment for malignant bone cancer, but progress in keyhole surgery and in chemotherapy and radiation mean that this can now be avoided in many cases.

Research focused on refining joint replacement techniques has continued since Charnley's work

He had this engineering bent and really redesigned nature.
Lady Jill Charnley
on her husband John Charnley

during the 1960s. Different types of metal, ceramics, and plastics have been trialed, and "resurfacing," which leaves patients with more of their original bone than a total joint replacement operation, is also now an option.

Surgeons are investigating cartilage transplantation and the use of tissue grown from stem cells to replace damaged tendons and ligaments in joints. While many of the mechanical principles and treatment aims of orthopedic surgery have remained the same over the centuries, the field has come a long way from the use of bark splints. ∎

John Charnley

Born in Bury, UK, in 1911, John Charnley served as a medical officer in the British Army during World War II. After the war, he became interested in the effect of compression on fractures and the lubrication of artificial joints.

Charnley knew it was vital to collaborate with mechanical engineers to achieve replacement joints that worked well. In 1958, he established a hip surgery center at Wrightington Hospital in Wigan. After experimenting unsuccessfully with Teflon for the hip socket material, he opted for polyethylene from 1962. Charnley continued to strive to improve hip operation outcomes for many years, and also made important contributions to the reduction of postoperative infections, for which he was awarded the prestigious Lister Medal in 1975. He died in 1982.

Key works

1950 *The Closed Treatment of Common Fractures*
1979 *Low Friction Arthroplasty of the Hip*

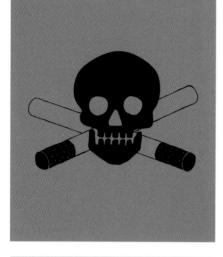

SMOKING KILLS

TOBACCO AND LUNG CANCER

World Health Organization data from 2018 showed lung cancer to be the most common cancer worldwide, accounting for 2.1 million diagnoses and 1.76 million deaths—22 percent of all cancer deaths. Tobacco smoking is responsible for around 80 percent of these deaths. For decades, the link between tobacco and lung cancer was strongly denied by cigarette companies, which funded and published research that supported their position and then employed statisticians to challenge any evidence to the contrary.

The British Doctors Study

In 1951, British epidemiologists Richard Doll and Austin Bradford Hill embarked on the British Doctors Study to establish the strength of the link between smoking and lung cancer. At that time, most British men smoked, including the majority of doctors. (Smoking among British women peaked at 45 percent in the mid-1960s.) Doll and Hill interviewed more than 40,000 physicians about their smoking habits and conducted follow-up surveys until 2001.

By 1965, the British Doctors Study clearly showed that smokers had a greater chance of contracting lung cancer and other diseases than nonsmokers. Those who had started smoking before World War II lost, on average, 10 years of life. Hill applied nine criteria (the Bradford Hill criteria) to the data to ensure that the correlation was robust enough to stand up to opposition from tobacco companies.

Triggering cancer

Environmental and occupational exposure to radon gas, asbestos, and air pollution can all cause lung cancer, and around 8 percent of cases are inherited due to

> Advancing knowledge ... does not confer upon us a freedom to ignore the knowledge we already have.
> **Austin Bradford Hill**
> **"The Environment and Disease: Association or Causation?", 1965**

The Bradford Hill criteria

Devised in 1965, the Bradford Hill criteria identify nine principles that should be considered when looking for the causes of a disease. Although genetics and molecular biology have provided new research tools, these criteria are still used.

Principle	Question
1. Strength	How strong is the link between cause and effect?
2. Consistency	Have other studies shown similar results?
3. Specificity	Are any other diseases present?
4. Temporality	Does the cause precede the effect?
5. Dose response	Does greater exposure increase the effect?
6. Plausibility	Is the relationship between cause and effect credible?
7. Coherence	Do laboratory tests fit with epidemiological knowledge?
8. Experiment	Can the disease be altered by experimental interventions?
9. Analogy	Has a strong enough cause-and-effect relationship been established for weaker evidence of a similar cause and effect to be accepted?

mutations on chromosomes 5, 6, or 15. Most cases, however, are the result of smoking. Tobacco smoke contains a cocktail of particulates and other carcinogens, which are cancer-triggering substances. These activate oncogenes (genes with the capacity to cause cancer), which drive abnormal cell proliferation or deactivate the body's natural tumor suppressor genes.

People with lung inflammation are also susceptible to lung cancer. Emphysema and bronchitis, for example, are caused by particulates entering the body's airways. These diseases make it more difficult for the lungs to remove such irritants, increasing the chances of a person contracting cancer.

Treating lung cancer
Lung cancer therapy has improved dramatically since American surgeon Evarts Graham carried out the first successful pneumonectomy (lung removal) in 1933. Radiotherapy was introduced as a treatment in the 1940s, and chemotherapy was added in the 1970s. Modern treatment involves a combination of radiotherapy and chemotherapy, often after surgery, but outcomes are still generally poor.

One recent development in the ongoing search for an effective treatment for lung cancer is TRAIL therapy. TRAIL, or CD253, is a cytokine, a protein secreted by cells in very small quantities, which binds to certain cancer cells and destroys them. TRAIL causes no harm to healthy tissue and can be delivered via an intravenous drip but oncologists have found that cancer cells quickly become resistant to TRAIL. Nevertheless, trials continue in the hope that new treatments may prove successful in curing many cancers. ∎

Anti-smoking legislation

Campaigns to raise public awareness of the dangers of smoking and government interventions, such as raising tobacco taxes, banning advertising, and outlawing smoking in public places, can be effective in reducing rates of cancer. In the UK, cigarette ads were banned on TV in 1965 and completely in 2005, and smoking was banned in enclosed public places in 2006. Smoking in the UK has fallen as a result, and with it the incidence of lung cancer.

In many parts of the world, smoking has not declined, and it is rising in some countries, including China, Brazil, Russia, and India. In China, a law to prohibit smoking in shopping malls, bars, restaurants, offices, and on public transportation was enacted in 2015. In the US, legislation varies between states, but awareness of the dangers of smoking is high, and the level of smoking and incidence of lung cancer in the US as a whole have fallen.

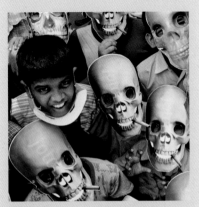

Children take part in a rally in Kolkata, India, on World No Tobacco Day, held every year at the end of May.

HELP TO LIVE UNTIL YOU DIE

PALLIATIVE CARE

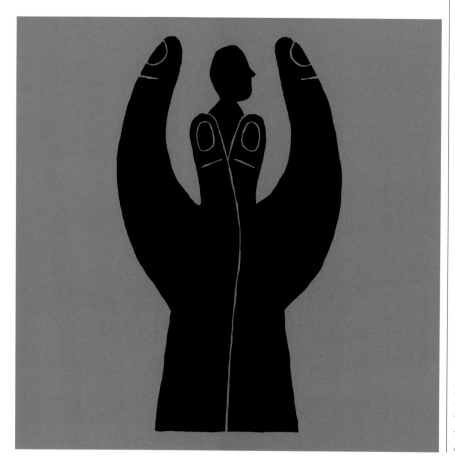

IN CONTEXT

BEFORE

1843 Jeanne Garnier sets up a facility to care for the dying in Lyon, France.

1879 Australia's first hospice, the Home of Incurables, is set up in a convent in Adelaide.

1899 St. Rose's Hospice opens in New York City to look after patients with incurable cancer.

1905 The Religious Sisters of Charity found St. Joseph's Hospice in Hackney, London.

AFTER

1976 Balfour Mount in Montreal, Canada, holds North America's first conference on palliative care.

1987 The UK, New Zealand, and Australia recognize palliative care as a sub-specialty of general medicine.

1990 A report by the World Health Organization (WHO) on palliative care says the "control of pain ... and of psychological, social, and spiritual problems is paramount."

The concept of palliative care—specialized support for the terminally ill—was pioneered by British nurse, social worker, and doctor Cicely Saunders. In 1967, Saunders founded the world's first custom-built hospice, St. Christopher's, in London.

Saunders believed that dying people should be treated with compassion, respect, and dignity, with access to painkilling medicine to alleviate their suffering. This ethos led to Saunders' theory of

See also: Ayurvedic medicine 22–25 ▪ Herbal medicine 36–37
▪ Hospitals 82–83 ▪ Anesthesia 112–117

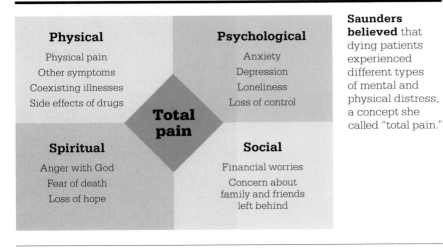

Physical	Psychological
Physical pain	Anxiety
Other symptoms	Depression
Coexisting illnesses	Loneliness
Side effects of drugs	Loss of control

Total pain

Spiritual	Social
Anger with God	Financial worries
Fear of death	Concern about family and friends left behind
Loss of hope	

Saunders believed that dying patients experienced different types of mental and physical distress, a concept she called "total pain."

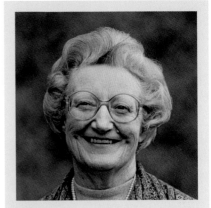

Cicely Saunders

The eldest of three children, Cicely Saunders was born in Hertfordshire, UK, in 1918. She studied politics and philosophy at Oxford University before training as a nurse during World War II, and later as a hospital-based social worker.

Saunders began to form her ideas on care for the dying while looking after Polish refugee David Tasma in 1948. Before his death, Tasma suggested to Saunders that she open a home for the dying and included a bequest for her to do so in his will. In 1967, 10 years after retraining as a doctor, Saunders opened St. Christopher's in London.

Saunders was awarded the prestigious Order of Merit in 1989. She died at St. Christopher's in 2005. Her publications on palliative care have since been translated into many languages.

Key works

1959 "Control of pain in terminal cancer"
1970 "An individual approach to the relief of pain"
1979 "The nature and management of terminal pain and the hospice concept"

"total pain"—the idea that a patient's physical pain was one aspect of overall distress that included emotional, social, and spiritual elements. After opening St. Christopher's Hospice, Saunders advocated that every terminally ill patient should be listened to as an individual, receive tailored medical treatment, and be given holistic care by a team of specialists up until their death.

Saunders developed her ideas during a time of great change in British healthcare. Founded in 1948, the National Health Service (NHS) provided free healthcare for all. In its early days, however, the NHS provided little in the way of care for the terminally ill. Such patients often spent their last hours in the hospital, with doctors administering generic pain medication.

Changing practices

Having a doctor present at a patient's deathbed is a modern phenomenon. Historically, doctors had focused purely on curing disease rather than aiding the terminally ill. In medieval Europe, an early death caused by disease or disaster was commonplace and often quick, but by the late 19th century, advances in medicine and science meant people were generally living longer. A longer life increased the chances of a longer death from diseases such as cancer and the possibility of a protracted period of pain and suffering. Having a doctor present, armed with judicious doses of opium or laudanum (a tincture of opium), became as important as having a priest at the deathbed.

In the early 20th century, doctors were still a long way from developing a process for identifying requirements for end-of-life pain relief. They usually gave all dying patients morphine and repeated the dose only when the effects of the previous one had worn off. Patients were in constant dread of the next wave of pain.

Another source of anxiety for dying patients was their isolation. Most patients wanted their lives to end at home, given the choice, but only the wealthy could afford to have a physician present. From 1948, NHS-funded hospitals became the place where most terminally ill people in Britain died. There » were also a small number of homes, called hospices, that tended to the needs of the dying, but they typically relied on older traditions of religious care and were almost entirely separate from the NHS. In some cases, hospices provided innovative ways of looking after the terminally ill, but their provision of care was not comprehensive, nor was it regulated.

Managing pain

Saunders set out to change this landscape for the dying. While working as a volunteer nurse at St. Luke's Hospital in London, she had become versed in the theories of its founder, Dr. Howard Barrett. Barrett instigated the policy of giving pain relief regularly to prevent the recurrence of pain, not just when the last dose ran out. Saunders imitated this approach after retraining as a doctor and working at St. Joseph's Hospice in east London. Finding that many patients felt deserted by their doctors at the end, she decided that doctors should make up only one part of a hospice team who would deliver holistic care and pain relief until a patient's death.

Reasoning that "constant pain needs constant control," Saunders discovered that by relieving a patient's anxiety about pain, the pain often receded faster, eliminating the need for long-term pain relief. She also established a system for identifying levels of pain—mild, medium, and severe—each of which was to be treated differently rather than with a one-size-fits-all medicine such as morphine.

This fed into Saunders' theory of "total pain." She believed that pain was made up of physical, psychological, social, and spiritual distress and that each patient's pain needed to be treated on an individual basis. She argued that doctors needed to listen to their patients describe their pain in order to understand their requirements. In Saunders' view, pain was a syndrome and needed the same attention as the underlying illness that was causing it.

Saunders' research culminated in the opening of St. Christopher's, where staff combined expert pain relief with holistic care that met the individual needs of patients, and also took those of their visiting

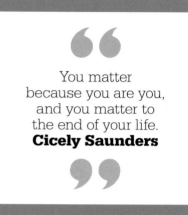

You matter because you are you, and you matter to the end of your life.
Cicely Saunders

family and friends into consideration. By 1970, St. Christopher's had gained enough recognition to receive financial support from the NHS and be the template for several new hospices that were then springing up around Britain.

The movement spreads

During the 1970s, end-of-life care became a talked-about medical issue, both in Britain and abroad. In 1972, the British government held a symposium on Care of the Dying in London that highlighted the haphazard and inadequate delivery of palliative care.

It was Canadian doctor Balfour Mount who coined the term "palliative care" in the mid-1970s. A supporter of Saunders, Mount used the term instead of "hospice," which had different connotations in French-speaking Quebec. Palliative care soon became the favored term, even by Saunders, who initially disliked it, and Mount opened the first palliative care ward in Quebec in 1975. It was based on St. Christopher's, but also embraced some of the teachings of Elisabeth Kübler-Ross, a Swiss American psychiatrist who urged the medical profession to treat the terminally ill with the utmost respect.

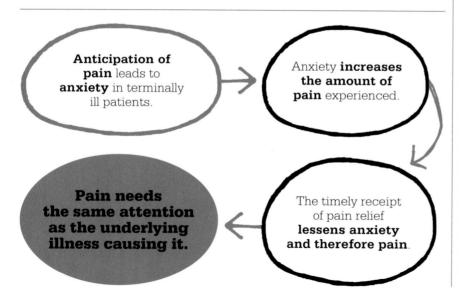

Anticipation of pain leads to **anxiety** in terminally ill patients.

Anxiety **increases the amount of pain** experienced.

The timely receipt of pain relief **lessens anxiety and therefore pain**.

Pain needs the same attention as the underlying illness causing it.

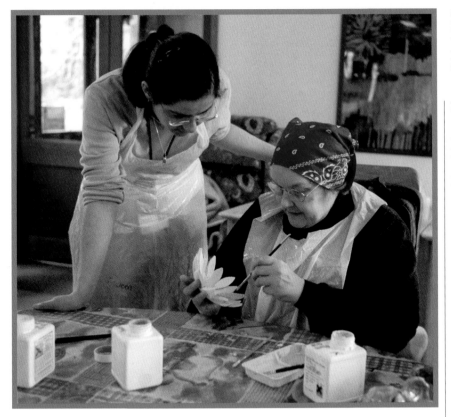

Staff at St. Christopher's Hospice, London, are trained not just to attend to the physical needs of terminally ill patients, but to engage with their lives and comfort them.

medication is usually a complex cocktail of medicines, including analgesics (opioid and nonopioid painkillers) and adjuvant drugs (drugs that are not painkillers but are useful in managing pain), such as antidepressants, muscle relaxants, and anti-anxiety pills, which form part of holistic programs. Such programs dedicated to the alleviation of suffering, alongside a wide network of hospices, form the basis of Cicely Saunders' legacy to medicine.

Palliative care benefits not only patients and their families, but the rest of the medical service, which is then freed up to do other vital work. Due to an aging global population, the need for palliative care is ever growing, with an estimated 40 million people worldwide in need every year. Yet there is a long way to go, as the WHO stated that in 2020 only 14 percent of people in need of such care currently receive it. ■

The palliative movement began to spread worldwide, and in 1987, Australia, New Zealand, and Britain all established palliative care as a specialized area of medicine. In that same year, oncologist Declan Walsh developed the Cleveland Cancer Center in Ohio, the first palliative care program in the US. The clinic was set up to address the needs of patients with incurable diseases that were not being met by existing health providers.

Modern care

Today, palliative care is considered a distinct branch of medicine in many countries. It is usually practiced by interdisciplinary teams that include doctors, nurses, care workers, chaplains, therapists, and social workers. Palliative medicine focuses on alleviating pain in patients with life-threatening illnesses. It is now broadly accepted that pain manifests itself in different but interlinked forms, just as Cicely Saunders had maintained in her theory of total pain.

The different forms of pain experienced by the terminally ill are variously defined as physical; psychosocial or interpersonal; emotional or psychological; and spiritual or existential. Palliative patients are asked to describe their pain to health professionals who make assessments based on examinations and conversations about a patient's history and situation. Their conclusions are then matched to pain severity assessment tools, provided by authorities such as the World Health Organization (WHO).

Far from the all-purpose pain relief medicines prescribed during the Victorian era, palliative pain

> 66
>
> The concept of "total pain" [and] her observation that patient and family need to be considered together as the unit of care … are Cicely's enduring contributions.
> **Balfour Mount**
>
> 99

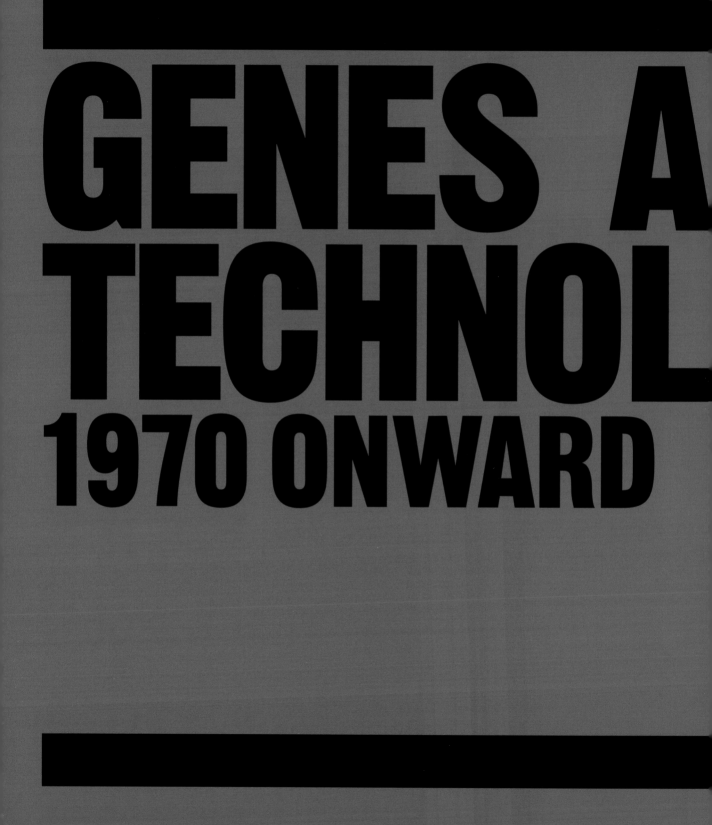

GENES A
TECHNOL
1970 ONWARD

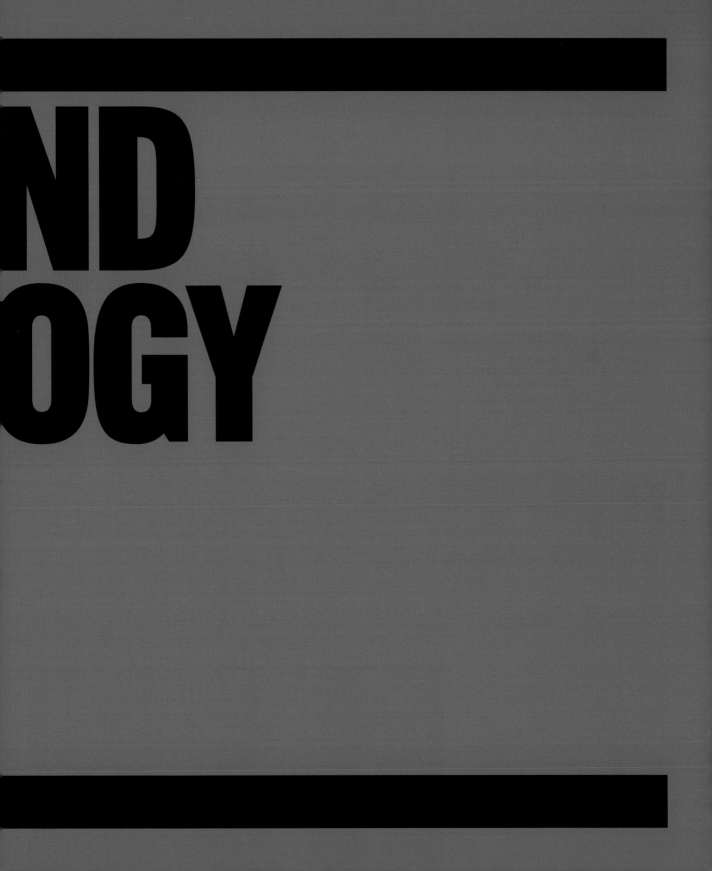

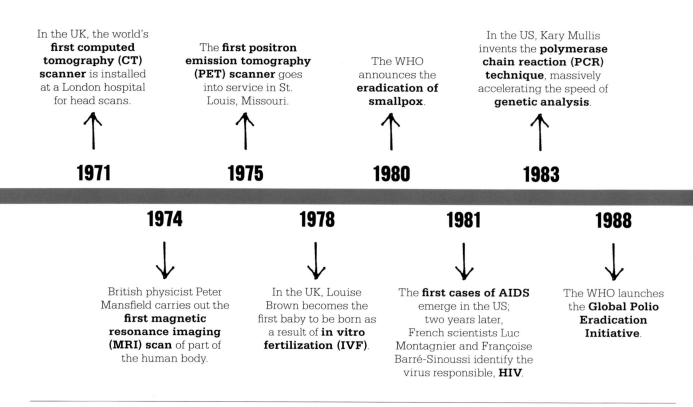

In the UK, the world's **first computed tomography (CT) scanner** is installed at a London hospital for head scans.

1971

The **first positron emission tomography (PET) scanner** goes into service in St. Louis, Missouri.

1975

The WHO announces the **eradication of smallpox**.

1980

In the US, Kary Mullis invents the **polymerase chain reaction (PCR) technique**, massively accelerating the speed of **genetic analysis**.

1983

1974

British physicist Peter Mansfield carries out the **first magnetic resonance imaging (MRI) scan** of part of the human body.

1978

In the UK, Louise Brown becomes the first baby to be born as a result of **in vitro fertilization (IVF)**.

1981

The **first cases of AIDS** emerge in the US; two years later, French scientists Luc Montagnier and Françoise Barré-Sinoussi identify the virus responsible, **HIV**.

1988

The WHO launches the **Global Polio Eradication Initiative**.

H uge advances in the fields of cell biology, genetics, and immunology have changed the landscape of medicine since the 1970s. Techniques that were once confined to the pages of science fiction have become medical reality. Scientists are able to clone cells, analyze and modify DNA, and grow body tissue, transforming diagnostic tests and treatments.

The ensuing decades have also presented unforeseen challenges. In 1970, no one could have forecast the deaths of more than 30 million people from a new virus called HIV, or the scale and speed at which bacteria causing some infections—including pneumonia and tuberculosis— would develop antibiotic resistance.

Many of the breakthroughs became possible because of the revolution in technology. The development of diagnostic tools, such as computed tomography (CT), magnetic resonance imaging (MRI), and positron emission tomography (PET), enabled physicians to view the body's interior in astonishing detail. Minimally invasive keyhole surgery made many operations safer, and laser technology made surgery easier. Robotic and telesurgery have allowed surgeons to perform surgery remotely, sometimes thousands of miles from the patient. In the not-too-distant future, nanomedicine—the diagnosis and treatment of disease at molecular level—should enable physicians to target individual cells.

Defeating disease

The World Health Organization (WHO) has led international efforts to eradicate some of the deadliest infectious diseases. In 1980, the WHO declared that smallpox had been eradicated, and eight years later, it instigated the Global Polio Eradication Initiative. By 2020, polio, a potentially fatal disease, was endemic in only two countries (Afghanistan and Pakistan). Various campaigns to eradicate malaria, a mosquito-borne illness affecting 228 million people and causing 405,000 deaths in 2018, continue.

Meanwhile, new diseases have emerged. HIV, the virus causing AIDS (acquired immunodeficiency syndrome), was discovered in 1983, by which time it was already spreading rapidly. The subsequent development of antiretroviral drugs has suppressed the development of AIDS in individuals, but no cure has so far been found: in 2018, almost 38 million people lived with the HIV infection, two-thirds of them

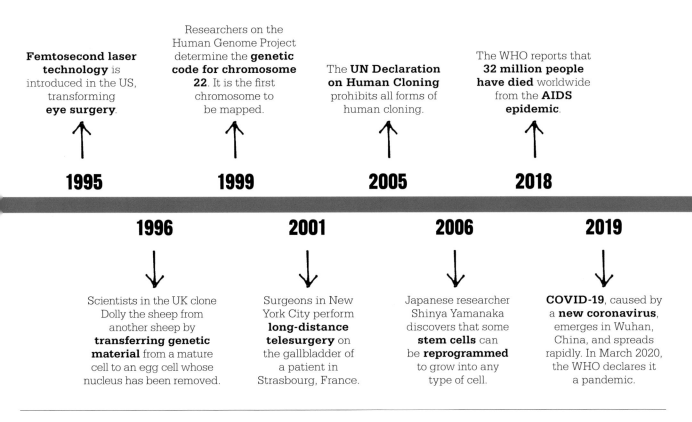

Femtosecond laser technology is introduced in the US, transforming **eye surgery**.

Researchers on the Human Genome Project determine the **genetic code for chromosome 22**. It is the first chromosome to be mapped.

The **UN Declaration on Human Cloning** prohibits all forms of human cloning.

The WHO reports that **32 million people have died** worldwide from the **AIDS epidemic**.

1995

1999

2005

2018

1996

2001

2006

2019

Scientists in the UK clone Dolly the sheep from another sheep by **transferring genetic material** from a mature cell to an egg cell whose nucleus has been removed.

Surgeons in New York City perform **long-distance telesurgery** on the gallbladder of a patient in Strasbourg, France.

Japanese researcher Shinya Yamanaka discovers that some **stem cells** can be **reprogrammed** to grow into any type of cell.

COVID-19, caused by a **new coronavirus**, emerges in Wuhan, China, and spreads rapidly. In March 2020, the WHO declares it a pandemic.

in sub-Saharan Africa. The danger of infectious diseases was again highlighted with the spread of the COVID-19 virus. Within nine months of the virus emerging in Wuhan, China, in December 2019, only 12 countries had no reported cases.

Transforming medicine
A host of new treatments in the last few decades have improved or saved millions of lives. In 1975, immunologists César Milstein and Georges Köhler discovered how to make unlimited, identical copies of the same antibody (monoclonal antibodies), leading to many new treatments. Monoclonal antibodies are used to help prevent the rejection of transplanted organs, to carry drugs or radiation to particular cells, and to fight autoimmune diseases such as rheumatoid arthritis.

Another breakthrough, in 1978, offered a solution to the problem of infertility. In vitro fertilization (IVF), in which a human egg is fertilized with sperm in a laboratory and then implanted into the womb as an embryo, led to more than 8 million births over the next 40 years.

Advances in microsurgery and immunosuppressant drugs have also extended the possibilities of transplant surgery. The first full face transplant, an intricate feat, was performed in France in 2008.

Some of the biggest medical advances have been made possible by the strides made in genetics since British biochemist Frederick Sanger developed a method for sequencing DNA. Sanger's work paved the way for the Human Genome Project, the complete mapping of human genes, allowing

scientists to identify genes linked to particular diseases and opening up the possibility of gene editing.

Revolutionary techniques can sometimes raise ethical dilemmas. Gene therapy, which involves introducing healthy DNA to a cell with defective DNA, potentially ending a range of genetic diseases, is particularly controversial. Critics point out that such techniques could be abused to "improve" humanity. Objections are also raised by the use of embryonic stem cells to grow tissue for regenerative medicine.

Balancing ethical concerns with the desire to save and improve lives has never been so pertinent. Stem cell research and genetic editing have the potential to transform health to an extent on par with the development of anesthesia, antibiotics, and vaccines. ■

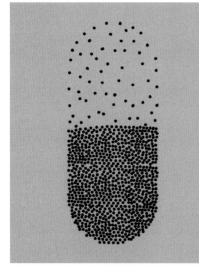

RANDOMIZE TILL IT HURTS

EVIDENCE-BASED MEDICINE

IN CONTEXT

BEFORE
c. 1643 Flemish physician Jan Baptista van Helmont proposes a randomized controlled clinical trial to determine the efficacy of bloodletting.

1863 In the US, physician Austin Flint offers 13 patients a dummy remedy (placebo) to compare its effects with those of an active treatment.

1943 The UK's Medical Research Council conducts the first double-blind controlled trial (where neither subjects nor researchers know who gets a specific therapy or treatment).

AFTER
1981 A series of articles by clinical epidemiologists at McMaster University, Canada, advises physicians how to assess medical literature.

1990 Physician Gordon Guyatt, at McMaster University, uses the term "evidence-based medicine" for the first time.

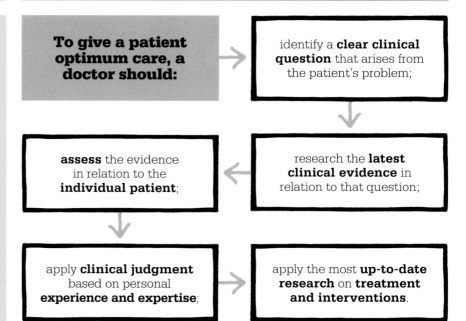

To give a patient optimum care, a doctor should:

identify a **clear clinical question** that arises from the patient's problem;

research the **latest clinical evidence** in relation to that question;

assess the evidence in relation to the **individual patient**;

apply **clinical judgment** based on personal **experience and expertise**;

apply the most **up-to-date research** on **treatment and interventions**.

E
vidence-based medicine (EBM) is concerned with using the best-quality, most up-to-date research available to find answers to medical questions and to give clinicians and patients the evidence they need to make informed choices about treatments.

Central to EBM are randomized controlled trials (RCTs) that measure the effectiveness of one or more interventions by allocating them at random (to avoid bias) to similar groups of people so that outcomes can be compared and measured. In 1972, Scottish epidemiologist Archie Cochrane's influential *Effectiveness and Efficiency* highlighted both the value of RCTs and the perils of ineffective treatments.

RCTs were pioneered in 1747 by James Lind, a Scottish naval surgeon. He selected 12 sailors, all sick with scurvy to a similar degree;

See also: Nosology 74–75 ▪ Case history 80–81 ▪ Preventing scurvy 84–85 ▪ Epidemiology 124–127 ▪ Vitamins and diet 200–203

Not all evidence in evidence-based medicine is given the same weight. The most valued evidence, at the top of the pyramid, is systematic reviews that evaluate and synthesize the results of carefully designed randomized controlled trials.

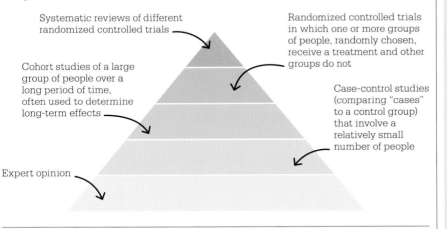

Systematic reviews of different randomized controlled trials

Randomized controlled trials in which one or more groups of people, randomly chosen, receive a treatment and other groups do not

Cohort studies of a large group of people over a long period of time, often used to determine long-term effects

Case-control studies (comparing "cases" to a control group) that involve a relatively small number of people

Expert opinion

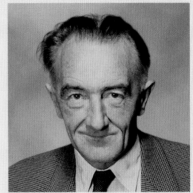

Archibald Cochrane

The son of tweed-makers, Archibald (Archie) Cochrane was born in 1909 in Galashiels, Scotland. He graduated from King's College, Cambridge, in 1930. He qualified as a doctor at University College Hospital, London, in 1938, having earlier volunteered with a British ambulance unit between 1935 and 1937 during the Spanish Civil War. In World War II, he served in the Royal Army Medical Corps before he was captured and interned.

In 1948, Cochrane joined the MRC at its Pneumoconiosis Research Unit in Wales. He left to take up a professorial post at the Welsh National School of Medicine in 1960 and, in 1969, he became director of a new MRC epidemiology unit in Cardiff, where he conducted several groundbreaking RCTs.

Cochrane was also an award-winning gardener and a collector of modern art and sculpture. He suffered cancer in his later years and died in 1988 at the age of 79.

Key work

1972 *Effectiveness and Efficiency: Random Reflections on Health Services*

divided them into six pairs; and ensured they had the same living conditions and followed the same daily diet. Each pair also received one of six daily treatments, which included seawater, vinegar, cider, and two oranges plus a lemon. The citrus fruits worked best, followed by cider, indicating that daily doses of vitamin C treat scurvy.

More trials and studies

Clinical trials progressed during the 19th century, but largely as the work of individual practitioners. In the 20th century, the establishment of national bodies such as the UK's Medical Research Council (MRC), founded in 1913, helped coordinate investigations, provide funding, and raise the standard of clinical trials.

Cochrane, who later joined the MRC, conducted his first RCT in Salonika, Greece, while a prisoner of war during World War II. To test which vitamin supplement might help treat ankle edema (swelling as a result of fluid retention), a common condition in the camp, he allocated daily doses of yeast (B vitamins) to six of those affected and vitamin C to a further six. The efficacy of the yeast treatment persuaded his captors to give all the prisoners daily yeast to improve their health.

After the war, Cochrane worked at an MRC research unit in Wales studying pneumoconiosis ("dust lung") in coal miners. In this and later research, Cochrane paid meticulous attention to the accuracy and standardization of the data he collected and its reproducibility.

World resource

Cochrane was passionate about improving scientific evidence to validate medical interventions. In 1993, the Cochrane Collaboration (now known simply as Cochrane) was founded in the UK to collect and disseminate reviews of clinical trials. Today, it operates in 43 countries, encouraging healthcare professionals to make clinical decisions based on the best evidence available. ▪

SEEING INSIDE THE BODY

MRI AND MEDICAL SCANNING

IN CONTEXT

BEFORE
1938 Polish American physicist Isidor Rabi discovers nuclear magnetic resonance, the basis for MRI.

1951 Robert Gabillard uses varying magnetic fields to locate the origin of radio waves emitted by the nuclei of atoms.

1956 David Kuhl builds a device for tracking radioactive isotopes in the human body.

AFTER
1975 The first PET scanner goes live at Washington University, in St. Louis.

1977 Peter Mansfield invents the echo-planar technique to speed up MRI scanning.

2018 Scientists in New Zealand develop the first 3D color medical scanner.

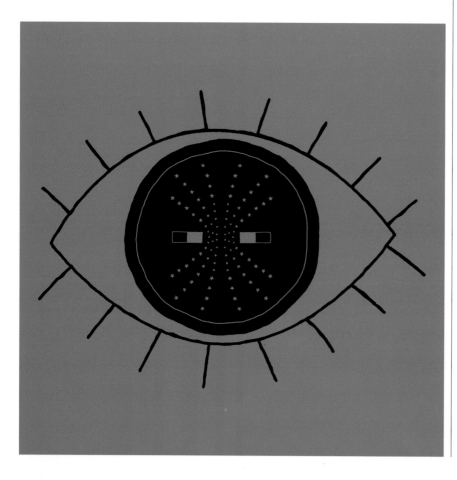

Medical scanning allows physicians to see inside the body, helping them diagnose and treat disorders. A variety of techniques are used, including X-rays, ultrasound, magnetic resonance imaging (MRI), computed tomography (CT), and positron emission tomography (PET). While X-rays were used from the end of the 19th century, most of the other methods developed in the late 1960s or early 1970s. These new techniques could differentiate between types of soft tissue, making the detection of injuries, tumors, and other abnormalities easier.

Experiments in physics

MRI is based on the principle of nuclear magnetic resonance (NMR)—the application of a magnetic field

Hydrogen is one of the most abundant elements in the human body. The **nuclei** of hydrogen atoms are like **tiny magnets**.

An MRI scanner produces a **magnetic field**, causing the nuclei to **align**. It then uses **radio waves** to **knock them out of alignment**.

When the radio waves are **turned off**, the **nuclei realign** and send out **radio signals**.

By **measuring these radio signals**, the scanner's computer can **create a detailed image** of the body part being examined.

to matter so that the nuclei of its hydrogen atoms release energy. Measuring this energy reveals the chemical structure of the matter.

NMR techniques had been used to analyze chemical samples since 1945. Chemist Paul Lauterbur and physician Raymond Damadian in the US and British physicist Peter Mansfield were all familiar with the technique when, in 1969, Damadian hypothesized that cancerous cells

could be distinguished from healthy cells using NMR. He reasoned that cancerous cells would show up because they hold more water and therefore have more hydrogen atoms. Two years later, he demonstrated this in experiments on dead rats.

In 1972, Lauterbur, then working at Stony Brook University in New York, showed that clear images could be produced by introducing gradients to NMR magnetic fields.

This made it possible to determine where each atom was in relation to the others and identify differences in the resonance signals more precisely. (This idea was first proposed by two physicists working independently, Robert Gabillard in France and Hermann Carr in the United States, but it had not been taken any further.) Lauterbur tried the technique on the contents of two test tubes, »

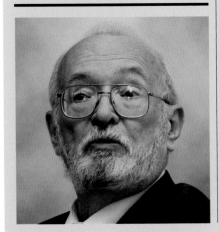

Paul Lauterbur

Born in 1929 in Sidney, Ohio, Paul Lauterbur was so enthusiastic about chemistry as a teenager that he built his own laboratory in his parents' house. He was awarded a doctorate from the University of Pittsburgh in 1962 and lectured in chemistry at Stony Brook University, New York, from 1963 to 1985.

Lauterbur worked with NMR technology for several years, but it was not until 1971 that he thought of using it to make images of human organs. The revelation happened while he was eating a burger in a Pittsburgh diner; he

quickly scribbled a model of the MRI technique on a paper napkin, then set about refining the idea.

In 2003, Lauterbur and Peter Mansfield were jointly awarded the Nobel Prize in Physiology or Medicine for their work on MRI. Lauterbur died in 2007.

Key work

1973 "Image formation by induced local interaction; examples involving nuclear magnetic resonance"

one holding regular water and the other heavy water (whose hydrogen atoms have a neutron as well as a proton, making it "heavier"). The heavy and regular water looked different from one another—the first time that imaging had shown this. Lauterbur also used the technique on a clam found by his daughter, clearly showing its tissue structure. He was convinced that his imaging method could be used to distinguish between different types of human tissue without harming the patient.

The first body scans

In 1974, Mansfield made the first MRI scan of a human body part—cross-sectional images of a student's finger. However, the scans took up to 23 minutes to create. To speed up the process, he developed the echo-planar imaging technique, which produced multiple nuclear NMR echoes from a single excitation of the protons. This meant that an entire MR image could be obtained in a fraction of a second. The advantage of echo-planar imaging is that it can image rapid physiological processes, such as respiration and cardiac rhythm.

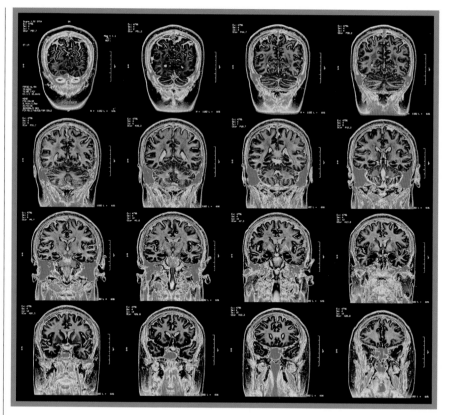

> We began to produce quite nice images ... as the 1980s ticked by, the quality became more and more acceptable to our clinical colleagues.
> **Peter Mansfield**

Mansfield used echo-planar imaging in his prototype scanner, which went into experimental use in 1978. In the US, Damadian unveiled the first whole-body MRI scanner in May 1977. The US Food and Drug Administration (FDA) approved it for use in 1984.

The big advantage of MRI is that it provides extremely detailed images. It is used for noninvasive examination of the brain and spinal cord, bones and joints, breasts, blood vessels, the heart, and other organs. One disadvantage is the cost of an MRI scanner—as high as $2 million (£1.5 million). The other disadvantage of MRI is that it cannot be used on patients with metallic implants. Despite this, there were more than 50,000 MRI scanners in service in 2018, with the highest concentration—55 per 1 million people—in Japan.

MRI allows doctors to view the brain in "slices" of 0.04–0.16 in (1–4mm). False color can be added to highlight particular features.

Scanners with powerful 3T (tesla) magnets produce very high-quality images of the minute details of the musculoskeletal and nervous systems. Engineers are building increasingly powerful scanners that will provide even more detailed images of the body faster.

CT scans

British electrical engineer Godfrey Hounsfield and American physicist Allan MacLeod Cormack developed CT (computed tomography)—also known as CAT (computerized axial tomography)—scanning for medical diagnosis. Hounsfield's first scanner, in 1968, took nine days to capture a full three-dimensional (3D) image

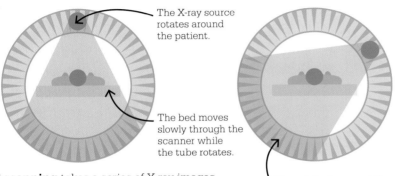

The X-ray source rotates around the patient.

The bed moves slowly through the scanner while the tube rotates.

X-ray detectors send the images to a computer, which creates a 3D image.

CT scanning takes a series of X-ray images from different angles while the patient lies flat. The process takes 10–20 minutes.

of a dead pig's brain. He later used X-rays and reduced the scanning time to nine hours. It worked by firing gamma rays as it rotated around the brain, one degree at a time, creating thousands of cross-sectional images. A computer program then assembled these "slices" (the word tomography derives from *tomei*, the Greek word for slice) to produce the 3D image.

The first head-scanning CT machine was installed at Atkinson Morley Hospital, London, in 1971. Its first scan was of the head of a patient with a frontal lobe brain tumor. The first whole-body CT scanner was introduced in 1976.

CT scans are used to detect tumors and bone fractures and to monitor changes in a disease such as cancer. Although CT scanners are much more sophisticated than they were in the 1970s, and quicker and quieter than MRI machines, their images of organs and soft tissues are not as clear. Importantly, CT radiation may be up to 1,000 times more than traditional X-ray. This is still small, but the doses may

A doctor examines a PET scan for chemical activity that indicates cancer. The tracer fluorodeoxyglucose (FDG) is usually used in such cases, as cancer cells absorb glucose at a faster rate.

accumulate if the body is scanned repeatedly, fractionally increasing a patient's risk of getting cancer.

PET scans

Positron emission tomography (PET) can reveal biochemical changes in tissue at cellular level, something that CT and MRI cannot do. The patient ingests or is injected with a radioactive drug called a radiotracer, which collects in areas of the body with greater chemical activity, often a sign of disease. The tracer emits subatomic particles called positrons. When these collide with electrons in the body tissue being examined, they produce gamma rays, which are detected by a ring of

receptors in the donut-shaped scanner. A computer then plots the gamma rays to produce a 3D image of tracer concentrations.

PET technology emerged in the US in 1956, when scientist David Kuhl developed a photoscanner based on the earlier work of physicist Benedict Cassen. It worked on the same principle as modern PET, creating images from radioactivity detected in the body. Development continued during the 1960s and 1970s, and the first clinically practical whole-body scanner, known as PET (III), was used to examine patients in 1975. Combined PET–CT scanning takes advantage of the great detail that is possible with CT scans to create 3D images of even greater clarity. Combined PET–MRI scanning is also possible.

PET scans are used to monitor cancer; to plan surgery; and to diagnose, manage, and treat neurological disorders, including Parkinson's disease, dementia, and epilepsy. They are, however, not given to pregnant women—the radiation emitted by the tracers is potentially damaging to fetuses—or to some diabetics, because the tracer is combined with glucose. ∎

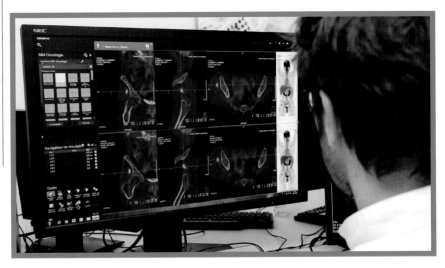

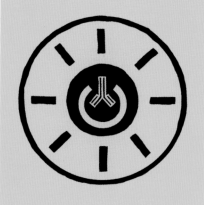

ANTIBODIES ON DEMAND
MONOCLONAL ANTIBODIES

Monoclonal antibodies (mAbs) are unlimited, identical copies of the same antibody that are produced artificially. They were first made in 1975 by two immunologists, César Milstein from Argentina and Georges Köhler from Germany, and although research is ongoing, they have already proved useful in many areas of medicine. They make up a high proportion of new drugs and diagnostic tests, from innovative treatments for cancers to identifying blood types.

Antibodies are proteins the body uses to target alien cells such as germs. There are millions of kinds, each matching a different alien protein (or antigen), and they latch on to their specific antigen either to neutralize it or to identify it as a target for the body's immune cells.

Paul Ehrlich coined the term "antibodies" in 1891, and went on to describe how they interact with antigens like lock and key. By the 1960s, scientists knew they are made by white blood cells called B-cells, or B-lymphocytes, each

---

Plasma cells produce a **mix of antibodies** in response to the **presence of a pathogen**.	**Myeloma** cancer cells can multiply **limitlessly**.

Scientists fuse a myeloma cell with a plasma cell just as it is producing **one type of antibody**, creating a **hybridoma**.

The **hybridoma can multiply** to produce **limitless supplies** of that one type of antibody.

See also: Vaccination 94–101 ▪ Cellular pathology 134–135 ▪ The immune system 154–161 ▪ Cancer therapy 168–175 ▪ Targeted drug delivery 198–199

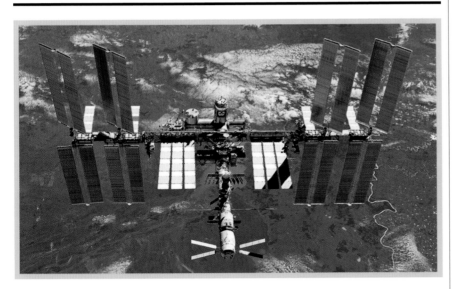

Experiments on the International Space Station aim to grow a crystalline form of a monoclonal antibody used in cancer treatment so it can be injected rather than delivered intravenously.

primed with its own antibody. When triggered by its matching antigen, a B-cell clones itself, producing multiple copies of plasma cells, which release floods of antibodies. As plasma cells produce more than one kind of antibody, the process is described as "polyclonal."

Harnessing immune cells

Milstein and Köhler's breakthrough was to create limitless copies of identical "monoclonal" antibodies using cells made in the lab called hybridomas. These are artificial fusions of plasma cells and myeloma cells (abnormal plasma cells that cause cancer) primed to produce the desired antibody. Plasma cells are short-lived, whereas myeloma cells reproduce indefinitely. By fusing them, Milstein and Köhler created an endlessly multiplying source of their chosen antibody.

Milstein's original intention was to find a way to make antibodies for research. But he and Köhler quickly realized that mAbs might also be a "magic bullet," offering tailor-made antibodies to target any disease.

Increasingly useful tool

Although monoclonal antibodies have not yet proved to be a magic cure-all, they are finding new uses all the time. They can even be used to detect biological weapons. In pregnancy tests, mAbs detect the hormone HCG, and in tissue typing, they help prevent a donor organ from being rejected by blocking the immune response. They can identify blood clots and rogue cells and are used in cancer treatment to carry drugs or radiation to targeted cells.

Monoclonal antibodies are also used to fight autoimmune diseases including rheumatoid arthritis, and new mAb drugs are in the pipeline for malaria, influenza, and HIV. In 2020, scientists found several mAbs that appear to neutralize the COVID-19 virus in cell cultures. ▪

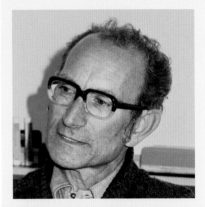

César Milstein

Born in Argentina in 1927, César Milstein studied at the University of Buenos Aires. After completing a doctorate, Milstein was invited to join the biochemistry department at Cambridge University in the UK. His main interest was in the body's defenses, and most of his professional career was devoted to antibody research.

At Cambridge, Milstein collaborated with biochemist Frederick Sanger (a double Nobel Prize recipient), and later Georges Köhler, with whom he carried out the groundbreaking work on monoclonal antibodies. Milstein and Köhler did not take out a patent on their discovery, so he did not benefit financially, but in 1984, they were awarded the Nobel Prize in Physiology or Medicine. Milstein went on to help develop the field of antibody engineering. He died in 2002.

Key works

1973 "Fusion of two immunoglobulin-producing myeloma cells"
1975 "Continuous cultures of fused cells secreting antibody of predefined specificity"

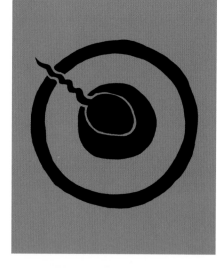

NATURE COULD NOT, SO WE DID

IN VITRO FERTILIZATION

IN CONTEXT

BEFORE

1959 Working in the US at the Worcester Foundation, Min Chueh Chang proves IVF is possible in mammal eggs by using it to conceive rabbits.

1969 Robert Edwards fertilizes a human egg outside the body.

1973 A team at Australia's Monash University achieves the first human IVF pregnancy, but this ends in a miscarriage.

AFTER

1979 The first IVF baby boy is born in Glasgow, Scotland, after treatment from Robert Edwards and Patrick Steptoe.

1981 Monash University announces the birth of nine babies following IVF.

1992 The first ICSI baby is born in Belgium.

2018 About 8 million children worldwide have been born using IVF and similar methods of assisted conception.

On July 25, 1978, the medical world celebrated the birth of Louise Brown, the first baby to be born as a result of in vitro fertilization (IVF). The pioneers of this groundbreaking event were British scientist Robert Edwards and gynecologist Patrick Steptoe.

The concept of IVF was not new. Austrian embryologist Samuel Schenk attempted IVF on rabbit eggs in 1878 and discovered that cell division could occur outside the body when sperm was added to an egg cell. In 1934, American doctor Gregory Pincus laid claim to

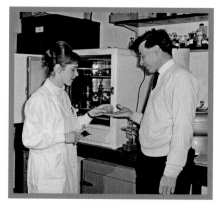

This image from 1968 shows Purdy passing Edwards a dish containing in-vitro-fertilized human egg cells. The UK's Medical Research Council refused to fund the work, deeming it unethical.

the first IVF pregnancy in a rabbit, but the fertilization probably took place *in vivo* ("in the body") rather than *in vitro* ("in glass," outside the body). Having shown in 1951 that spermatozoa needed to reach a certain stage of maturity before being capable of fertilizing an egg, Chinese American scientist Min Chueh Chang successfully used IVF to impregnate a rabbit in 1959.

British breakthrough

In 1968, Edwards teamed up with Steptoe, who was an early expert in laparoscopy (keyhole surgery), a technique that could be used to collect eggs without abdominal surgery. Many of Steptoe's patients in Oldham, Lancashire, agreed to donate eggs to aid the research. With the help of Jean Purdy, an embryologist, the team achieved fertilization of eggs, followed by cell division, in a Petri dish. But their goal of successfully implanting an embryo into a woman's uterus remained elusive.

British couple John and Lesley Brown approached Edwards and Steptoe in 1976. They had been trying to conceive for nine years but had failed due to blocked fallopian tubes. In November 1977, timing

See also: Midwifery 76–77 ▪ Inheritance and hereditary conditions 146–147 ▪ Birth control 214–215 ▪ Ultrasound 244 ▪ Genetics and medicine 288–293 ▪ Minimally invasive surgery 298

Stages in IVF treatment

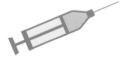 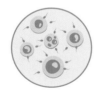 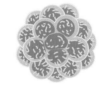 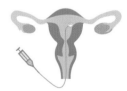

1. The mother takes fertility drugs to stimulate production of eggs. Mature eggs are collected from her ovaries, and a semen sample is taken from the father.

2. The egg and sperm cells are mixed in a Petri dish and left in an incubator for several hours to allow fertilization to take place.

3. The eggs that are fertilized are monitored closely as they begin to divide. Each egg becomes a hollow ball of cells called an embryo.

4. After several days, the selected embryo is placed into the mother's uterus. If the embryo implants successfully, it is likely to develop into a baby.

the process with Lesley Brown's natural ovulation cycle, Edwards and Steptoe collected one of her eggs and added it to a Petri dish containing her husband's sperm. Closely watched by Purdy, the fertilized egg began to divide. After two and a half days, Edwards and Steptoe transferred the resulting eight-cell embryo into Lesley Brown's uterus. Nine months later, Louise Brown was born.

Although a medical milestone, the birth of baby Louise was not universally popular. Many balked at the idea of a "test-tube baby," which they considered unnatural. But as more and more healthy babies were born as a result of IVF treatment, attitudes began to change. By the time Edwards was awarded the Nobel Prize in 2010 for his pioneering work, more than 4.5 million IVF babies had been born.

IVF today

Assisted-conception techniques continue to evolve, as do people's reasons for undergoing treatment. More and more same-sex couples, single women, and surrogates are using fertility services to conceive children. In most modern treatment cycles, the mother is given fertility drugs to stimulate the maturation of multiple eggs and therefore increase the chance of achieving one or more viable embryos after fertilization. Unused embryos, as well as eggs and sperm, can be frozen for use in later cycles. Intracytoplasmic sperm injection (ICSI), in which a single sperm is injected into an egg, is a common treatment for male infertility. Once the subject of fierce opposition, IVF is now safer, more successful, and more popular than ever. ▪

Robert Edwards

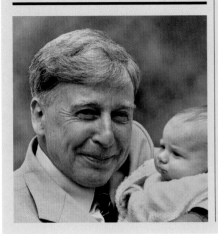

Born in Yorkshire, England, in 1925, Robert Edwards served in the army during World War II before studying agricultural science, and later zoology, at the University of Wales, Bangor. In 1951, he studied artificial insemination and mouse embryos for his doctorate in genetics at Edinburgh University.

After moving to Cambridge in 1963, Edwards set himself the goal of removing human eggs and fertilizing them in vitro. But it was not until he met Patrick Steptoe in 1968 that Edwards was able to attain this goal. Following the birth of Louise Brown, the pair set up the world's first IVF clinic at Bourn Hall, near Cambridge, in 1980. Edwards received the Nobel Prize in 2010, and was knighted a year later. He died in 2013.

Key works

1980 *A Matter of Life: The Story of a Medical Breakthrough*
2001 "The bumpy road to human in vitro fertilization"
2005 "Ethics and moral philosophy in the initiation of IVF, preimplantation diagnosis and stem cells"

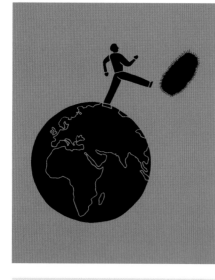

VICTORY OVER SMALLPOX
GLOBAL ERADICATION OF DISEASE

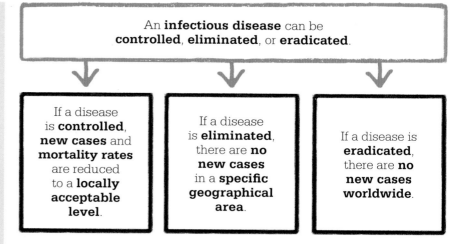

An **infectious disease** can be **controlled**, **eliminated**, or **eradicated**.

If a disease is **controlled**, **new cases** and **mortality rates** are reduced to a **locally acceptable level**.

If a disease is **eliminated**, there are **no new cases** in a **specific geographical area**.

If a disease is **eradicated**, there are **no new cases worldwide**.

On May 8, 1980, the World Health Organization (WHO) declared smallpox to be eradicated—the first major disease, and the only human disease to date, to have been beaten. For centuries, smallpox had been a major scourge, killing millions of people a year. As recently as the 1950s, more than 50 million people every year were infected by the disease.

British physician Edward Jenner had discovered a vaccine in 1796, and smallpox deaths slowly reduced as vaccinations became widespread. As well as providing immunity to individuals, vaccines can protect the whole community. The more who are vaccinated and gain immunity, the fewer hosts the germ can find, and the less the disease can spread.

However, intense opposition to mass vaccination programs was sparked as vaccines accidentally became contaminated on occasion with other germs, such as syphilis. In the 1890s, British physician Sydney Copeman introduced the technique of storing a vaccine in glycerine, dramatically improving its safety. Trust in vaccination rose, and by 1953, smallpox had been eliminated from the US and Europe.

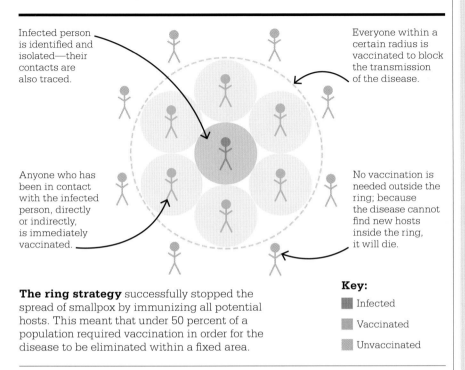

Infected person is identified and isolated—their contacts are also traced.

Everyone within a certain radius is vaccinated to block the transmission of the disease.

Anyone who has been in contact with the infected person, directly or indirectly, is immediately vaccinated.

No vaccination is needed outside the ring; because the disease cannot find new hosts inside the ring, it will die.

The ring strategy successfully stopped the spread of smallpox by immunizing all potential hosts. This meant that under 50 percent of a population required vaccination in order for the disease to be eliminated within a fixed area.

Key:
▪ Infected
▪ Vaccinated
▪ Unvaccinated

Extending vaccination programs to tropical regions was difficult, as the vaccine spoiled within a few days in warm conditions. Then two major innovations progressed the fight against smallpox. First, British scientist Leslie Collier found a way to freeze-dry the vaccine, enabling it to be stored as powder for up to six months, even in hot weather. Then the bifurcated (two-pronged) needle was invented by American microbiologist Benjamin Rubin, enabling the powdered vaccine to be simply pricked into the skin.

The road to eradication

In 1967, the WHO launched the Smallpox Eradication Program in South America, Asia, and Africa. Key to the campaign's success was its "ring" strategy, which involved containing outbreaks within a set zone, or ring, of immunity in order to prevent further transmission.

An infected person was isolated and all potential contacts were immediately tracked, traced, and vaccinated. If that failed, everyone within a given radius would be given the vaccine. This avoided the need for mass vaccination programs.

In 1975, a 3-year-old from Bangladesh became the last person to naturally contract the severe variant of smallpox; in 1977, the last case of the minor variant was identified in Somalia. In both cases, the ring strategy was used, and the battle against smallpox was won.

So far, only the animal disease rinderpest has also been eradicated, in 2011. The success with smallpox led the WHO's global immunization program to target other vaccine-preventable diseases, such as measles, tetanus, diphtheria, and whooping cough. It is hoped that polio and Guinea worm disease may soon be eradicated. ▪

War on vectors

The first major efforts at disease eradication were led by epidemiologist Fred Soper at the Rockefeller Foundation in the US. Yet rather than focusing on vaccines, Soper's campaigns targeted disease vectors—organisms such as flies, mosquitoes, and parasitic worms that pass diseases on to humans.

The three priorities were the vector-borne diseases hookworm, yellow fever, and malaria, and eradication focused on eliminating their vectors. These programs had considerable success but were mired in controversy during the late 1950s by the widespread use of insecticides such as DDT, which posed severe risks to human health and the environment.

The WHO estimates vector-borne diseases make up more than 17 percent of infectious diseases today and cause 700,000 deaths globally a year. Efforts to eradicate malaria, one of the key threats to public health, now include genetic programs to prevent the mosquitoes from breeding.

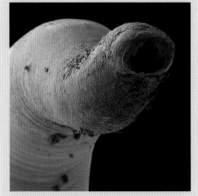

This species of the parasitic hookworm, *Ancylostoma duodenale*, is one of the most common causes of hookworm infestation in humans.

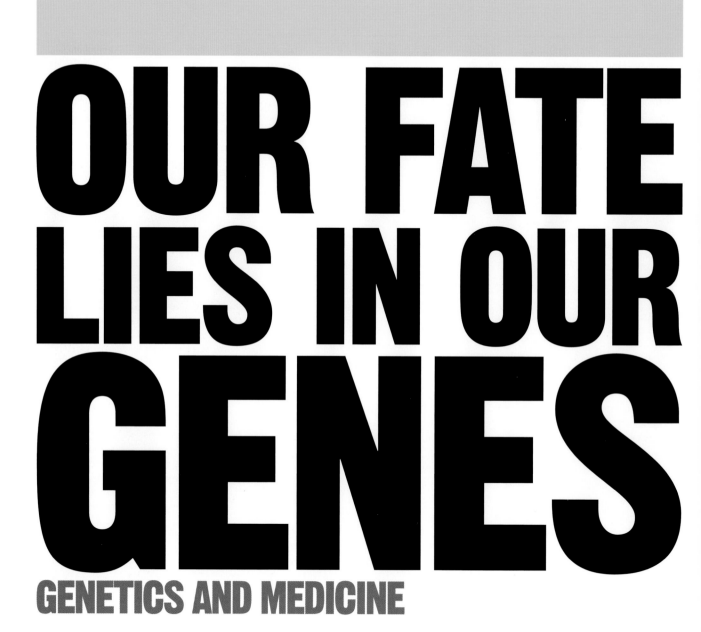

OUR FATE LIES IN OUR GENES

GENETICS AND MEDICINE

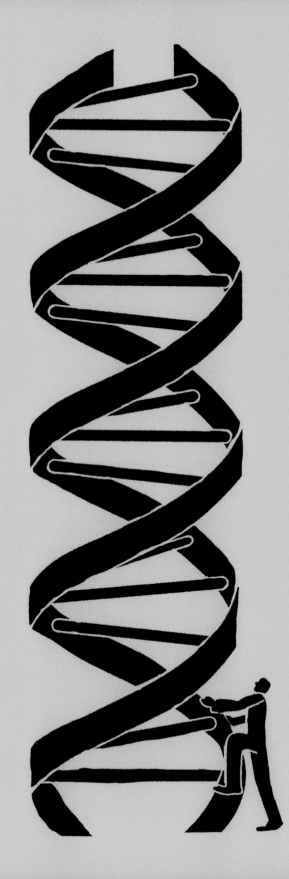

IN CONTEXT

BEFORE

1842 Swiss botanist Carl Wilhelm von Nägeli discovers chromosomes in plants.

1865 Gregor Mendel outlines the laws of inheritance after experimenting with pea plants.

1869 Swiss physiologist Friedrich Miescher discovers the molecule DNA but does not understand its role.

1879 Walther Flemming observes threadlike material, later called chromosomes, in the cells of vertebrate animals as the cells divide.

AFTER

1999 The genetic code for chromosome 22 is mapped.

2003 The Human Genome Project—aiming to map all human genes—is completed.

In 1983, American biochemist Kary Mullis invented a way of rapidly cloning small segments of DNA (deoxyribonucleic acid), the molecules that are packed into chromosomes in the nucleus of cells and carry genetic instructions. The technique, called polymerase chain reaction (PCR), was later refined by fellow American Randall Saiki. This development revolutionized the study of genetics and opened up new areas of medical research and diagnostics. PCR is used to detect hereditary mutations of genes that can cause many serious medical disorders, including Huntington's disease, cystic fibrosis, and sickle cell anemia.

Building understanding

The development of PCR built on the huge strides made in the field of genetics since the early 1940s. The hereditary role of DNA in chromosomes ("the transforming principle") had been recognized in 1944 by a team of American chemists led by Oswald Avery at

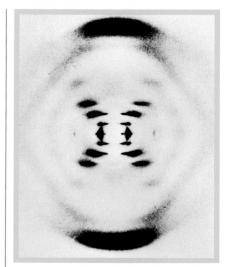

The first image of a strand of DNA, known as Photo 51, revealed the structure of DNA for the first time. The X-shape proves that DNA has a double-helix structure.

New York's Rockefeller Institute. It had previously been assumed that proteins in the chromosomes were responsible for passing on hereditary traits.

Scientists' understanding of genetics quickly accelerated. In the early 1950s, Austrian-born biochemist Erwin Chargaff showed that the composition of DNA varies between species, and in 1952, British chemist Rosalind Franklin (co-working with physicist Maurice Wilkins) photographed DNA for the first time. The following year, two molecular biologists, James Watson from the US and Francis Crick in Britain, modeled DNA's structure at the Cavendish Laboratory in Cambridge, UK, as two connected strands that form a double helix. Watson then discovered the pairing

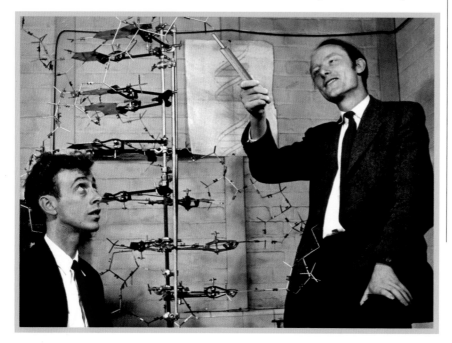

James Watson (left) and Francis Crick with their 3D model of DNA. Based on all available research into DNA at the time, its metal rods are arranged in a spiral around a stand.

See also: Inheritance and hereditary conditions 146–147 ▪ Alzheimer's disease 196–197 ▪ Chromosomes and Down syndrome 245 ▪ In vitro fertilization 284–285 ▪ The Human Genome Project 299 ▪ Gene therapy 300

structure of the four chemical bases that form the "rungs" in a DNA molecule: guanine always pairs with cytosine, and adenine always pairs with thymine. In 1962, Watson, Crick, and Wilkins received the Nobel Prize in Physiology or Medicine for their work on nucleic acids and how these carried information.

Mapping DNA

British biochemist Frederick Sanger spent 15 years trying to discover a rapid way to reveal the sequence of the bases in a strand of DNA. In 1977, he and his team published a technique called the dideoxy or Sanger method that uses chemical reactions to sequence up to 500 base-pairs per reaction. It was the start of a revolution in the mapping of DNA. The modern technique of pyrosequencing can read up to 20 million bases per reaction.

Sequencing has helped identify the genes responsible for certain disorders, including Huntington's disease, an inherited condition that results in the progressive death of brain cells. The disease, whose

symptoms begin with a decline in coordination and gradually progress to language problems and dementia, had been known since at least the medieval era but was described in detail by American physician George Huntington, after whom it was named, in 1872. In 1979, the Hereditary Disease Foundation began to analyze the DNA of 18,000 people in two Venezuelan villages that had a very high incidence of Huntington's. They discovered the approximate position (a genetic marker) of the gene responsible, then pinpointed it precisely in 1993. This enabled scientists to develop the first presymptomatic genetic test for Huntington's disease.

A medical game-changer

The invention of PCR by Kary Mullis in 1983 enabled easier and more targeted analysis of DNA, massively improving the diagnosis of disease. PCR has been called molecular photocopying. It involves heating a DNA sample so that it splits into two pieces of single-stranded DNA. An enzyme »

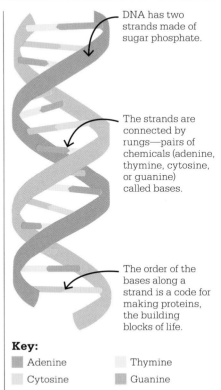

DNA has two strands made of sugar phosphate.

The strands are connected by rungs—pairs of chemicals (adenine, thymine, cytosine, or guanine) called bases.

The order of the bases along a strand is a code for making proteins, the building blocks of life.

Key:
■ Adenine ■ Thymine
■ Cytosine ■ Guanine

The DNA molecule, which makes up our genes, looks like a spiral staircase, a shape known as a double helix. Each strand of DNA contains a unique sequence (code) of genetic information.

Kary Mullis

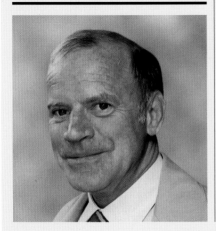

Born in the foothills of the Blue Ridge Mountains, North Carolina, in 1944, Mullis became interested in chemistry while building home-made solid-fuel rockets as a teenager. After gaining a doctorate in biochemistry from the University of California, Berkeley, in 1973, he spent a brief time writing science fiction before taking up research posts at various universities.

In 1979, Mullis joined the Cetus biotech corporation in California. It was here that he invented the PCR technique, for which he was awarded the Nobel Prize in

Chemistry in 1993. Mullis later invented an ultraviolet-sensitive ink and worked as a consultant on nucleic acid chemistry.

Some of Mullis's views were controversial: he questioned the evidence for climate change and ozone depletion and disputed the link between HIV and AIDS. Mullis died in 2019.

Key work

1986 "Specific enzymatic amplification of DNA in vitro: The polymerase chain reaction"

(*Taq* DNA polymerase) then builds two new strands, using the original pair as templates. A biochemist can then use each new strand to make two new copies in a machine called a thermocycler; if the process is repeated 12 times, there will be 2^{12} as much DNA as at the start of the process—more than 4,000 strands. Repeated 30 times, there will be 2^{30} (over 1 billion) strands. PCR duplication speeds up the detection of viruses and bacteria, the diagnosis of genetic disorders, and DNA fingerprinting—a technique used to link biological evidence to suspects in forensic investigations.

It was PCR that made the Human Genome Project physically possible. Between 1990 and 2003, researchers mapped almost all of the base-pairs that make up human DNA—some 3 billion in total. It was an enormous scientific undertaking. Clinicians also use PCR for tissue typing—to match donors with recipients prior to organ transplantation and for the early diagnosis of blood cancers such as leukemia and lymphomas.

Prenatal screening

The invention of PCR has facilitated screening for many serious genetic conditions, even prebirth. In 1989,

British geneticist Alan Handyside pioneered preimplantation genetic diagnosis (PGD). The following year, Handyside and clinicians Elena Kontogianni and Robert Winston successfully used the technique at Hammersmith Hospital, London.

Parents who are at high risk of having children with an inherited disease can now opt for IVF with genetic analysis so that only embryos without genetic mutations are implanted in the womb. Nearly 600 genetic disorders can now be detected using PGD, including cystic fibrosis and sickle cell anemia. In the case of a non-IVF pregnancy, prenatal genetic diagnosis can be conducted on an embryo in the uterus by taking cells from the placenta or fetus. If genetic mutations are found to be present, parents and medical professionals can then discuss options. In the future, it may be possible to reverse some inherited conditions before birth.

PGD can also be used to screen embryos for hereditary breast and ovarian cancers. Most cases of these cancers are not inherited, but in 1994 and 1995, scientists identified the two genes (*BRAC1*

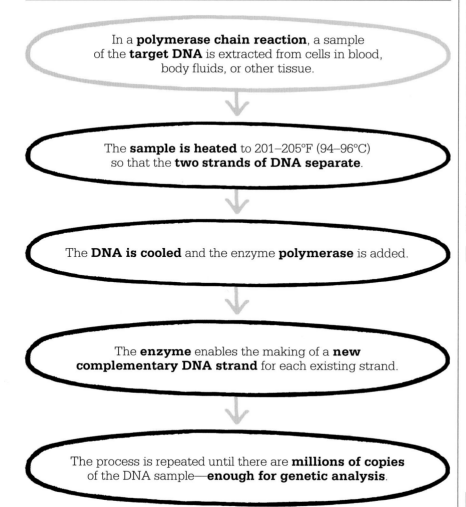

In a **polymerase chain reaction**, a sample of the **target DNA** is extracted from cells in blood, body fluids, or other tissue.

The **sample is heated** to 201–205°F (94–96°C) so that the **two strands of DNA separate**.

The **DNA is cooled** and the enzyme **polymerase** is added.

The **enzyme** enables the making of a **new complementary DNA strand** for each existing strand.

The process is repeated until there are **millions of copies** of the DNA sample—**enough for genetic analysis**.

Beginning with a single molecule of the genetic material DNA, the PCR can generate 100 billion similar molecules in an afternoon.
Kary Mullis
Scientific American, **1990**

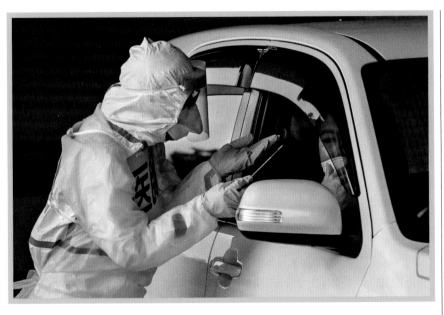

A medical worker in Japan takes a nasal swab for a PCR test for COVID-19. PCR is used to identify the genes of viruses.

and BRAC2) responsible for the hereditary forms. Women who carry mutations in these genes have a 50–85 percent chance of developing breast cancer and a 15–50 percent chance of getting ovarian cancer. Men who carry these mutations run an increased risk of prostate and breast cancer. Having a mutation of the BRAC2 gene also increases the chance of getting skin, esophageal, stomach, pancreatic, and bile duct cancers.

Fighting viruses

In 1986, Chilean biochemist Pablo Valenzuela, working at the University of California, San Francisco, used genetic engineering to develop the world's first recombinant vaccine (one that stimulates cells in the immune system) to protect children from hepatitis B. This virus, first identified by American geneticist Baruch Blumberg in 1965, attacks the liver and causes cirrhosis and liver cancer. It is one of the world's biggest killers. According to the WHO, 2 billion people have been infected with hepatitis B worldwide: 260 million live with a chronic form of the disease and around 887,000 people die from hepatitis B each year. The most common route of transmission is from an infected mother to her child at birth.

Valenzuela isolated the noninfectious part of the virus that makes the surface protein HBsAg and put it into yeast cells. When the cells multiplied, they produced many copies of the protein, which was then used in the vaccine. The vaccine causes the baby's immune system to produce its own protection against the disease.

The search goes on

Great advances have been made in understanding the relationship between genetics and health, but much remains unknown. At least 70 percent of cases of Alzheimer's disease are thought to be inherited, but the mechanism of inheritance is not fully understood. Researchers have, however, linked early-onset Alzheimer's with mutations in three genes, on chromosomes 1, 14, and 21, that cause the production of abnormal proteins.

Scientists also know that most cases of late-onset Alzheimer's relate to the APOE (apolipoprotein E) gene on chromosome 19. This is involved in making a protein that helps carry cholesterol and other fats in the bloodstream. APOE comes in one of three forms, or alleles. Two are not linked with Alzheimer's, but one, APOE4, has been shown to increase the risk of developing the disease. About 25 percent of people carry one copy of this allele and 2–3 percent carry two copies, but some people with APOE4 never get the disease, and many who develop it do not have the allele.

Determining and understanding the genetic variants of early- and late-onset Alzheimer's disease may be the first step in developing an effective treatment for cases that have a genetic basis. While drugs today are only able to manage (rather than cure) symptoms, gene research could potentially lead to earlier detection and treatments that slow or even stop the onset of Alzheimer's and other disorders. ∎

Genomics is … exciting science with the potential for fantastic improvements in prevention, health protection and patient outcomes.
Sally Davies
UK's Chief Medical Officer, 2017

THIS IS EVERYBODY'S PROBLEM

HIV AND AUTOIMMUNE DISEASES

IN CONTEXT

BEFORE
1950s US medical researcher Noel Rose's experiments with rabbits prove the previously rejected notion of autoimmunity.

1974 In Britain, Gian Franco Bottazzo and Deborah Doniach discover that type 1 diabetes has an autoimmune basis.

1981 The first cases of AIDS emerge among previously healthy gay men in California and New York City.

AFTER
1996 Antiretroviral therapy (HAART) is introduced as an anti-HIV treatment.

2018 New Zealand becomes the first country in the world to fund PrEP (preexposure prophylaxis) drugs for the prevention of HIV in people at high risk of catching the virus.

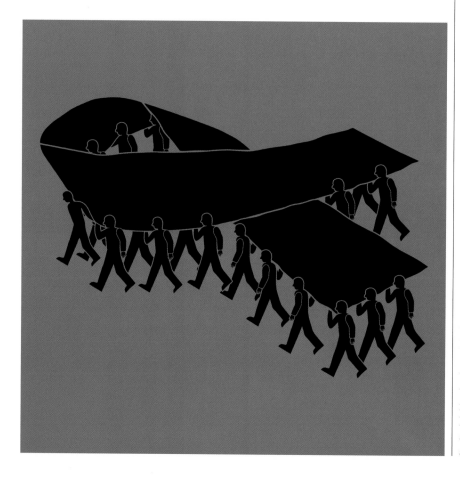

In May 1983, French virologists Luc Montagnier and Françoise Barré-Sinoussi announced in the journal *Science* their discovery of the virus that causes AIDS (acquired immunodeficiency syndrome). It was a retrovirus, a type of virus with RNA as genetic material (rather than the usual DNA). It converts the RNA into DNA, which it then integrates into the host cell's DNA to replicate.

AIDS had already killed more than 500 people in the US, and by the end of 1983, the number had risen to more than 1,000. The French team isolated the virus from a patient with swollen lymph nodes and physical tiredness, the classic

See also: Epidemiology 124–127 ▪ The immune system 154–161 ▪ Virology 177 ▪ The nervous system 190–195 ▪ Diabetes and its treatment 210–213 ▪ Steroids and cortisone 236–239

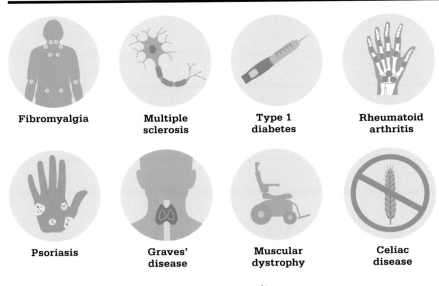

Fibromyalgia   **Multiple sclerosis**   **Type 1 diabetes**   **Rheumatoid arthritis**

Psoriasis   **Graves' disease**   **Muscular dystrophy**   **Celiac disease**

There are more than 80 known autoimmune diseases, most of which can only be managed, not cured. Many are characterized by alternating periods of flare-up and remission.

symptoms of AIDS. Montagnier and Barré-Sinoussi named the virus lymphadenopathy associated virus (LAV), but it was renamed HIV (human immunodeficiency virus) three years later. Their discovery unlocked the mystery of one of the deadliest immune disorders the world has known.

Abnormal responses

Immune disorders—when the natural production of antibodies to fight infection is disrupted—present some of the most intractable problems in medicine. They include many chronic and deadly diseases, whose triggers and pathogenesis (development in the body) are only slowly being understood.

There are two main categories of immune disorders: those that cause overactivity of the immune system and those that produce immune deficiency. Overactivity can make the body overreact to harmless substances in the environment (an allergic response) or attack and damage its own tissues and organs (an autoimmune response). Immune deficiency reduces the body's ability to fight infection and disease, as in AIDS.

Autoimmune diseases

The concept of autoimmunity—that antibodies produced by the body to fight disease could be directed against the body itself—was first postulated by Alexandre Besredka at the Pasteur Institute in Paris in 1901. His ideas were largely rejected, and it was not until the mid-20th century that scientists began to accept the premise of autoimmune diseases and understand some of their complex mechanisms.

Many common diseases are thought to have an autoimmune basis, including type 1 diabetes, rheumatoid arthritis, inflammatory bowel disease, lupus, and psoriasis.

Multiple sclerosis (MS)—which affects 2.3 million people worldwide and produces symptoms such as tiredness, poor coordination, and mobility problems—was identified as an autoimmune disease in the 1960s. Neurologists know that it is, at least in part, the result of the body's immune system attacking the cells (oligodendrocytes) that produce myelin, a fatty protein that forms a protective sheath around the neurons (nerve cells) of the nervous system.

Graves' disease, another autoimmune disorder, interferes with the thyroid gland, which controls how the body uses energy. The immune system makes antibodies called TSIs that bind to thyroid cell receptors, the "docking stations" for thyroid-stimulating hormone (TSH). By binding there, the TSIs trick the thyroid into producing high and damaging levels of hormone, causing insomnia, muscle wastage, heart palpitations, heat intolerance, and double vision.

For many years, physicians recognized autoimmune diseases without knowing their cause. British physician Samuel Gee described »

> The challenge of AIDS can be overcome if we work together as a global community.
> **World Economic Forum, 1997**

the symptoms of celiac disease, a condition triggered by eating gluten, in 1887, but its autoimmune basis was not understood until 1971. In sufferers of celiac disease, the body mounts an immune response that attacks the fingerlike villi that line the small intestine, reducing the body's ability to absorb nutrients. This can cause growth problems in children and increased chances of coronary artery disease and bowel cancer in adults.

HIV and AIDS

There are two categories of immune deficiency diseases: primary disorders, which are hereditary, and secondary disorders caused by environmental factors. HIV, the retrovirus responsible for AIDS, is now believed to have originated in nonhuman primates in West Africa, crossing over to humans in the early 20th century after coming into contact with infected blood (a process called zoonosis). In 1983, Montagnier and Barré-Sinoussi discovered that the virus attacked and destroyed the body's infection-fighting T-helper cells (also known as CD4+ cells), a type of white blood cell. A healthy person has a T-helper cell count of 500–1,500

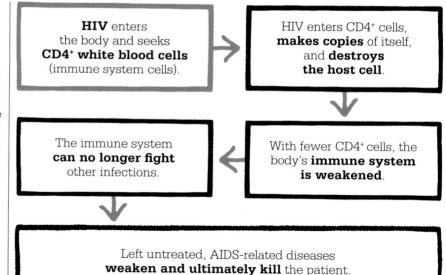

HIV enters the body and seeks **CD4+ white blood cells** (immune system cells).

HIV enters CD4+ cells, **makes copies** of itself, and **destroys the host cell**.

With fewer CD4+ cells, the body's **immune system is weakened**.

The immune system **can no longer fight** other infections.

Left untreated, AIDS-related diseases **weaken and ultimately kill** the patient.

per mm³. Someone with HIV has a T-helper cell count below 500 per mm³—if it drops below 200 per mm³, the immune system is severely weakened, and there is a high risk of infection from bacteria and viruses.

Left untreated, a person with HIV is unlikely to live more than 10 years, and often much less. In the early years of the epidemic, Kaposi's sarcoma (KS) was a recognized illness in people with advanced HIV. Kaposi's sarcoma is caused by a virus (HHV-8). While the virus is carried by many people who do not develop Kaposi's sarcoma, the cancer can develop in those with a weakened immune system. The virus attacks genetic instructions controlling cell growth, resulting in tumors and skin lesions.

The spread of AIDS

HIV passes from person to person in certain bodily fluids, such as blood, semen, and breast milk. Since many of the early cases involved gay men, damaging misinformation suggested AIDS was confined to this group, even describing it as a

"gay plague." This tended to limit knowledge about HIV in other sections of the population, who thought it was irrelevant to them. However, by 1984, scientists had confirmed that female partners of HIV-positive men could contract the disease through sexual contact and drug users could transmit it by sharing needles.

The spread of HIV was dramatic. In 1985, just over 20,000 cases were known, the vast majority in the

History will surely judge us … if we do not respond with all the energy and resources that we can … in the fight against HIV/AIDS.
Nelson Mandela

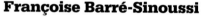

HIV has shown the way to go in the field of science. You can't be isolated in your laboratory. You need to work with others.
Françoise Barré-Sinoussi

US, but in 1999, the World Health Organization (WHO) estimated that 33 million people were living with the virus. By then, AIDS-related diseases had become the fourth-biggest cause of deaths worldwide, and the largest in Africa, having killed 14 million people since the epidemic began. In 2018, the WHO announced that since the start of the epidemic, 74.9 million people had become infected and 32 million had died of AIDS-related illnesses. By 2019, 38 million people had HIV, including 1.8 million children; two-thirds of people with HIV were living in sub-Saharan Africa.

Virus suppression

The majority of people who are HIV positive are now receiving antiretroviral treatment (ART). This treatment helps people live longer, healthier lives and dramatically reduces the risk of transmission. In 1996, highly active antiretroviral therapy (HAART), the most effective treatment to date, was introduced. This uses a combination of drugs, drawing on various antiretroviral (ARV) drugs that each work in a different way. They target HIV at different stages of its life cycle: entry inhibitors prevent it from entering a CD4$^+$ cell; "nukes" (nucleoside reverse transcriptase inhibitors) and "non-nukes" (non-nucleoside reverse transcriptase inhibitors) prevent HIV from translating its RNA to the DNA necessary to multiply; integrase inhibitors stop HIV from inserting its DNA into the chromosome of a CD4$^+$ cell; and protease inhibitors prevent the virus from maturing. By using a combination of drugs from at least two of these classes, HAART reduces the problem of drug resistance, and it has been very successful in suppressing HIV in those carrying the virus, thereby reducing their viral load and their chance of spreading the virus.

Like other immune disorders, AIDS has not yet been conquered, but research into immune diseases and their development in the body is advancing rapidly. One day, physicians will not just treat the symptoms and manage the progress of these debilitating diseases, but deliver effective cures. ∎

Men on a Gay Pride march in New York City in 1983 demand medical research into AIDS. Congress approved funding for research in July 1983, having refused it the previous year.

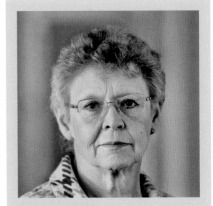

Françoise Barré-Sinoussi

Born in Paris, France, in 1947, Barré-Sinoussi was fascinated by nature as a child. She considered pursuing a career in medicine but opted to study life sciences at the University of Paris, while also working at the Pasteur Institute, initially as a volunteer. After gaining a doctorate for her research on retroviruses and leukemia in 1974, she went to work at the laboratory of virologist Luc Montagnier. Their discovery of HIV in 1983 earned them the Nobel Prize in Physiology or Medicine in 2008.

Barré-Sinoussi spent more than 30 years trying to find a cure for AIDS. In 1996, she became head of the Retrovirus Biology Unit at the Pasteur Institute, and she headed the International AIDS Society from 2012 to 2014. In 2013, Barré-Sinoussi was made Grand Officer of the Légion d'honneur, one of France's highest accolades.

Key work

1983 "Isolation of a T-lymphotropic retrovirus from a patient at risk for AIDS"

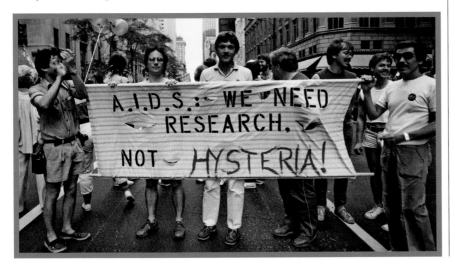

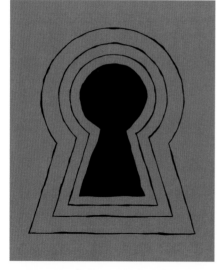

A REVOLUTION THROUGH THE KEYHOLE
MINIMALLY INVASIVE SURGERY

IN CONTEXT

BEFORE
1805 German army surgeon Philipp Bozzini invents the first endoscope to view inside the body; his "light conductor" is a candle in a leather tube.

1901 Georg Kelling, a German surgeon, inserts a cystoscope through a dog's abdominal wall after pumping gas into its stomach to prevent bleeding.

1936 Swiss gynecologist P. F. Boesch performs the first laparoscopic sterilization, using an electrical current to cauterize the fallopian tubes.

AFTER
1997 Surgeons in the US use keyhole procedures to bypass large, diseased blood vessels in the abdomen and groin—aortofemoral bypass surgery.

2005 The US Food and Drug Administration (FDA) approves the da Vinci robotic system for keyhole hysterectomy.

The first minimally invasive procedures known as keyhole surgery emerged in the early 20th century, but the landmark moment was 1981, when German gynecologist Kurt Semm performed the first appendectomy (appendix removal) using the keyhole technique. At first deemed unethical and dangerous, keyhole procedures became increasingly accepted from the mid-1980s and now include not only laparoscopic (abdominal) but also joint (arthroscopic) and chest (thoracoscopic) surgeries.

In 1910, Swedish surgeon Hans Jacobaeus described the first use of diagnostic laparoscopy, performed by inserting a cystoscope through the patient's abdominal wall. He recognized the dangers but also the potential of the technique. In the US, internist John Ruddock popularized its practice in the 1930s, when the first surgical laparoscopies were carried out, but progress was slow.

Technological advances in the 1980s—especially the advent of 3D videoscopic imaging—made keyhole surgery safer and more precise, so

> Laparoscopy is … a highly perfected technique … [that] has revolutionized the science of gynecology.
> **Hans Troidl**
> **President of the 1988 International Congress on Surgical Endoscopy**

that most abdominal surgical procedures can now be carried out using keyhole techniques; in areas such as urology, robot-assisted laparoscopy is also widely used.

Keyhole surgery has several advantages over open surgery: it requires a single incision of just 0.2–0.6 in (5–15 mm); it causes less pain and bleeding; a local anesthetic is usually sufficient; and the patient recovers quickly. ■

See also: Scientific surgery 88–89 ▪ Anesthesia 112–117 ▪ Orthopedic surgery 260–265 ▪ Robotics and telesurgery 305

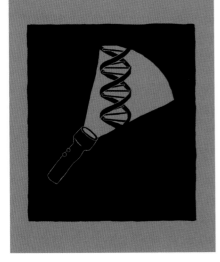

THE FIRST GLIMPSE OF OUR OWN INSTRUCTION BOOK

THE HUMAN GENOME PROJECT

A genome is an organism's complete set of genetic instructions, in the form of the chemical DNA. In 1990, the Human Genome Project (HGP) was launched to map human DNA. By 2003, researchers had sequenced the whole genetically active region of the human genome—92.1 percent. Scientists could begin to identify genes linked to disease and study how genetic engineering could modify genes to prevent disease.

While the HGP was progressing, scientists led by Ian Wilmut at the Roslin Institute in Scotland were investigating a cloning technique called somatic cell nuclear transfer (SCNT), in which genetic material from a somatic (mature) cell is transferred to an egg cell whose nucleus has been removed. In 1996, the team inserted the nucleus of a cell from a sheep's udder into an unfertilized egg cell of another

sheep, creating Dolly, a replica of the donor sheep. This paved the way for research into therapeutic cloning—the possibility of using a patient's own cells to treat their disease.

While both the Human Genome Project and SCNT have led to new fields of research, they have also raised social, ethical, and legal concerns about who has access to genome data and the risk of discrimination against those who carry gene mutations. ∎

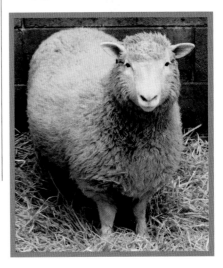

Dolly the sheep, the first successful clone of an adult mammal, was grown into an embryo in a laboratory and then transferred to a surrogate mother.

See also: Cancer therapy 168–175 ▪ In vitro fertilization 284–285 ▪ Genetics and medicine 288–293 ▪ Gene therapy 300 ▪ Stem cell research 302–303

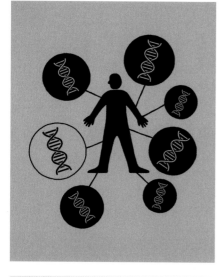

FIXING A BROKEN GENE
GENE THERAPY

Gene therapy involves the delivery of healthy DNA into a cell with defective DNA to cure a disorder. In 1990, American geneticist William French Anderson first used it successfully to treat a girl with severe combined immunodeficiency (SCID), who lacked the enzyme (adenosine deaminase, or ADA) required to make infection-fighting white blood cells. Only three treatment options were available at the time: enzyme injections, which did not always work; a bone marrow transplant from a compatible donor; or isolation in an artificial germ-free environment.

Anderson's team took white blood cells from the girl's blood, inserted the ADA gene using a viral vector, then injected the modified cells back into her bloodstream. Within six months, the child's white blood cell count rose to normal levels. The technique offered promise, but as it does not place the new DNA in its natural position within the host's genome, the cell's functioning can be disrupted. This disruption triggered leukemia in some later recipients.

Geneticists have since found ways to put the introduced DNA in the right place, and also to conduct "in-body" gene editing. These offer the prospect of curing a range of genetic conditions, but they also raise ethical questions about what constitutes a disability and whether gene editing might be abused to "improve" the human race. For now, gene therapy is still risky and is used only if there is no other cure. ∎

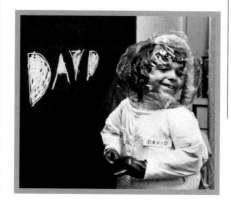

Before gene therapy, children with SCID had limited options. Born in 1971, American "bubble baby" David Vetter lived for 12 years in a sterile bubble.

See also: The immune system 154–161 ▪ Genetics and medicine 288–293 ▪ HIV and autoimmune diseases 294–297 ▪ Stem cell research 302–303

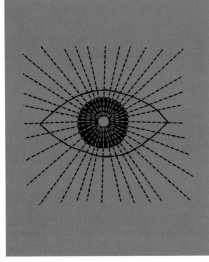

THE POWER OF LIGHT
LASER EYE SURGERY

Lasers are used as a surgical knife in many areas of medicine—including ophthalmology, from repairing the retina to correcting eyesight. But it was the development of femtosecond laser technology in 1995–1997 by American biomedical engineers Tibor Juhasz and Ron Kurtz that made laser eye surgery safer, more precise, and more predictable.

Ophthalmic surgeons have been using the LASIK technique since the mid-1990s to treat far- and nearsightedness. Originally, this involved using a microkeratome precision blade to create a flap in the surface of the cornea and a laser to reshape the cornea beneath, but increasingly, femtosecond lasers are being used for both parts of the procedure. These ultrafast lasers work by emitting very short pulses of light that disrupt the eye tissue, enabling incredibly precise incisions to be made without a blade.

Femtosecond technology is also transforming how surgeons deal with cataracts—cloudy patches that develop on the lens of an eye,

The ability to restore vision is the ultimate reward.
Patricia Bath
African American eye surgeon
(1942–2019)

resulting in impaired vision. About 30 million cataract surgeries are performed every year, but untreated cataracts are still the main cause of blindness globally. In femtosecond laser-assisted cataract surgery, a laser makes tiny incisions in the cornea and then a circular opening in the front of the capsule that surrounds the lens. The cataract is then broken up and an artificial lens implant is inserted. The incisions in the cornea heal naturally. ■

See also: Scientific surgery 88–89 ▪ Ultrasound 244 ▪ Minimally invasive surgery 298 ▪ Robotics and telesurgery 305

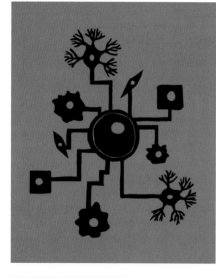

HOPE FOR NEW THERAPIES
STEM CELL RESEARCH

In 1998, James Thomson, an American cell biologist, and his team in Wisconsin isolated some human embryonic stem cells (ESCs) from embryos that had been donated for experimentation. This was a giant step, enabling the creation of almost any type of cell in the body. Stem cells are the nonspecialist cells that can give rise to all other cells with specialist roles. After a cell divides, each new daughter cell can either remain a stem cell or become one of more than 200 types of specialist cells. Embryonic stem cells are pluripotent: they can be programmed to develop into almost any specialist cell. That makes them incredibly valuable for researchers. However, most adult stem cells are multipotent; they can give rise to other types of cells, but—unlike pluripotent stem cells—these are of limited variety.

The only clinical use of adult stem cells began in the 1960s, before Thomson's discovery, when oncologists began carrying

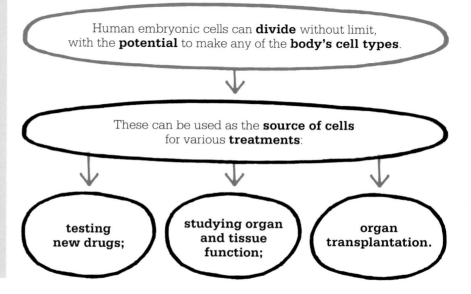

out bone marrow transplants as a cure for a variety of blood cancers. In this procedure, hematopoietic stem cells (HSCs, which give rise to all blood cells) are removed from the pelvis marrow of the patient, or a compatible donor, and stored while high doses of radiation eradicate any cancerous blood cells in the bone marrow. The HSCs are then injected back into the bloodstream.

A controversial procedure

Thomson's work used only embryos from donors who no longer wanted to use them for children. The US Food and Drug Administration agreed that the project could go ahead, but the Catholic Church opposed it. In 2001, US president George W. Bush prohibited the creation of new cell lines, although this policy was later partly reversed by his successor, Barack Obama.

Today, stem cell research is still mired in controversy. An embryo from which cells are extracted is unable to develop. While opponents of the research insist that embryos have the right to life, others debate

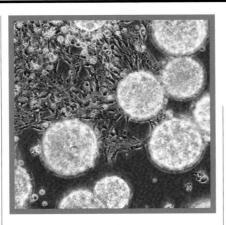

at what stage an embryo gains human status and believe in a moral duty to develop treatments that could potentially offer cures for terminal diseases and debilitating or degenerative conditions.

Developing the science

In 2006, Shinya Yamanaka, a researcher from Japan, found a way to genetically alter multipotent stem cells and convert them into pluripotent cells. This key discovery means that stem cells can now be taken from other body parts, not just embryos, and reprogrammed to produce the kind of cells required.

A light micrograph shows stem cells (pink) during the process of division, or mitosis. By directing this process, scientists can cause cells to specialize into a particular cell type.

However, scientists have not yet established whether these cells have the same potential as ESCs, so both are still used in research.

When a pluripotent stem cell undergoes mitosis (division into two daughter cells), one of the daughter cells may be of a more specialized type. This process repeats, the cells becoming more specialized each time until they reach maturity. For use in therapy, scientists must first convert these stem cells into the desired cell types. This procedure, known as directed differentiation, allows researchers to grow cell and tissue types—such as heart muscle, brain, and retinal—and to coat synthetic organs to avoid tissue rejection by the body. Reprogrammed stem cells are also used in clinical trials for the treatment of heart disease, as well as neurological conditions, retinal disease, and type 1 diabetes. ▪

James Thomson

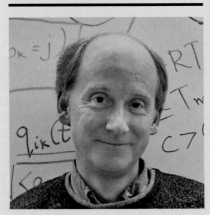

Born in Chicago in 1958, James Thomson graduated from the University of Illinois with a degree in biophysics before studying at the University of Pennsylvania. He was awarded a doctorate in veterinary medicine in 1985, and later another in molecular biology.

Thomson worked as the chief pathologist for the Wisconsin Regional (now National) Primate Research Center, after conducting key research into stem cell development in rhesus monkeys. The next step was to work with human embryos, which resulted in

his 1998 breakthrough. In 2007, he described a way to convert human skin cells into pluripotent cells that closely resembled embryonic stem cells but could potentially free research from ethical controversies over the use of human embryos.

Key works

1998 "Embryonic stem cell lines derived from blastocysts"
2007 "Induced pluripotent stem cell lines derived from human somatic cells"

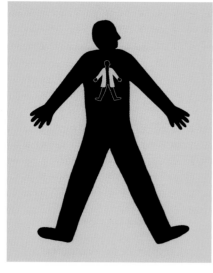

SMALLER IS BETTER
NANOMEDICINE

Nanomedicine is the use of materials on an atomic scale to monitor, repair, build, and control body systems. Nanostructures measure less than 100 nanometers (nm) in at least one dimension—a sheet of paper is about 100,000 nm thick. Nanotechnology has been used for years in fields ranging from food packaging to electronics, but it was not until 1999, when American nanotechnologist Robert Freitas published his first volume of *Nanomedicine*, that the concept of using nanotechnology in medicine became mainstream.

Quantum dots

Nanoscientists are exploring fields applicable to medicine. One is the investigation of quantum dots (QDs) as biomarkers for diagnosis and treatment. QDs are nanoparticles, tiny crystals (less than 20 nm across) of semiconducting materials. They are sensitive to light, so if "excited" by certain wavelengths, they emit tiny packets of light called photons. Larger QDs emit red or orange light, and smaller ones show blue or green.

Most QDs are fabricated from toxic chemicals such as zinc sulfide, so have to be coated in a polymer to shield the body. This "coat" mimics receptors on body cells, enabling QDs to bind them. Coated QDs can be used as biomarkers to highlight the presence of target cells, such as cancer cells, before symptoms show. Scientists are also working on using QDs to deliver drugs to target cells. Such precise delivery would avoid damage to healthy cells. ∎

> " We have come much further than I would have predicted just a few years back when the research resembled science fiction.
> **Karen Martinez, 2011** "

See also: The immune system 154–161 ▪ Cancer therapy 168–175 ▪ Genetics and medicine 288–293 ▪ Gene therapy 300 ▪ Stem cell research 302–303

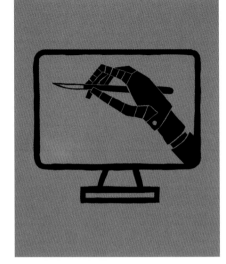

THE BARRIERS OF SPACE AND DISTANCE HAVE COLLAPSED
ROBOTICS AND TELESURGERY

IN CONTEXT

BEFORE
1984 Surgeons in Vancouver, Canada, use a robotic support ("Arthrobot") to reposition a patient's leg during surgery.

1994 The FDA (Food and Drug Administration) approves the use of AESOP, the first robotic camera operator, in the US for laparoscopy (keyhole surgery).

1995 A prototype of the ZEUS system is unveiled in the US.

1998 The first robot-assisted heart bypass is performed in Germany, using the da Vinci system developed in the US.

2000 American cardiac surgeon Stephen Colvin uses telesurgery to repair the valve of a patient's heart.

AFTER
2018 Surgeons in Cleveland, OH, perform the first robotic single-port kidney transplant, using just one incision in the patient's abdomen.

In 2001, French surgeon Jacques Marescaux and his team performed the first long-distance telesurgery on a woman in Strasbourg, France, from a building in New York City. They guided the arms of a ZEUS medical robot to remove the patient's gallbladder using minimally invasive surgery.

Work on medical robots began in the 1980s. In the UK, medical robotics engineer Brian Davies developed a robot (PROBOT) with some autonomous functions, which was used in a clinical trial in 1991 to operate on a patient's prostate. AESOP, designed in the US, soon followed; it could maneuver an endoscope inside the body during surgery. Then in 1998, the ZEUS system performed the first robotic coronary artery bypass surgery. By the time Marescaux used it, ZEUS was equipped to manipulate 28 different surgical implements.

There are three types of robotic surgery system. Shared-control robots steady a surgeon's hand and manipulate instruments but do not act autonomously. Telesurgical

robots like ZEUS are controlled from a remote console: the robot's arms work as scalpels, scissors, graspers, and camera operators. Supervisory controlled robots are the most autonomous: a surgeon inputs data into the robot, which then carries out controlled motions to accomplish the surgery. At present, they are limited to simple operations, but in the future, sophisticated autonomous robotic surgeons may be able to perform complex operations. ∎

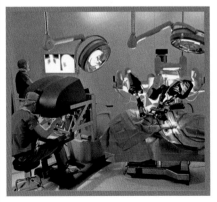

This surgeon is using the da Vinci telesurgical system to perform heart surgery. Da Vinci robots assist in more than 200,000 operations annually.

See also: Plastic surgery 26–27 ▪ Transplant surgery 246–253 ▪ Orthopedic surgery 260–265 ▪ MRI and medical scanning 278–281 ▪ Minimally invasive surgery 298

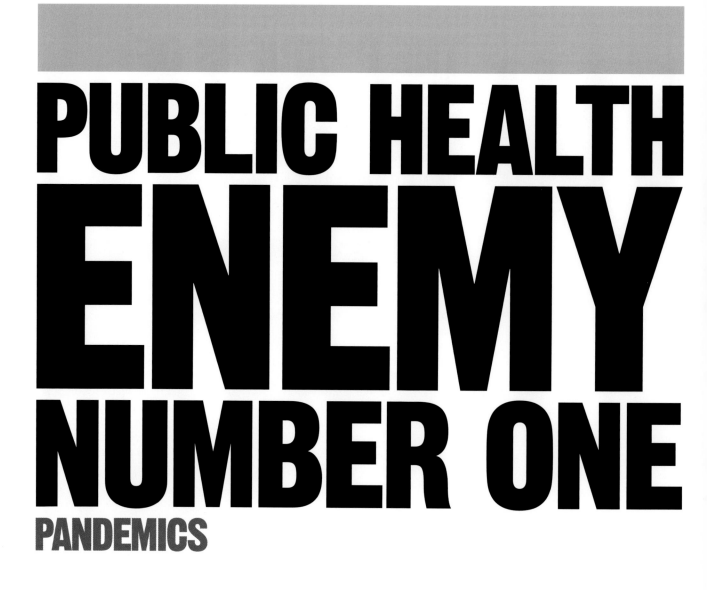

PUBLIC HEALTH ENEMY NUMBER ONE

PANDEMICS

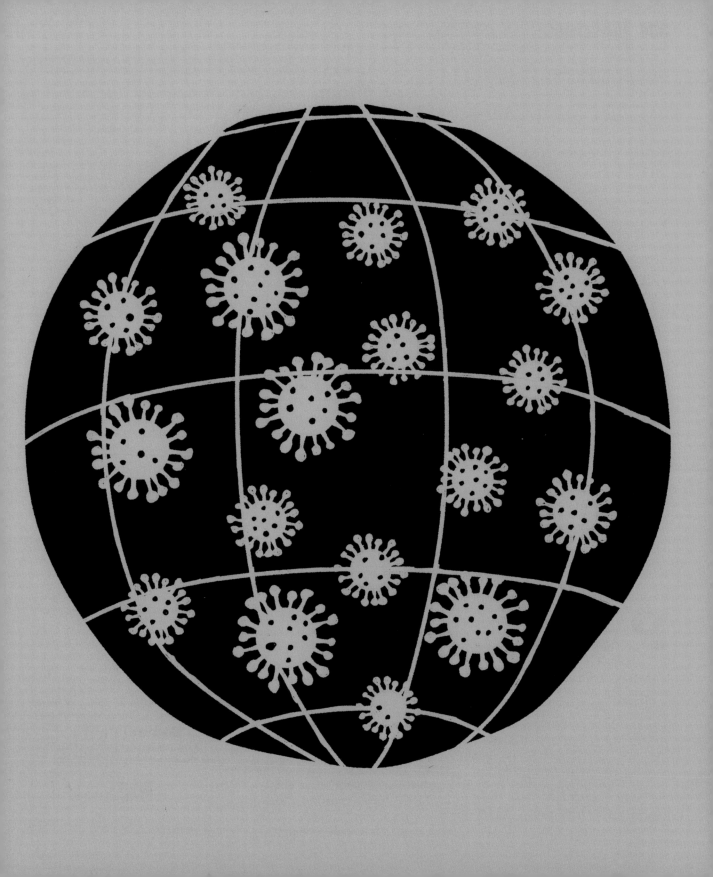

IN CONTEXT

BEFORE

165–180 CE The Antonine Plague kills a quarter of the Roman Empire's population.

1347 The Black Death reaches Europe from Asia, spreading westward via trading ships.

c. 1500 In Central and South America, European explorers introduce diseases that kill 90 percent of Indigenous people.

1918 The Great Influenza pandemic begins, killing an estimated 50 million people worldwide by 1920.

1981 HIV starts to spread; by 2018, 32 million people globally have died from the disease.

AFTER

2013 An outbreak of Ebola virus in West Africa raises fears of a pandemic.

2019 The COVID-19 virus appears in Wuhan, China, and spreads across the world; it is declared a pandemic in March 2020.

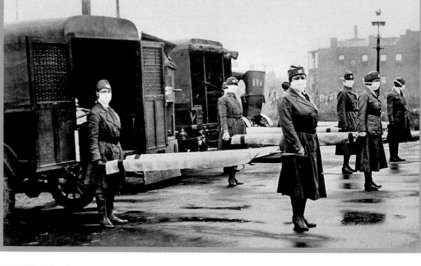

Little has changed since 1918 in terms of the medical response to a pandemic. Wearing face masks, these American National Red Cross nurses are waiting to collect flu patients.

Pandemics are outbreaks of infectious disease spread over multiple countries. Some spread rapidly but are less damaging, such as the pandemic swine flu of 2009. Others spread slowly but are highly dangerous, such as Ebola. A few spread quickly and make many who catch it very ill. The COVID-19 outbreak that erupted in 2020 is one such pandemic.

The Great Influenza was one of the most devastating pandemics in history, killing 50 million people in the wake of World War I. Like COVID-19, this was a virus—now identified as a deadly strain of the H1N1 influenza virus. One of the great discoveries in the century between these two outbreaks is that all it can take to trigger a pandemic is a tiny chance mutation in a virus, especially an influenza virus or a coronavirus such as COVID-19. That chance mutation conceals the virus's identity, leaving the human body defenseless. The proximity of people and animals in the modern world makes such mutations highly likely.

Pandemics are complex global threats that test to the limits how people and governments behave. Epidemiologists have made much progress in understanding how an epidemic spreads from one area to multiple countries (at which point it becomes a pandemic), and experts provide detailed protocols for taking action. Yet vaccines remain the one proven weapon against such outbreaks. In 2005—more than 80 years after the Great Influenza pandemic—American virologist Jeffery Taubenberger revealed the complete genetic structure of the 1918 H1N1 virus, enabling it to be reconstructed and analyzed. This was a landmark achievement in increasing scientists' ability to pin down the exact nature of a mutant virus and provide the necessary data to create a vaccine quickly.

In the early days of humankind, infectious diseases were probably rare. Hunter-gatherers were too scattered for germs to spread. They did not stay long enough near water sources to pollute them, nor did

> **Bodies were left in empty houses, and there was no one to give them a Christian burial.**
> **Samuel Pepys**
> **English diarist (1633–1703), on the Great Plague of 1665–1666**

they keep animals that today harbor germs. The rise of farming around 10,000 BCE provided food for a population explosion, but bringing people and animals close together promoted the conditions for infectious diseases to thrive.

Breeding grounds

Domestic animals share germs with humans directly. Tuberculosis (TB), smallpox, and measles originally came from cattle, and the common cold possibly from birds. Flu may have come from chickens or pigs, or possibly humans passed it to them. As farming intensified, manure-polluted water allowed diseases such as polio, cholera, typhoid, and hepatitis to thrive, while irrigation water provided breeding grounds for the parasites that cause malaria and schistosomiasis.

As each infection struck, survivors acquired resistance. Short-term immunity to many diseases was passed from mothers to children in the womb or through breast milk. But waves of new epidemics spread across the globe as populations grew and people moved around.

> There have been as many plagues as wars in history, yet always plagues and wars take people equally by surprise.
> **Albert Camus**
> *The Plague*, 1947

In 189 CE, the Antonine Plague (probably smallpox) flared up again, killing about 2,000 people per day in the city of Rome. Around 1300, the Black Death (a bubonic plague pandemic) began to sweep across Eurasia and Africa, culminating in 1347–1351, when at least 25 million people died in Europe alone and whole villages were wiped out.

Virgin populations are especially vulnerable to infectious diseases. When European settlers arrived in the Americas in the 16th and 17th centuries, they brought smallpox and swine flu. This devastated Indigenous peoples, who had no past exposure to these diseases and therefore no natural immunity.

The Great Influenza

In 1918, the Great Influenza struck. It probably started in the trenches of World War I, where millions of soldiers crammed together in the mud with pigs there to provide food. The flu virus may have become more virulent as it passed among soldiers. It is often called the Spanish flu, since news of it first came out in Spain, but in reality, it appeared almost everywhere globally at about the same time.

This pandemic left the world in a state of shock, and no one could identify the killer. It was assumed to be bacteria, not a virus. Viruses are so tiny they could not even be seen before the invention of the electron microscope in 1931. It was not until 1933 that Wilson Smith, Christopher Andrewes, and Patrick Laidlaw at the National Institute for Medical Research in London, UK, »

Some hospitals set up "pneumonia porches" in the hope that fresh air would help reduce transmission.

Killer flu

The Great Influenza began in 1918 and spread with devastating speed across a world already ravaged by war, infecting around a third of the global population. This horrific disease was nothing like a winter flu. Those who were worst affected suffered acute pain; rib-cracking coughing fits; and profuse bleeding from their skin, eyes, and ears. Their lungs became inflamed, starving the blood of oxygen and giving their skin a deep blue hue—a condition called cyanosis. Very quickly, over the space of a few hours or a few days at best, their lungs filled up with fluid and they suffocated. This is now known as acute respiratory distress syndrome (ARDS), but doctors at the time called it "atypical pneumonia."

Unlike most flu strains, which are dangerous for young children and the elderly, the 1918 strain proved most fatal to those aged between 20 and 40. As more people developed immunity, the virus could no longer spread, and the pandemic ended in 1920.

deliberately infected ferrets with influenza and proved it to be a virus: a near-invisible disease-causing agent that can be filtered but not cultured in a dish (as bacteria can).

Many people hoped the Great Influenza was a never-to-be-repeated aberration. But as soldiers crowded into barracks again at the onset of World War II in 1939, doctors feared there might be a new outbreak. In the United States, Thomas Francis and Jonas Salk at the Commission on Influenza developed the first flu vaccine, which was used to immunize US troops. What Francis and Salk did not know is that a flu vaccine only works against the strains it is made for. Their vaccine was based on existing strains from the 1930s, so when a new mutation appeared in 1947, the vaccine proved useless. Fortunately, the 1947 flu epidemic was mostly mild in effect.

The chameleon virus

It was soon discovered that the flu virus is more variable than anyone imagined. There are several kinds. Type C (IFCV) is the mildest, causing coldlike symptoms. Type B brings the classic seasonal flu, which can be severe but can only

> **Better a vaccine without an epidemic than an epidemic without a vaccine.**
> **Edwin Kilbourne, 1976**

be passed from human to human. Type A is the most dangerous. It is essentially a bird virus but can acquire the ability to cross into humans, either via a host animal, such as a pig, or directly from birds. When it does, people may have so little resistance that another pandemic is a real possibility.

In 1955, American scientists Heinz Fraenkel-Conrat and Robley Williams found that viruses can be single strands of the genetic material RNA wrapped in a shell (capsid). The genetic material in human body cells is double-helix

DNA, as James Watson and Francis Crick had discovered in 1953. Influenza and coronaviruses are both RNA viruses.

Shifting identity

When DNA is copied, it is copied near perfectly. But when RNA viruses such as coronaviruses and flu replicate themselves in order to infect other cells, there are often misprints. This creates problems for immune systems, which identify a virus by matching up antibodies with antigens (markers) on the virus's shell. If a misprint in RNA changes the shell enough, antibodies may no longer recognize it, so the virus can enter the body undetected.

This "antigenic drift" is why flu comes around again and again. With viral diseases like measles, people usually only get it once, since the first attack primes the body with antibodies to fight measles viruses. Flu viruses, however, are rarely the same, so antibodies built up after one year's winter flu fail to identify the next year's version. Even so, they are recognizable enough for the body to mount a defense and eventually defeat it. This is why, for most people, seasonal flu is mild.

Human activity brings people into **close contact with animals**. →

Prolonged contact with animals increases the chances of **mutations** that **allow viruses to jump between animals and humans**. →

Humans **may have no resistance** to a mutant animal virus, so the virus can **multiply in the body** and **cause dangerous illness**. ↓

Once a mutant virus is able to **multiply in one human host**, it can **spread rapidly** from person to person. ←

Global connectivity and air travel make it possible for a virus to be transported around the world in a matter of hours, **leading to a pandemic**.

How viruses mutate

Antigenic drift

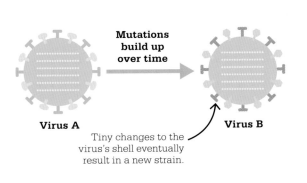

Mutations build up over time

Virus A

Virus B

Tiny changes to the virus's shell eventually result in a new strain.

When a flu virus copies itself, mutations cause minute changes in the hemagglutinin (H) and neuraminidase (N) antigens on the virus's surface. This process creates winter flu strains, to which most people have some resistance.

Antigenic shift

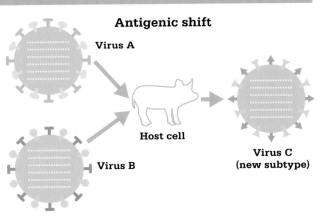

Virus A

Host cell

Virus B

Virus C (new subtype)

When two different viruses infect the same cell in a host species (such as a pig), they form an entirely new subtype, which can jump between species and may spread rapidly as populations have no immunity.

In 1955, Australian virologist Frank Macfarlane Burnet suggested that more radical changes can occur if different flu viruses colonize the same cell, letting their genes swap certain sections. If this reshuffling involves the genes that code for the virus's shell, their antigens may become completely unrecognizable, leaving people with little or no protection against the new virus. This dramatic change is called an "antigenic shift."

Two years later, in 1957, another pandemic broke out. Dubbed Asian flu, it spread widely and rapidly and vaccines had no effect. For most, symptoms were mild, yet over 2 million died. Over the next decade, virologists including Christopher Andrewes and American medical researcher Edwin Kilbourne showed that the virus had had an antigenic shift of the kind Burnet suggested.

Identity spikes

Under an electron microscope, it is possible to see minute spikes on the flu virus's shell of the protein hemagglutinin (H) and the enzyme neuraminidase (N). H spikes bind to host cells so the virus can invade, while N spikes dissolve cell walls to create the virus's escape route. Crucially, though, both H and N are antigens that identify the virus to the host body. Andrewes and Kilbourne showed that in the Asian flu virus, both H and N had changed. Consequently, the Great Influenza virus was dubbed H1N1 and the Asian flu H2N2. Since then, scientists have discovered that there are 16 versions of H and 9 of N, which come together in different combinations.

These advances shed little light on what made the 1918 H1N1 virus so deadly. In 1951, Johan Hultin, a Swedish microbiologist, had gained permission to excavate the burial site at Brevig Mission in Alaska, where 72 of the village's 80 mostly Inuit inhabitants had died from the flu in 1918. The frozen ground preserved bodies well, and Hultin extracted a sample of lung tissue, but with the technology of the time, he could not find much information from it.

In 1997, Taubenberger, working at the Armed Forces Institute of Pathology in the US, described a partial analysis of the 1918 virus based on a fragment of lung tissue taken from an American serviceman who died from the disease. Hultin saw the paper and returned to Brevig. This time, he obtained a sample from the body of a young Inuit woman who he called "Lucy."

The killer resurrected

From Hultin's sample, Taubenberger and his colleague Ann Reid at last unlocked the 1918 H1N1 virus's full genome in 2005. Their sequencing was so complete that later that year, American microbiologist Terrence Tumpey managed to create a live version. The resurrected virus is securely contained at the Centers for Disease Control and Prevention.

Studying Tumpey's resurrected virus proved it originated in birds rather than pigs, with telltale H spikes similar to the bird flu virus that sparked a panic in 2005. There is no real understanding yet of why one mutant flu virus is deadly and »

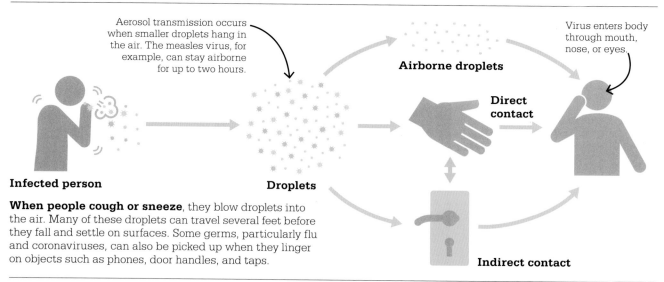

Aerosol transmission occurs when smaller droplets hang in the air. The measles virus, for example, can stay airborne for up to two hours.

Airborne droplets

Virus enters body through mouth, nose, or eyes.

Direct contact

Infected person

Droplets

Indirect contact

When people cough or sneeze, they blow droplets into the air. Many of these droplets can travel several feet before they fall and settle on surfaces. Some germs, particularly flu and coronaviruses, can also be picked up when they linger on objects such as phones, door handles, and taps.

another not, but Tumpey and his colleagues concluded that no one genetic component of the 1918 virus made it so lethal; rather, it was a particular combination of genes that made this strain of the virus so deadly. Even so, increasing knowledge of how viruses work helps speed up the creation of a vaccine each time a new and dangerous mutation emerges.

Coronaviruses

Just as scientists were getting a handle on flu viruses, coronaviruses emerged as a major pandemic threat. Coronaviruses were first identified in the 1930s in chickens and named by Scottish virologist June Almeida in 1967, when she made the first electron microscope images. The corona (from the Latin for "crown") described the virus's fringe of bulbous projections.

In 2003, Carlo Urbani, an Italian doctor working in Hanoi, Vietnam, realized that a patient admitted to the hospital did not have flu, as suspected, but was suffering from an entirely new disease, now known as SARS, or severe acute respiratory syndrome, from the way it attacks the lungs.

The World Health Organization (WHO) issued an alert at once, and SARS victims, already identified as far away as Toronto, Canada, were isolated. Guangdong in China, where the disease originated, was subjected to a huge public hygiene operation, and SARS was brought in check within a year. The virus was identified as a coronavirus and traced to animals in Guangdong such as the masked civet and ferret badger used in Chinese medicine.

There are many coronaviruses. Most circulate among animals such as pigs, camels, bats, and cats. Seven are known to jump to humans in a "spillover" event and

> We have rung the alarm bell loud and clear.
> **Tedros Adhanom Ghebreyesus**
> **WHO director-general (2017–)**

cause disease. With four of these, symptoms are mild, but the other three can be fatal. SARS appeared in 2002; followed by MERS (Middle East respiratory syndrome) in 2012, which was probably transmitted from camels; and then COVID-19, which was identified in 2019.

Zoonotic diseases

Urbanization, intensive agriculture, and deforestation create breeding grounds for viral diseases. As humans disrupt ecosystems and come into ever closer contact with animals, they are exposed to more "zoonotic" pathogens—germs that can be transmitted from vertebrate animals to humans. Around three-quarters of new infectious diseases come from wildlife, and there is an increasing probability of one mutating to create a pandemic killer.

Besides flu and coronaviruses, a range of viral diseases has recently emerged in the tropics, including Ebola, Lassa fever, dengue, West Nile virus, hantavirus, and HIV. Some of these are entirely "novel" mutations, but others have been brought out of hiding by human activity. The COVID-19 virus is likely to have originated in bats,

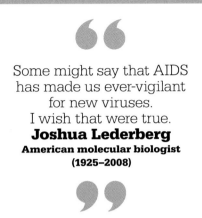

driven from forest habitats into close proximity to humans and other animals.

Although scientists now know that mutant viruses are responsible for pandemics, there is no telling where or when one will emerge, or how deadly it will be. But by studying past outbreaks intently, epidemiologists can plot just how far and fast they spread. This has given them the tools to predict how a disease will develop once it reaches a certain stage.

The WHO has devised a six-phase timetable to guide the global response to a pandemic in the early stages. The first three phases involve monitoring viruses that are circulating among animals and identifying any that may present a threat to humans or that have already mutated and infected humans. Once human-to-human infection has been established at community and then national level (phases 4–5), rapid containment and national pandemic responses are called for, culminating in a pandemic being declared (phase 6) once human-to-human infection has been reported in at least two WHO regions.

If an emerging disease is spotted early, it may be possible to isolate victims and carriers before the disease spirals out of control. This is what happened with SARS in 2003, but not with COVID-19. If a pandemic does break out, scientists expect it to run around the globe in two or three waves. Each may last several months and may be up to four months apart, but they peak locally after about five weeks.

Limiting the spread

Globalization and air travel have increased the threat of pandemics. In the time of the Black Death, an outbreak could take years to spread across the globe. COVID-19 emerged in Wuhan, China, in late 2019. By March 2020, cases had been recorded in at least 140 countries.

Growing knowledge of viruses improves the chances of a vaccine being found, but however quickly this happens, it will still be well after the first wave. Antiviral drugs might ameliorate symptoms in some cases, and antibiotics may help treat secondary infections.

Many hospitals are well equipped to support severely ill patients, with machines to help breathing, for example. But the most effective measures for tackling a pandemic remain as they have always been: to limit the spread of the disease and prevent people catching it.

When the threat of a bird flu pandemic loomed in 2005, the UK's NHS informed the public: "Since vaccines and antiviral drugs are likely to be in limited supply … other public health and 'social' interventions may be the only available countermeasures to slow the spread of the disease. Measures such as hand washing, and limiting nonessential travel and mass gatherings of people may slow the spread of the virus to reduce the impact and 'buy' valuable time." COVID-19 proved this right. ∎

Milan's Duomo is deserted in March 2020 after Italy's government enforced a strict COVID-19 lockdown. Limiting the movement of people and closing churches, businesses, and schools helped slow the spread of the virus.

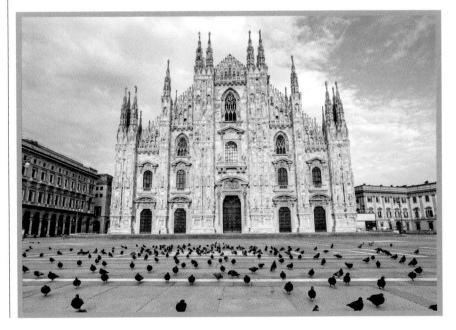

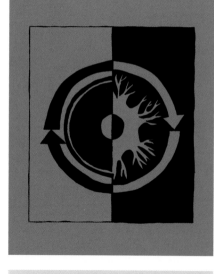

TO REPROGRAM A CELL
REGENERATIVE MEDICINE

IN CONTEXT

BEFORE
1962 British biologist John Gurdon demonstrates that the genetic material of a mature cell can be reprogrammed.

1981 Martin Evans and Matt Kaufman, biologists at the University of Cambridge, successfully culture embryonic stem cells from mice.

2003 An inkjet printer in the US is modified by biomedical engineer Thomas Boland to build cell arrays and place them in successive layers—a crucial step toward printing complex tissue types.

AFTER
2012 German researchers use bioprinted skin tissue to heal wounds on mice.

2019 Researchers at Tel Aviv University, Israel, print a miniature 3D heart from human cells—the first to be printed complete with blood cells, vessels, and chambers.

Organ transplantation is often hindered by organ availability and the problem of tissue rejection. The relatively new science of "regenerating" human cells and tissues aims to overcome such obstacles, paving the way for growing organs to order.

In 2006, Japanese researcher Shinya Yamanaka made the crucial discovery that multipotent stem cells (those with the capacity to develop into a range of specialized cell types within a specific organ) can be reprogrammed to become pluripotent cells (those with the potential to grow into any cell type). Yamanaka's vital work reversed the development of multipotent cells, turning them back into immature cells with the potential to grow into a range of different body cells.

In 2015, using the techniques pioneered by Yamanaka, researchers working at Heriot-Watt University in Edinburgh, Scotland, developed a 3D printing process that can print human stem cells derived from a donor's own tissue. This paved the way for making laboratory-grown human tissue available for wider use, both in transplantation and in pharmaceutical research.

Brazilian researchers in 2019 reprogrammed human blood cells to form hepatic organoids, in effect "mini livers" to mimic the functions of a normal liver, such as storing vitamins, producing enzymes, and secreting bile. Only miniature livers have been produced so far, but the technique could be used to produce entire organs for transplantation. ∎

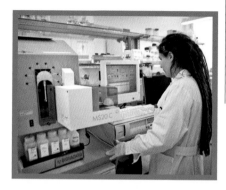

A bioprinter at Zurich University of Applied Sciences is used to print 3D human tissue. The tissue is then matured in a cell culture.

See also: Histology 122–123 ▪ Cellular pathology 134–135 ▪ Transplant surgery 246–253 ▪ Genetics and medicine 288–293 ▪ Stem cell research 302–303

THIS IS MY NEW FACE
FACE TRANSPLANTS

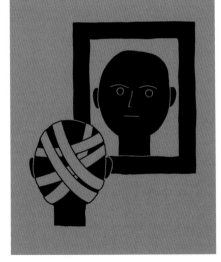

IN CONTEXT

BEFORE

1597 Italian surgeon Gaspare Tagliacozzi describes skin grafts to repair noses that have been sliced off in duels.

1804 Giuseppe Baronio, an Italian physician, discovers small grafts survive with no blood supply as they reattach.

1874 Using thinly cut skin to make large grafts, German surgeon Karl Thiersch enables the treatment of extensive burns for the first time.

1944 Key techniques, such as the walking skin graft, are developed by New Zealand plastic surgeons Harold Gillies and Archibald McIndoe.

AFTER

2011 Belgian surgeon Phillip Blondeel performs the first face transplant using 3D printing.

2017 At the Cleveland Clinic, surgeon Frank Papay does the first face transplant using augmented reality.

P lastic surgery is an ancient art, first recorded by the Egyptians around 1600 BCE. The development of microsurgery techniques in the 1970s enabled the complex reattachments of skin and body parts, complete with nerves and blood supply. In 1994, the successful reattachment of the face of a 9-year-old girl in India gave plastic surgeons confidence to try face transplants.

Transplantation

In 2005, French surgeon Bernard Devauchelle made the first partial transplant by rebuilding the face of a woman. Another French plastic surgeon, Laurent Lantieri, claimed the first full face transplant on a 30-year-old man in 2008. In 2010, Spanish doctors declared they had carried out a more complex, "fuller" face transplant, but Lantieri remains a pioneer in this field. His team performed eight of the world's 42 face transplants by 2020—including a second operation on the 2008 patient after his body rejected the first transplant in 2018.

> Faces help us understand who we are and where we come from.
> **Royal College of Surgeons, 2004**

Face transplants rely on "free tissue transfer," where a donor's tissue has its blood supply cut off and is then reconnected to the blood supply of the recipient. 3D printing can create models of both donor and recipient for surgeons to follow. In the US in 2017, surgeons used augmented reality computer visualizations to guide them in a facial transplant. As yet, there is no certainty of long-term success, and immunosuppressive drugs to prevent rejection increase the risk of dangerous infections. ■

See also: Plastic surgery 26–27 ▪ Skin grafts 137 ▪ The immune system 154–161 ▪ Transplant surgery 246–253 ▪ Regenerative medicine 314

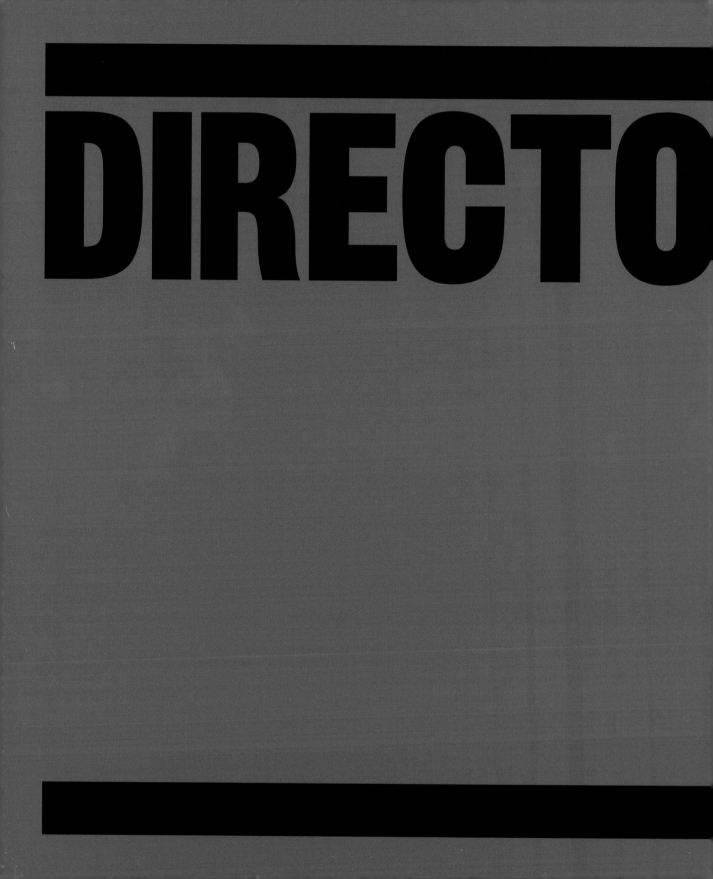

DIRECTORY

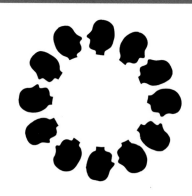

Far more people have made crucial contributions to the development of medical science than those featured in detail in this book. The following pages acknowledge some of the other individuals who have played a vital role in improving human health. Whether scientists, physicians, or patients, they have influenced the practice of medicine, the technologies associated with that practice, or knowledge of how our bodies are constructed and function. Some achieved fame during their lifetimes, although many are scarcely known outside their own specialties. Others contributed unwittingly or posthumously as organ or tissue donors or subjects for study, or played a part as authors of seminal texts and advocates of health reforms that still benefit us today.

AMMAR AL-MAWSILI
c. 996–c. 1020

An innovative ophthalmologist, Ammar al-Mawsili was born in Mosul, in present-day Iraq, and later moved to Egypt. His only known writing, a treatise on eye diseases, describes his pioneering use of a syringe to perform cataract surgery. His method of using a thin, hollow needle to remove cataracts by suction became an established practice among Islamic oculists.
See also: Islamic medicine 44–49

HILDEGARD OF BINGEN
1098–1179

Born into German nobility, Hildegard of Bingen entered the convent of Disibodenberg, Germany, aged 14, eventually becoming its prioress. She combined her deep theoretical and practical knowledge of herbal medicine in two key texts: *Physica*, which described the properties of plants and minerals, and *Causae et Curae*, which set out causes, as well as treatments, for diseases

and injuries. In 2012, more than 800 years after her death, she was canonized and made a doctor of the Church, one of only four women ever to have been accorded this distinction.
See also: Herbal medicine 36–37 ▪ Medieval medical schools and surgery 50–51 ▪ Pharmacy 54–59

HIERONYMUS FABRICIUS
1537–1619

Often described as the "father of embryology," Fabricius was a highly influential teacher of surgery and anatomy at the University of Padua in Italy. By dissecting animals, he investigated the formation of the fetus and determined the structure of the intestines, stomach, and esophagus; described the cerebral fissure between the brain's frontal and temporal lobes; and discovered the valves within veins. In 1594, he designed the first public-viewing operating theater, transforming the teaching of anatomy.
See also: Anatomy 60–63 ▪ Blood circulation 68–73 ▪ Scientific surgery 88–89 ▪ Physiology 152–153

NICHOLAS CULPEPER
1616–1654

A botanist, herbalist, physician, and political radical, Culpeper is best known for his systematic appraisal of herbal medicine in *The English Physician* (or *Culpeper's Herbal*), published in 1653 and still in print today. This work popularized astrological botany—the belief that plants' medical properties are linked to the movements of the planets and stars. A reformer, opposed to bloodletting, Culpeper believed that medicine should be based on reason rather than received wisdom and that it should be available to all, regardless of wealth.
See also: Herbal medicine 36–37 ▪ Midwifery 76–77

STEPHEN HALES
1677–1761

British parish priest Stephen Hales developed a fascination with biology after attending lectures given by Italian chemist Giovanni Francisco Vigani at Cambridge University.

Although an amateur, Hales came to be considered one of the great physiologists of his day. He was the first to measure blood pressure and to describe the roles of the aortic and mitral valves. In 1733, many of his discoveries were published in *Haemastaticks*. In the third edition of the book (1740), he suggested that electricity plays a role in enabling nerves to control muscle function—long before Luigi Galvani was able to prove this in 1791.
See also: Blood circulation 68–73
▪ The nervous system 190–195

JAMES BARRY
c. 1789–1865

Because women were barred from accessing higher education, Irish-born Margaret Bulkley disguised herself as a man and took the name James Barry to enroll at Edinburgh University in Scotland. In 1813, Barry joined the British Army as a surgeon, traveling widely and rising to the rank of general. As well as treating soldiers and their families, Barry campaigned for better sanitation; fought to improve conditions for slaves, prisoners, and those with leprosy; and performed one of the first described caesarean sections. In 1857, Barry was posted to Canada as the inspector-general of military hospitals there.
See also: Battlefield medicine 53
▪ Midwifery 76–77 ▪ Women in medicine 120–121 ▪ Nursing and sanitation 128–133

THOMAS WAKLEY
1795–1862

After running a medical practice in London for a number of years, British surgeon Thomas Wakley turned to journalism. In 1823, he founded *The Lancet*, with the primary aim of exposing the nepotism, secrecy, and incompetence of the medical establishment. *The Lancet* also campaigned against many social injustices, including flogging, workhouses, and the adulteration of food. In 1835, Wakley was elected as a Member of Parliament, and he was largely responsible for the 1859 Medical Act, which introduced medical registration for doctors.
See also: Scientific surgery 88–89
▪ Epidemiology 124–127

JOHN HARRIS
1798–1849

In 1827, American physician John Harris began preparing would-be doctors for medical college at his home in Bainbridge, Ohio. By including dentistry, a specialty often ignored at the time, Harris pioneered education in this field and inspired several of his students to become skilled dentists. One, his brother Chapin, founded the first American college of dental surgery in Baltimore in 1840. Another, James Taylor, set up the Ohio College of Dental Surgery five years later.
See also: Scientific surgery 88–89

KARL ROKITANSKY
1804–1878

A pioneering pathologist, Rokitansky helped establish the New Vienna School, Austria, as a medical center of excellence, and anatomical pathology—the study of tissues and organs to diagnose disease—as a medical science. His vast practical experience, gained through more than 30,000 autopsies, was distilled in his influential *Handbook of Pathological Anatomy*, published between 1842 and 1846. By linking the symptoms of disease with the abnormalities observed at autopsy, Rokitansky advanced understanding of how the body can malfunction.
See also: Anatomy 60–63
▪ Cellular pathology 134–135

CAMPBELL DE MORGAN
1811–1876

Based on more than 30 years of observations at London's Middlesex Hospital, British surgeon Campbell de Morgan described in a series of papers (1871–1874) how cancer arises locally and then spreads, first to the lymph nodes, then elsewhere. His explanation of metastasis effectively ended a decades-long debate about whether cancer has a generalized or focal origin. He stressed the importance of prompt treatment, also warning that patients often have no signs of illness at the onset of cancer.
See also: Cancer therapy 168–175
▪ Cancer screening 226–227

HENRY DUNANT
1828–1910

While traveling in Italy in 1859, Swiss businessman Henry Dunant witnessed the bloody aftermath of the Battle of Solferino. Horrified by the treatment of the injured, he campaigned for the creation of a neutral body to help those wounded on the battlefield. His work led to the establishment of the International Committee of the Red Cross in 1863 and the first Geneva Convention the following year. The latter decreed that all wounded soldiers and prisoners of war should be given the best treatment, regardless of nationality, and that the safety of

medical personnel should be guaranteed on the battlefield.
See also: Battlefield medicine 53 ▪ Triage 90

JOHN MARSHALL HARLAN
1833–1911

In 1905, US Supreme Court justice John Marshall Harlan delivered the landmark *Jacobson* v. *Massachusetts* verdict that the state had the right to enforce a compulsory vaccination program. An outbreak of smallpox in Massachusetts posed a serious threat to public safety, but resident Henning Jacobson had argued that vaccination infringed his personal liberty. The Supreme Court ruling established that the obligation to maintain public health can override individual freedoms.
See also: Vaccination 94–101 ▪ Global eradication of disease 286–287

ORONHYATEKHA
1841–1907

A Mohawk born on the Six Nations reserve near Brantford, in Canada, Oronhyatekha ("Burning Cloud") was invited to study at Oxford University, in the UK, after impressing visiting British royal physician Henry Acland in 1860. Oronhyatekha returned to Canada in 1863 to complete his studies at the Toronto School of Medicine, becoming one of the first doctors from North America's First Nations. He established a successful medical practice and, in 1871, was appointed consulting physician to the Mohawk people of Tyendinaga, Ontario. A scholarship fund in his name continues to support First Nations medical students.
See also: The World Health Organization 232–233

DANIEL HALE WILLIAMS
1856–1931

African American surgeon Daniel Hale Williams was a pioneer of open-heart surgery. In 1891, he opened the Provident Hospital in Chicago, which was the first American hospital with interracial medical staff. Two years later, he became one of the first surgeons to operate successfully on a patient's heart, repairing damage caused by a severe stab wound. In 1913, he became a founding member of the American College of Surgeons.
See also: Transplant surgery 246–253 ▪ Pacemakers 255

THEODOR BOVERI
1862–1915

In 1914, German biologist Theodor Boveri published *Concerning the Origin of Malignant Tumours*, which became the foundation for future cancer research. He explained that chromosomal defects cause cancers and that tumors arise from single cells. His pioneering genetic work on chromosomes also proved that inheritance plays a role in an individual's susceptibility to cancer.
See also: Cellular pathology 134–135 ▪ Inheritance and hereditary conditions 146–147 ▪ Cancer therapy 168–175

HARVEY CUSHING
1869–1939

Trailblazing American neurosurgeon Harvey Cushing developed many of the techniques responsible for reducing the mortality rate during and after neurosurgery. The world's leading teacher of neurosurgery in the early 20th century, he taught and practiced at Johns Hopkins, Harvard, and Yale universities. Cushing was the foremost expert on the diagnosis and treatment of brain tumors and a leading authority on the pituitary gland, identifying its role in the disease named after him.
See also: Cancer therapy 168–175 ▪ Hormones and endocrinology 184–187

ALFRED ADLER
1870–1937

The first psychologist to emphasize the need to understand individuals within their social context, Austrian psychiatrist Alfred Adler founded the field of "individual psychology." Believing that disabling feelings of inferiority arise from factors such as low social status, neglect during childhood, or physical disability, Adler advocated therapy to build an individual's self-esteem. His ideas had particular influence on child and educational psychology.
See also: Psychoanalysis 178–183 ▪ Behavioral and cognitive therapy 242–243

OSWALDO CRUZ
1872–1917

A Brazilian epidemiologist who studied bacteriology at the Pasteur Institute in Paris, France, Oswaldo Cruz became director general of the Federal Serum Therapy Institute in Rio de Janeiro in 1902, turning it into a world-class institution. After he became Brazil's director general of public health in 1903, he waged a series of successful campaigns to tackle yellow fever, bubonic plague, and malaria, as well as instituting a smallpox vaccination program.
See also: Vaccination 94–101

ANTÓNIO EGAS MONIZ
1874–1955

In 1927, Portuguese neurologist António Egas Moniz developed the brain imaging technique cerebral angiography. He injected dyes that block radiation into the arteries of the brain, then used X-rays to reveal abnormalities. Moniz also devised a surgical procedure (lobotomy) to isolate the brain's frontal lobe to treat psychosis. While this gained him a Nobel Prize in Physiology or Medicine in 1949, lobotomy fell out of use due to its serious side effects.
See also: Humane mental health care 92–93 ▪ MRI and medical scanning 278–281

CARL JUNG
1875–1961

The founder of analytic psychology, Swiss psychiatrist Carl Jung worked closely with German psychoanalyst Sigmund Freud between 1907 and 1912, but increasingly disagreed with what he viewed as Freud's overemphasis on sexuality in the development of personality. Jung introduced the idea of introvert and extrovert personalities, archetypes, and the power of the unconscious. He also defined four functions of the mind that affect personality: feeling, thinking, sensation, and intuition.
See also: Psychoanalysis 178–183 ▪ Behavioral and cognitive therapy 242–243

UGO CERLETTI
1877–1963

Italian neurologist Ugo Cerletti devised electroconvulsive therapy (ECT) after seeing a similar process used to anesthetize pigs before they were butchered. The treatment involves passing an electric current through the brain to induce a short-term seizure as a way of managing mental disorders that do not respond to other therapies. Cerletti began to apply ECT to patients at Sapienza University in Rome from 1938. ECT is still in use today for those with severe depression who have not responded to other treatments.
See also: Lithium and bipolar disorder 240 ▪ Chlorpromazine and antipsychotics 241

HAROLD GILLIES
1882–1960

Described as "the father of plastic surgery," Gillies was born in New Zealand but trained as a surgeon in the UK. After witnessing the horrific facial wounds suffered by soldiers in France during World War I, he returned to the UK and persuaded the authorities to open Queen's Hospital, Sidcup, the world's first hospital dedicated to facial reconstruction. There, Gillies pioneered new skin-grafting techniques while treating men disfigured by gunshot and shrapnel.
See also: Plastic surgery 26–27 ▪ Skin grafts 137 ▪ Face transplants 315

WILLIAM AUGUSTUS HINTON
1883–1959

The son of freed slaves, Hinton overcame racism and poverty to become a leading pathologist and the first African American professor at Harvard University. In 1927, he created a test for diagnosing syphilis whose accuracy dramatically cut the number of false positive results generated by earlier tests. In 1934, the Hinton test was adopted by the US Public Health Service, and Hinton became the first African American to publish a medical textbook, with *Syphilis and its Treatment*.
See also: Germ theory 138–145 ▪ Antibiotics 216–223

LINUS PAULING
1901–1994

A prolific researcher and writer, American scientist Linus Pauling received two Nobel Prizes—one in chemistry and one for his peace activism. In 1949, he became the first person to advance the concept of a molecular disease when he showed that the inherited disorder sickle cell anemia is caused by the presence of abnormal hemoglobin proteins in red blood cells. The start of molecular genetics, this showed that the specific properties of proteins can be inherited, and has fueled modern genome research.
See also: Inheritance and hereditary conditions 146–147 ▪ Genetics and medicine 288–293

CHARLES RICHARD DREW
1904–1950

An African American pioneer in preserving blood for transfusion, Drew turned his attention from surgery to blood storage when he won a postgraduate fellowship to study at Columbia University in New York City. Drew developed a method for processing and preserving blood plasma—blood without cells—which lasts much longer than whole blood. In 1940, as head of the "Blood for Britain" program in World War II, Drew initiated a blood banking process, collecting, testing, and transporting blood plasma from the US to the UK to alleviate shortages of blood for transfusion. Drew was appointed director of the American Red Cross Blood Bank in 1941 but resigned when the blood of African Americans was segregated from that of white Americans.

See also: Blood transfusion and blood groups 108–111

HENRIETTA LACKS
1920–1951

In 1951, aged 31, African American Henrietta Lacks underwent a biopsy at the Johns Hopkins Hospital in Baltimore, Maryland, and was diagnosed with cervical cancer. Some of her cells were sent to pathologist George Gey, whose research required live tumor cells. Usually, Gey couldn't keep cells alive for more than a short time, but Lacks' cells divided rapidly and could be kept alive long enough to allow more in-depth examination. These "immortal" cells, known as the HeLa cells, have been used in countless research projects—from the development of the polio vaccine to the investigation of AIDS. Lacks died months after her diagnosis, but her cell line lives on and continues to aid the progress of medical science.

See also: Cancer therapy 168–175 ▪ Cancer screening 226–227 ▪ HIV and autoimmune diseases 294–297

PETER SAFAR
1924–2003

Of Jewish ancestry, Peter Safar evaded the Nazis in wartime Vienna, Austria, then moved to the US in 1949 and trained in surgery at Yale University. In 1958, while head of anesthetics at the Johns Hopkins Hospital in Baltimore, Maryland, Safar developed the procedure of cardiopulmonary resuscitation (CPR). In order to train people how to clear an airway and give mouth-to-mouth resuscitation, he persuaded a Norwegian doll company to design and produce mannequins, versions of which have been used to teach the lifesaving method ever since.

See also: Triage 90

JAMES BLACK
1924–2010

Scottish pharmacologist James Black was interested in the way hormones affect blood pressure, particularly in people suffering from angina. When blood oxygen levels are low, adrenaline and other hormones instruct the heart to beat faster, and if the circulation cannot keep up, pain results. From 1958, Black sought a way to break the cycle while working as a chemist at pharmaceutical company ICI. Six years later, the company launched the beta-blocker drug propranolol; it is still used today to reduce high blood pressure. Black also helped develop drugs to prevent some types of stomach cancers and treat peptic ulcers, and was awarded the 1988 Nobel Prize in Physiology or Medicine.

See also: Hormones and endocrinology 184–187

EVA KLEIN
1925–

Inspired by Marie Curie, Jewish-born Eva Klein (née Eva Fischer) studied medicine at the University of Budapest, where she hid during the Nazi occupation. She left Hungary in 1947 to work at the Karolinska Institute in Stockholm, Sweden. In the early 1970s, she led the discovery of a new type of white blood cell. Later named natural killer (NK) cells, they form a vital part of the immune system, responding quickly to kill virus-infected cells and identify cancer cells. Klein also developed cell lines derived from Burkitt lymphoma biopsies.

See also: The immune system 154–161 ▪ Cancer therapy 168–175

GILLIAN HANSON
1934–1996

After graduating in 1957, British physician Gillian Hanson spent her entire working life at Whipps Cross Hospital, London. An authority on lung disease, kidney failure, and other acute metabolic disorders, she was appointed head of the hospital's new intensive care unit in 1968. Under her direction, the unit gained an international reputation for excellence and innovation and established the field of intensive care as a medical specialty.

See also: Diabetes and its treatment 210–213 ▪ Dialysis 234–235

DOLORES "DEE" O'HARA
1935–

After working as a surgical nurse in Oregon, O'Hara joined the US Air Force, and in 1959, she was assigned to Project Mercury, America's first human space flight program, at Cape Canaveral, Florida. There, she developed the field of "space nursing" for NASA, conducting the preflight and postflight physical examinations of every astronaut on the Mercury,

Gemini, and Apollo space missions to determine fitness for participation and the effects of space on the human body.
See also: Nursing and sanitation 128–133

GRAEME CLARK
1935–

The son of a deaf father, Australian ear surgeon Graeme Clark began researching the possibility of an implantable, electronic hearing device in the mid-1960s. In 1978, he installed the first cochlear implant in a patient in Melbourne. The "bionic ear" converts sound into electric impulses that stimulate the auditory nerve, sending messages to the brain. Clark's device has improved the hearing of thousands of people with profound deafness.
See also: The nervous system 190–195

ROBERT BARTLETT
1939–

During the 1960s, American thoracic surgeon "Bob" Bartlett developed a lifesaving extracorporeal membrane oxygenation (ECMO) machine. This supports patients whose heart and lungs cannot provide sufficient oxygen exchange to sustain life. In 1975, Bartlett had his first neonatal success using ECMO when he saved the life of newborn "Baby Esperanza," who was experiencing severe breathing difficulties; after three days, she made a full recovery. ECMO is now an established tool for supporting patients with life-threatening conditions such as heart attacks or severe lung disease.
See also: Transplant surgery 246–253 ▪ Pacemakers 255

HIDEOKI OGAWA
1941–

In 1993, Japanese immunologist and dermatologist Hideoki Ogawa argued that the chronic skin disorder atopic dermatitis (eczema) results from a defect in the permeability of skin, as well as abnormalities in the immune system. The latter was already recognized, but his "barrier defect" theory has helped clinicians better understand this as-yet incurable condition, which affects more than 10 percent of children and up to 3 percent of adults.
See also: Cellular pathology 134–135 ▪ The immune system 154–161

DENIS MUKWEGE
1955–

Described as the world's leading expert on repairing injuries caused by rape, Congolese gynecologist Denis Mukwege trained as a pediatrician, gynecologist, and obstetrician before devoting himself to helping female victims of sexual violence. In 1999, he founded Panzi Hospital, Bukavu, in the Democratic Republic of the Congo. The hospital has treated more than 85,000 women with gynecological damage and trauma, 60 percent of them victims of violence inflicted as a weapon of war. He addressed the United Nations on rape as a war strategy in 2012, and created the Mukwege Foundation in 2016, to "advocate for an end to wartime sexual violence." He and fellow campaigner Nadia Murad (an Iraqi Yazidi survivor of rape) were jointly awarded the Nobel Peace Prize in 2018.
See also: The World Health Organization 232–233

FIONA WOOD
1958–

British-born Australian plastic surgeon Fiona Wood invented and patented "spray-on skin" in 1999. The treatment involves taking a small patch of healthy skin and dissolving the cells with an enzyme to create a solution that is sprayed across the damaged skin. The technique allows regenerated skin to heal more quickly and creates less scarring than traditional skin grafting and meshing. Although the technique had not yet been fully tested in clinical trials, Wood successfully used this method to treat burn victims from the Bali bombings in 2002. It has since been approved for use in a number of countries.
See also: Skin grafts 137 ▪ Regenerative medicine 314

JOANNA WARDLAW
1958–

Scottish clinical neurologist Joanna Wardlaw established the Brain Research Imaging Centre in Edinburgh in 1997. By 2020, it was an international center of excellence for neuroimaging, with one of the largest groups of academic radiologists in Europe. A world authority on brain scanning; brain aging; and the prevention, diagnosis, and treatment of strokes, Wardlaw has conducted pioneering research into the small strokes and dementia caused by damage to the brain's smallest blood vessels.
See also: Alzheimer's disease 196–197 ▪ Electroencephalography 224–225 ▪ MRI and medical scanning 278–281

GLOSSARY

In this glossary, terms defined within another entry are identified with *italic* type.

Acute Describes a condition that begins abruptly and may last for a short time. See also *chronic*.

AIDS The abbreviation for acquired immunodeficiency syndrome, a deficiency of the *immune system* that can occur as a result of *HIV*.

Analgesia A form of pain relief.

Anatomy 1) The body's structure. 2) The study of that structure through *dissection*. See also *histology*.

Anesthetic A drug or mixture of drugs that either numbs part of the body (local anesthesia) or renders the patient unconscious (general anesthesia).

Antibiotic A drug that is used to kill or inhibit the growth of *bacteria*, usually those causing *infections*.

Antibody A *protein* produced in the body by *white blood cells* to mark foreign particles or *antigens* and stimulate the *immune* response.

Antigen A foreign substance that stimulates the body to produce *antibodies* and an *immune* response.

Antiseptic Antimicrobial chemical applied to skin or wounds to kill *microbes* that may cause *infection*.

Antitoxin An *antibody* that counteracts a *toxin*, or poison.

Apothecary A term used in medieval times to refer not only to the place where remedies were dispensed, but also to the person who dispensed them.

Artery A blood *vessel* that carries blood away from the heart.

Autoimmune disease A disease that occurs when the body's *immune system* attacks healthy *tissue*.

Autopsy The examination of a dead body to establish the cause of death and/or the nature of disease.

Bacterium (plural: **bacteria**) A single-*celled microorganism* that does not have a nucleus or other specialized membrane-bound structures and is too small to see with the naked eye.

Bile 1) A dark green/yellowish fluid produced by the liver that aids the digestion of fats in the small intestine. 2) Yellow or black "bile," two of the four *humors* in ancient and medieval medicine.

Biopsy The taking of a *tissue* or fluid sample for analysis.

Blood group/type system The presence or absence of certain *antibodies* and *antigens* in blood, which may mean that it clots and clumps when mixed with blood of a different type. Among more than 30 systems, the two most important are ABO and Rhesus (Rh).

Bloodletting The removal of blood from a patient to treat disease, used today to treat certain disorders that cause excess iron in the blood.

Blood pressure The pressure exerted by blood on the walls of blood *vessels* as it is pumped around the body by the heart. Blood pressure is measured to assess cardiovascular health and to *diagnose* disease.

Cancer The abnormal growth of *cells* in body *tissues* that causes disease.

Capillary A minute blood *vessel* with thin walls through which nutrients and waste products pass to and from body *tissues*.

Cell The smallest functional unit in the human body. As well as forming *tissues* and *organs*, cells take in nutrients, fight invaders, and contain genetic material. The body has 35–40 trillion cells of at least 200 different types.

Central nervous system (CNS) The part of the *nervous system* that consists of the brain and *spinal cord* and controls the body's activities.

Chemotherapy Treatment that uses drugs to target and kill *cancer cells*.

Chromosome A structure made of *DNA* and *protein* that contains a *cell's* genetic information (in the form of *genes*); human cells usually have 23 pairs of chromosomes.

Chronic Describes a medical condition that lasts several months and may result in long-term change in the body. See also *acute*.

Circulatory system The continuous movement of blood around the body via the heart and blood *vessels*.

Clinical medicine The study and practice of medicine based on direct examination of the patient to *diagnose*, treat, and prevent disease.

Computed tomography (CT) An imaging technique that uses weak *X-rays* to record thin 2D slicelike views through the body, then combines them to make 3D images. Also known as computerized axial tomography (CAT).

Congenital Describes a physical abnormality or condition that is present from birth and may be the result of genetic factors.

Contagious Describes an *infectious* disease that is spread by direct or indirect contact.

Coronavirus A common type of *virus* that causes upper respiratory *infections* in humans and animals.

Cytokine A small *protein* that is secreted by a specific *cell* of the *immune system* and has an effect on other cells.

Diagnosis Identification of an illness from its symptoms (what the person describes) and signs (what is observed).

Dissection Cutting apart a dead body to study its internal structure.

DNA (Deoxyribonucleic acid) The long, thin, double-helix-shaped molecule that makes up the *chromosomes* found in almost all body *cells*. It contains hereditary material called *genes*.

Endocrine system The *glands* and *cells* that make and control the production of the body's chemical messengers—*hormones*.

Endoscope A viewing instrument that is inserted into the body though an orifice or a surgical incision.

Enzyme A molecule, usually a *protein*, that acts as a catalyst to speed up chemical reactions in the body.

Epidemic An outbreak of a *contagious* disease in which the incidence rate is much higher than expected, but, unlike a *pandemic*, is confined to a particular region.

Epidemiology The study of how often diseases occur in different groups of people and why.

Functional magnetic resonance imaging (fMRI) A *magnetic resonance imaging* technique that measures brain activity by detecting changes in blood flow.

Gene The basic unit of heredity, passed from parents to offspring as a section of *DNA* that provides coded instructions for a specific trait.

Germ A *microbe*, such as a *virus* or *bacterium*, that causes disease.

Gland A group of *cells* or an *organ* that produces a chemical substance with a specific function in the body, such as a *hormone* or an *enzyme*.

Histology The study of the microscopic structure of *cells*, *tissues*, and *organs*.

HIV The abbreviation for human immunodeficiency *virus*, which causes *AIDS*.

Homeostasis The process of maintaining a stable internal environment within the body.

Hormone A chemical produced in an *endocrine gland* to control a process or activity in the body.

Human genome The complete set of *genes* for a human—there are approximately 20,000 genes.

Humors In early medicine, four chief body fluids or temperaments (blood/sanguine, yellow *bile*/choleric, black bile/melancholic, and phlegm/phlegmatic). Physicians believed that good health depended on these humors being in balance.

Immune system The body's natural defense network that protects against *infection* and disease.

Immunity The ability of the body to resist or fight a particular *infection* or *toxin* by the action of *antibodies* or *white blood cells*.

Immunization Rendering a person resistant to attack from *microbes* that cause an *infectious* disease, usually by *inoculation*.

Immunosuppressant A drug that reduces the workings of the *immune system*, such as to prevent the rejection of *transplanted organs*.

Immunotherapy The treatment of disease, usually *cancer*, with substances that stimulate the body's *immune* response.

Implant An item surgically inserted into the body. It may be living (for example, bone marrow), mechanical (hip replacement), electronic (heart pacemaker), or a combination of all three.

Infection A disease caused by invading *microbes* such as *bacteria*, *viruses*, or similar life forms.

Inflammation The body's *immune* response to damage such as injury, *infection*, or *toxins*.

Inheritance Characteristics passed on by parents to offspring through *genes*.

Inoculation In *immunization*, the introduction of disease-causing *microbes* into the body in a mild form to stimulate the production of *antibodies* that will provide future protection against the disease.

Insulin A *hormone* that regulates the level of glucose in the blood. Lack of it causes type 1 diabetes; the body's inability to use it can result in type 2 diabetes.

Keyhole surgery Minimally invasive surgery performed through a very small incision using special instruments and an *endoscope*.

Laser surgery Surgery performed with a laser beam—for example, reshaping the cornea in order to improve eyesight.

Laparoscopy A form of *keyhole surgery* that is used to examine *organs* inside the abdomen.

Lymph The excess fluid that collects in the *tissues* as *blood circulates* through the body; its contents include *white blood cells*.

Lymphatic system An extensive network of *tissues* and small *organs* that drains *lymph* from body *tissues* into the blood and transports the *infection*-fighting *white blood cells* contained in lymph around the body.

Lymphocyte A *white blood cell* that protects against *infection*, for example, by producing *antibodies*.

Magnetic resonance imaging (MRI) Computerized scanning that uses a powerful magnetic field and radio pulses to visualize 2D slices through the body, then combines them to create a 3D image.

Metabolism Biochemical processes in *cells* that are necessary for life. Some convert nutrients into energy; others use that energy to produce the *proteins* that build body *tissue*.

Metastasis The spread of *cancer cells* from the primary *tumor* where they first formed to other body parts.

Microbe/Microorganism A living organism too small to be seen by the naked eye, such as a *bacterium*.

Microsurgery Surgery requiring a specialized microscope to operate on minute structures of the body such as blood *vessels* and *nerves*.

Nerve A sheathed bundle of nerve *cells* (neurons) that carry electrical impulses between the brain, *spinal cord*, and body *tissues*.

Nervous system The system of the brain, *spinal cord*, and *nerves* that receives stimuli and transmits instructions to the rest of the body.

Obstetrics The field of medicine concerned with the care of women during pregnancy and childbirth.

Oncology The branch of medicine concerned with *cancer*.

Ophthalmology The study and treatment of disorders and diseases of the eye.

Organ A main body part with a specific function—for example, the heart, brain, liver, or lungs.

Orthopedics The study and treatment of the musculoskeletal system's bones, joints, and muscles.

Palliative care Relieving pain and other distressing symptoms to improve the quality of life of patients with life-threatening, and usually incurable, diseases.

Pandemic An outbreak of a *contagious* disease that affects the populations of multiple countries.

Pathogen A *microbe* or organism that causes disease or other harm.

Pathology The study of disease: its causes, mechanism, and effects on the body.

Parasite An organism that lives in or on another living creature and causes harm.

Pediatrics The *diagnosis* and treatment of disorders in children.

Penicillin An *antibiotic*, or group of antibiotics, produced naturally by certain blue molds but now mainly produced synthetically.

Pharmacology The study of drugs and how they act on the body.

Physiology The study of biological processes at every level, from *cells* to whole body systems, and how they interact with each other.

Plasma The liquid part of the blood in which the blood *cells* are suspended. It also carries *proteins*, *antibodies*, and *hormones* to different cells in the body.

Positron emission tomography (PET) An imaging technique that tracks radioactive tracers injected into the body to detect *metabolic* changes that indicate the onset of disease in *organs* or *tissues*.

Protein A large molecule made up of chains of amino acids. Proteins are the building blocks of the body, required for the structure, function, and regulation of *tissues* and *organs*.

Psychotherapy A talking therapy to treat mental health problems via psychological rather than medical means. This umbrella term covers a vast range of practices, from psychoanalysis to CBT, to help people overcome their problems.

Pulmonary/respiratory system The airways, lungs, and *vessels* involved in breathing, which takes oxygen into the body's *circulatory system* and expels carbon dioxide from the body.

Pulse 1) The rate at which the heart beats, reflected in the rhythmic expansion and contraction of an *artery* as blood is pumped through it. 2) The *diagnostic* measurement of this expansion and contraction per minute.

Radiotherapy The treatment of disease, especially *cancer*, using localized *X-rays* or similar forms of radiation.

Red blood cells The most common type of blood *cell*, containing hemoglobin, an oxygen-carrying *protein* that is delivered to body *tissue* via the *circulatory system*.

Respiratory system See *pulmonary system*.

RNA (Ribonucleic acid) A molecule that decodes *DNA's* instructions to make *proteins* or itself carries genetic instructions.

Spinal cord The bundle of *nerves* running from the brain down through the spinal column. It makes up part of the *central nervous system*.

Stem cell A nonspecialist *cell* from which all specialist cells are generated. Stem cells provide new cells as the body grows and replace damaged cells.

Steroids A class of chemical compounds that includes some *hormones*, such as testosterone, and anti-*inflammatory* medicines.

Telesurgery Surgery carried out by a robot that is operated from a remote console.

Tissue Groups of similar *cells* that carry out the same function, such as muscle tissue, which can contract.

Tissue typing The identification of *antigens* in the *tissue* of a donor and a recipient before procedures such as an *organ transplantation* take place, in order to minimize the possibility of rejection due to antigenic differences.

Toxin A poisonous substance, especially one produced by certain *bacteria*, plants, and animals.

Transfusion The transfer of blood from a donor to a recipient.

Transplant The taking and *implanting* of *tissue* or *organs* from one part of the body to another or from a donor to a recipient.

Tumor A growth of abnormal *cells* that may be malignant (*cancerous*) and spread throughout the body or benign (noncancerous) with no tendency to spread.

Ultrasound scan An image of a fetus, *organ*, or other *tissue*; this image is produced by passing high-frequency sounds into the body and analyzing reflected echoes.

Vaccination The administering of a *vaccine* to provide *immunity* against a disease.

Vaccine A preparation containing a weakened or killed form of a disease-causing *virus*, *bacterium*, or *toxin* to stimulate the body's *immune* response without actually causing the disease.

Vector An organism that transmits disease, such as a *virus*, *bacterium*, or some species of mosquitoes that carry malaria.

Vein A blood *vessel* that carries blood from the body back to the heart.

Vessel A duct or tube carrying blood or other fluid through the body.

Virus One of the smallest types of harmful *microbe*, consisting of genetic material in a protective coating; it can only multiply by invading other living *cells*.

White blood cells Colorless blood *cells* that play a part in the body's defensive *immune system*.

X-ray A photographic or digital image of inside part of the body, taken with X-rays, a form of electromagnetic radiation that penetrates soft *tissues*.

INDEX

QUOTE ATTRIBUTIONS

ACKNOWLEDGMENTS

Dorling Kindersley would like to thank Debra Wolter, Ankita Gupta, and Arushi Mathur for editorial assistance; Alexandra Black for proofreading; Helen Peters for indexing; Stuti Tiwari for design assistance; Senior DTP Designer Harish Aggarwal; Jackets Editorial Coordinator Priyanka Sharma; Managing Jackets Editor Saloni Singh; and Assistant Picture Research Administrator Vagisha Pushp.

PICTURE CREDITS

The publisher would like to thank the following for their kind permission to reproduce their photographs:

(Key: a-above; b-below/bottom; c-center; f-far; l-left; r-right; t-top)

19 Alamy Stock Photo: Prisma Archivo (bl). **Getty Images:** Mira Oberman / AFP (tr). **20 Alamy Stock Photo:** William Arthur (br). **21 SuperStock:** DeAgostini (tr). **23 Alamy Stock Photo:** Dinodia Photos RM (tr). **25 akg-images:** Gerard Degeorge (tl). **27 Alamy Stock Photo:** Photo Researchers / Science History Images (tl). **29 Alamy Stock Photo:** Fine Art Images / Heritage Images (br); Photo12 / Archives Snark (tl). **34 Alamy Stock Photo:** Science History Images (tl); View Stock (br). **37 Getty Images:** DEA / A. Dagli Orti (bc); **Science Photo Library:** Middle Temple Library (tl). **41 Alamy Stock Photo:** PhotoStock-Israel (bl). **42 Alamy Stock Photo:** Classic Image (tl). **43 Alamy Stock Photo:** The Print Collector (tl). **46 Alamy Stock Photo:** Pictures From History / CPA Media Pte Ltd (crb). **48 Alamy Stock Photo:** Pictures From History / CPA Media Pte Ltd (br). **49 Alamy Stock Photo:** Chronicle (tl); **Rex by Shutterstock:** Gianni Dagli Orti (br). **51 Alamy Stock Photo:** Fine Art Images / Heritage Image Partnership Ltd (tl); Werner Forman Archive / National Museum, Prague / Heritage Image Partnership Ltd (br). **53 Science Photo Library:** Sheila Terry (cr). **56 Alamy Stock Photo:** PhotoStock-Israel (br). **57 Alamy Stock Photo:** The History Collection (tr). **58 Alamy Stock Photo:** World History Archive (tl). **59 Alamy Stock Photo:** Zoonar GmbH (tr). **62 Bridgeman Images:** Christie's Images. **63 Alamy Stock Photo:** Oxford Science Archive / Heritage Images / The Print Collector (bl); **Wellcome Collection:** De humani corporis fabrica libri septem (tr). **70 Getty Images:** DeAgostini. **72 Wellcome Collection:** (tc). **73 Alamy Stock Photo:** Oxford Science Archive / Heritage Images / The Print Collector (cb); Timewatch Images (tl). **74 Alamy Stock Photo:** Photo12 / Ann Ronan Picture Library (bc). **75 Alamy Stock Photo:** Science History Images (bl). **77 Alamy Stock Photo:** Album / British Library (tl). **79 Alamy Stock Photo:** The Keasbury-Gordon Photograph Archive / KGPA Ltd (bc). **80 Alamy Stock Photo:** The Picture Art Collection (bc). **81 Wellcome Collection:** Hermann Boerhaave. Line engraving by F. Anderloni after G. Garavaglia (bl). **83 Getty Images:** Hulton Archive (tl). **84 Alamy Stock Photo:** Robert Thom (bc). **85 Alamy Stock Photo:** Science History Images (tr). **87 123RF.com:** ivdesign (tc/Salicylic acid); **Dreamstime.com:** Alptraum (tr); Evgeny Skidanov (tl); Levsh (tc); **Getty Images:** SeM / Universal Images Group (tr). **89 Alamy Stock Photo:** Hamza Khan (bl); **Dreamstime.com:** Georgios Kollidas (tl). **91 Alamy Stock Photo:** Garo / Phanie (crb). **93 Wellcome Collection:** Tucker, George A. (bc); Philippe Pinel/

Lithograph by P. R. Vignéron (tr). **96 Science Photo Library:** CCI Archives. **97 Alamy Stock Photo:** Fine Art Images / Heritage Image Partnership Ltd (bc). **99 Alamy Stock Photo:** The Print Collector / Heritage Images (bl); **Getty Images:** Christophel Fine Art / Universal Images Group (tr). **100 Alamy Stock Photo:** Ann Ronan Picture Library / Heritage-Images / The Print Collector (tr). **101** Global number of child death per year—by cause of death: https://ourworldindata. org/vaccination. **103 Getty Images:** DeAgostini (cr). **109 Wellcome Collection:** (tl). **110 Getty Images:** Keystone-France / Gamma-Keystone (bl). **111 Alamy Stock Photo:** Patti McConville (br); **Getty Images:** Aditya Irawan / NurPhoto (bl). **114 Alamy Stock Photo:** Granger Historical Picture Archive (bl). **115 Bridgeman Images:** Archives Charmet (tl). **116 Dreamstime.com:** Alona Stepaniuk (tl). **117 Alamy Stock Photo:** Medicshots (bl); Photo Researchers / Science History Images (tr). **118 Getty Images:** Johann Schwarz / SEPA.Media (bc). **119 Alamy Stock Photo:** Pictorial Press Ltd (bl). **121 Alamy Stock Photo:** Mary Evans / Library of Congress / Chronicle (tr); **Getty Images:** Topical Press Agency (bl). **123 Alamy Stock Photo:** Historic Images (bl); **Science Photo Library:** Science Source (tc). **126 Alamy Stock Photo:** Pictorial Press Ltd (bl). **127 Alamy Stock Photo:** GL Archive (bl); Photo Researchers / Science History Images (bc). **131 Alamy Stock Photo:** Pictorial Press Ltd (bl). **132 Wellcome Collection:** Diagram of the causes of mortality in the army (bl). **133 Alamy Stock Photo:** David Cole (bl); World Image Archive (tr). **135 Alamy Stock Photo:** Pictorial Press Ltd (tr). **136 Alamy Stock Photo:** Mashuk (br). **140 Alamy Stock Photo:** INTERFOTO / History (br). **141 Alamy Stock Photo:** Science History Images (tl). **142 Alamy Stock Photo:** Lebrecht Music & Arts (tr); **Science Photo Library:** Dennis Kunkel Microscopy (bl). **144 Alamy Stock Photo:** Photo12 / Ann Ronan Picture Library (bc). **145 Alamy Stock Photo:** GL Archive (bl); **Dreamstime.com:** Helder Almeida (tc/hand); Mikhail Rudenko (bl/nose); Valentino2 (tr). **147 Alamy Stock Photo:** FLHC 52 (tl). **149 Alamy Stock Photo:** GL Archive (bl); **Getty Images:** Bettmann (tr). **151 Alamy Stock Photo:** IanDagnall Computing (br); **Dreamstime.com:** Coplandj (tl). **152 Alamy Stock Photo:** Pictorial Press Ltd (br). **153 Alamy Stock Photo:** Granger Historical Picture Archive (tr). **157 Internet Archive:** L'immunité dans les maladies infectieuses (tl); **Science Photo Library:** National Library of Medicine (br). **159 Alamy Stock Photo:** Juan Gaertner / Science Photo Library (tr); **Rex by Shutterstock:** AP (bl). **160 Alamy Stock Photo:** Geoff Smith (bl). **161 Dreamstime.com:** Juan Gaertner (br). **162 Alamy Stock Photo:** The History Collection (tr). **163 Alamy Stock Photo:** Pictorial Press Ltd (tr). **171 Alamy Stock Photo:** Photo Researchers / Science History Images (tc); **Wellcome Collection:** (tr). **172 Unsplash:** nci (bl). **174 Alamy Stock Photo:** Everett Collection Inc (bl). **175 Science Photo Library:** Steve Gschmeissner (tl). **176 Alamy Stock Photo:** Science History Images (cr). **180 Alamy Stock Photo:** Granger Historical Picture Archive (br). **181 Alamy Stock Photo:** World History Archive (tl). **183 Alamy Stock Photo:** Heeb Christian / Prisma by Dukas Presseagentur GmbH (cb); **Pictorial Press Ltd** (tr). **185 Alamy Stock Photo:** GL Archive (tr). **187 Science Photo Library:** LENNART NILSSON, TT (tr). **189 Alamy Stock Photo:** Granger Historical Picture Archive (bl); World History Archive (tr). **193 Alamy Stock Photo:** Archive Pics (tr); Granger, NYC. /

Granger Historical Picture Archive (bl). **195 Science Photo Library:** Zephyr (br). **196 Alamy Stock Photo:** Science Photo Library / Juan Gaertner (br). **197 Alamy Stock Photo:** Colport (tl). **198 Alamy Stock Photo:** Granger Historical Picture Archive (bc). **199 Alamy Stock Photo:** World History Archive (tr). **203 Getty Images:** The LIFE Images Collection / Herbert Gehr (tc, bl). **204 Science Photo Library:** LEE D. SIMON (bc). **205 Alamy Stock Photo:** The Picture Art Collection (tr). **208 Getty Images:** Keystone-France\Gamma-Rapho (tr). **209 Alamy Stock Photo:** Niday Picture Library (tl). **211 Alamy Stock Photo:** Everett Collection Historical (tr); **Dreamstime.com:** Vichaya Kiatyingangsulee (tl); Reddogs (tl/1). **213 Getty Images:** Chris Ware / Keystone Features (bl). **215 Alamy Stock Photo:** Everett Collection Historical (tl); Everett Collection Historical (tr). **218 Alamy Stock Photo:** Keystone Pictures USA / Keystone Press (bl); **Getty Images:** Bettmann (tr). **220 Alamy Stock Photo:** Alpha Stock (tr); **Science Photo Library:** Corbin O'grady Studio (bl). **221 University of Wisconsin, Madison:** Dr. Cameron Currie (bl). **222 Alamy Stock Photo:** Science Photo Library (tl). **225 Getty Images:** Science & Society Picture Library (tl); **Science Photo Library:** SOVEREIGN, ISM (bc). **227 Alamy Stock Photo:** Everett Collection Inc (tr); **Wellcome Collection:** (tl). **233 Szeming Sze Estate:** (tr). **235 Alamy Stock Photo:** INTERFOTO (bl). **237 Science Photo Library:** (tl). **239 Alamy Stock Photo:** Granger Historical Picture Archive (bl). **243 Alamy Stock Photo:** Granger Historical Picture Archive (bl). **245 Alamy Stock Photo:** WENN Rights Ltd (cr). **249 Science Photo Library:** Jean-Loup Charmet. **251 Alamy Stock Photo:** Pictorial Press Ltd (bl). **252 Getty Images:** Rodger Bosch / AFP (tl). **255 Dreamstime.com:** Kaling Megu (tr). **257 Alamy Stock Photo:** Photo Researchers / Science History Images (tr). **262 Alamy Stock Photo:** Cultural Archive (tr). **263 Alamy Stock Photo:** The Reading Room (br). **264 Dreamstime.com:** Sebastian Kaulitzki (tc). **265 Alamy Stock Photo:** Mike Booth (tl). **267 Getty Images:** Dibyangshu Sarkar / AFP (br). **269 Alamy Stock Photo:** PA Images (tr). **271 Alamy Stock Photo:** BH Generic Stock Images (tl). **277 Cardiff University Library:** Cochrane Archive, University Hospital Llandough.: (tr). **279 Alamy Stock Photo:** DPA Picture Alliance (bl). **280 Alamy Stock Photo:** Science Photo Library (tr). **281 Getty Images:** BSIP / Universal Images Group (tr). **283 Getty Images:** Bettmann (tr); **NASA:** (tl). **284 Getty Images:** Central Press / Hulton Archive (cb). **285 Alamy Stock Photo:** PA Images / Rebecca Naden (bl). **287 Science Photo Library:** David Scharf (br). **290 Alamy Stock Photo:** Photo Researchers / Science History Images (tr); **Science Photo Library:** A. Barrington Brown, © Gonville & Caius College (bl). **291 Rex by Shutterstock:** Karl Schoendorfer (bl). **293 Getty Images:** Tomohiro Ohsumi (tl). **297 Getty Images:** AFP / Stephane De Sakutin (tr); Barbara Alper (bl). **299 Getty Images:** Handout (tr). **300 Alamy Stock Photo:** Science History Images (bc). **303 PLOS Genetics:** © 2008 Jane Gitschier (bl); **Science Photo Library:** NIBSC (tc). **305 Science Photo Library:** Peter Menzel (crb). **308 Alamy Stock Photo:** Everett Collection Historical (bl). **309 Alamy Stock Photo:** Everett Collection Inc (bl). **313 Alamy Stock Photo:** Cultura Creative Ltd / Eugenio Marongiu (br). **314 Alamy Stock Photo:** BSIP SA (cb).

For further information see: www.dkimages.com